CHARLES NICOLLE
PASTEUR'S IMPERIAL MISSIONARY

Rochester Studies in Medical History

Senior Editor: Theodore M. Brown
Professor of History and Preventive Medicine
University of Rochester

ISSN 1526–2715

The Mechanization of the Heart:
Harvey and Descartes
Thomas Fuchs
Translated from the German by Marjorie Grene

The Workers' Health Fund in Eretz Israel
Kupat Holim, 1911–1937
Shifra Shvarts

Public Health and the Risk Factor:
A History of an Uneven Medical Revolution
William G. Rothstein

Venereal Disease, Hospitals and the Urban Poor:
London's "Foul Wards," 1600–1800
Kevin P. Siena

Rockefeller Money, the Laboratory and Medicine
in Edinburgh 1919–1930: New Science in an Old Country
Christopher Lawrence

Health and Wealth:
Studies in History and Policy
Simon Szreter

Charles Nicolle, Pasteur's Imperial Missionary:
Typhus and Tunisia
Kim Pelis

CHARLES NICOLLE PASTEUR'S IMPERIAL MISSIONARY

Typhus and Tunisia

Kim Pelis

UNIVERSITY OF ROCHESTER PRESS

Copyright © 2006 Kim Pelis

All Rights Reserved. Except as permitted under current legislation, no part of this work may be photocopied, stored in a retrieval system, published, performed in public, adapted, broadcast, transmitted, recorded, or reproduced in any form or by any means, without the prior permission of the copyright owner.

First published 2006
Transferred to digital printing 2013

University of Rochester Press
668 Mt. Hope Avenue, Rochester, NY 14620, USA
www.urpress.com
and Boydell & Brewer Limited
PO Box 9, Woodbridge, Suffolk IP12 3DF, UK
www.boydellandbrewer.com

ISSN: 1526-2715

Hardcover ISBN: 978-1-58046-197-9
Paperback ISBN: 978-1-58046-465-9

Library of Congress Cataloging-in-Publication Data
Pelis, Kim, 1963-
  Charles Nicolle, Pasteur's imperial missionary : typhus and Tunisia / Kim Pelis.
    p. ; cm. – (Rochester studies in medical history, ISSN 1526-2715 ; 7)
  Includes bibliographical references and index.
  ISBN 1-58046-197-2 (hardcover : alk. paper)
  1. Nicolle, Charles, 1866-1936. 2. Institut Pasteur de Tunis–History. 3. Bacteriologists–France–Biography. 4. Typhus fever–Tunisia–History. [DNLM: 1. Nicolle, Charles, 1866-1936. 2. Institut Pasteur de Tunis. 3. Bacteriology–France–Biography. 4. Bacteriology–Tunisia–Biography. 5. Bacteriology–history–France. 6. Bacteriology–history–Tunisia. 7. Typhus, Epidemic Louse-Borne–history–France. 8. Typhus, Epidemic Louse-Borne–history–Tunisia. WZ 100 N654p 2006] I.Title. II. Series.
  QR31.N53P45 2006
  579.3092–dc22

2005033032

A catalogue record for this title is available from the British Library.

This publication is printed on acid-free paper.
Printed in the United States of America

for my grandmother,
Veronica Skierkowski
Sto lat (and more)

Does this mean that we must despise our accomplishments and turn back toward the harbor of some unspecified Golden Age? The Golden Age has always been a country of chimeras. The Ancients located it in the past because they believed it to be very old and because it is natural for old men to adorn the days of youth with flowers. We, who no longer respect a past that we measure with our sciences, place this ideal era in the future. The error is the same. The Golden Age would be the age in which one lives, if we knew how to savor it.

—Charles Nicolle, *Nature*, 1934

Contents

List of Illustrations	ix
Acknowledgments	x
List of Abbreviations	xiii
Prelude: The Substance of Shadows	xv
Introduction: The Door of the Sadiki	1

Part One
Thesis: Embracing Missions

1 Staring at the Sea: Nicolle and the Pasteur Institute of Tunis	17
2 The Threshold of Civilization: Typhus in Tunisia	47

Part Two
Rupture: Things Fall Apart

3 Light & Shadow: Lousy War and Fractured Peace	77

Part Three
Antithesis: Mosaics of Pieces

4 Alliances: "Emperor of the Mediterranean?"	113
5 Invisible Forces: or, Action at a Distance	144

Part Four
Synthesis: Mosaics of Power

6 Reservoir Docs: Birth, Life, and Death of Infectious Disease 173
7 Mosaics of Power: Confronting Paris 208

Part Five
Denouement

8 At Home with My Shadows: *Patrie de Nomade* 239

Appendix A 255
Appendix B 257
Notes 259
Bibliographic Note 347
Bibliography 351
Index 373

ILLUSTRATIONS

Figures

Following page 236:
1 Nicolle at his microscope
2 Young Nicolle
3 Dr. Eugène Nicolle
4 Schedule for Nicolle's Microbiology Course, Rouen
5 The Pasteur Institute of Tunis
6 Nicolle before the Door of his Institute, ca. 1909
7 Alfred Conor Administering Vaccines at the IPT
8 Georges Blanc in Serbia, World War I
9 Personnel of the IPT, World War I
10 The *AIPAN*
11 Nicolle and Hélène Sparrow in Mexico, 1931
12 Nicolle and the Ruins in Dougga
13 Nicolle in the Bled, Tunisia
14 Nicolle, Reflecting
15 Personnel of the IPT, ca. 1935
16 Nicolle
17 Nicolle standing before a sign warning against lice

ACKNOWLEDGMENTS

This project has its own long and complex history. Its origins extend back to the late 1980s, with dissertation work conducted at the Johns Hopkins University. In this first phase of its existence, it was supported not only by the Institute of the History of Medicine (under the sage guidance of Prof. Gert Brieger), but also by a Rockefeller Foundation research grant and a Fulbright dissertation support grant. From my years at Hopkins, I continue to be grateful to Ed Morman and the late Linda Bright, who cheerfully helped me find my often-obscure sources; and, in a later stage of this project's existence, to Coraleeze Thompson. Research in Paris, Tunis, and Rouen was not only facilitated but generally made delightful by the staffs of the related archives. In particular, I wish to thank Denise Ogilvie, Annick Perrot, and Daniel Demellier at the Pasteur Institute of Paris; and, in Tunis, the director of the IPT, Prof. Koussay Dellagi, as well as former director Amor Chadli. Also in Tunis, both Jeanne Jeffers M'rad and Ridha Mabrouk were of invaluable assistance. Further, I would like to thank those at the U.S. Embassy in Tunis who helped me with a host of concerns. In Paris, I am grateful to Nicolle "insiders" Maurice Huet, J.-J. Hueber, and Jean-Paul Giroud, all of whom generously shared their knowledge with me. More recently, Prof. Giroud has kindly allowed me to use the marvelous photographs his father took of Nicolle in the 1930s. These photographs may be found in Rouen's Archives Départementales de la Seine-Maritime, which has generously permitted me to reproduce these and other photographs from its Nicolle collection to illustrate this book.

For ever-patient assistance on matters scientific and military, I am indebted to Dr. Robert Joy at the Uniformed Services University. At Johns Hopkins, the late Dr. Thomas Turner took time out of his busy schedule to help a confused history graduate student to understand the relations between typhus varieties. Moreover, a number of Hans Zinsser's former collaborators, particularly the late Morris Shaffer, were immensely helpful.

I completed my dissertation on Charles Nicolle and the Pasteur Institute of Tunis in the autumn of 1994. Subsequently, at the University of Iowa and the (then) Wellcome Institute for the History of Medicine in London, my ever-collegial colleagues encouraged me to continue my research and invited to give a number of papers on the subject. A second project on "British blood," however, began to make completion of the Nicolle book difficult. I set French bacteriology aside for several years.

When I returned to Nicolle in 2003, I found that I still had a great deal of work ahead of me. Once again, I was fortunate in my abundant support. Kelly Mullally helped me organize my life so as to free up enough time to complete this project. Elizabeth Fee's History of Medicine Division at the National Library of Medicine has often seemed like a second home, made particularly welcoming by Stephen Greenberg. The Countway Library of the Harvard Medical School not only provided me with a travel grant to consult its archives, but offered the friendly and expert assistance of Thomas Horrocks and Jack Eckert. A return trip to France introduced me to many new and helpful staff members in Paris and Rouen. In particular, I am grateful to Stéphane Kraxner, now the archivist at the IPP, and currently conducting his own important research on the early pastorians.

I would like to thank the editors and readers at the University of Rochester Press. I would also like to thank the Johns Hopkins University Press for permission to use parts of my article, "Prophet for Profit" (*BHM* 71 [1997]: 583–622), in this book.

In the long process leading up to the publication of this book, I have come to learn that true mentoring is a lifetime commitment: and sometimes extends still further. Phillip Sloan, Emil Hofman, and the enduring examples of Stephen Rogers and Roy Porter have taught me this important lesson. I can only hope that, one day, I will myself be able to give to my students even a small part of what these mentors have so generously given to me. Then, there are the mentors who also provided direct and invaluable assistance on this book. Without Daniel Todes, my dissertation advisor and friend, this book, quite literally, would not exist. Anne Marie Moulin gave me a template not just for understanding the Pastorians, but for living a meaningful and generous life. (I fear I have often been better at applying the former than the latter.) She has rescued me on more occasions than I can begin to recount, and I will be forever grateful. And, to Dale Smith, who, in my "dark night of the soul," offered grace: any elegance that may have found its way into these pages is here because of you.

I have been blessed with friends at once wise, brilliant, and patient. I am grateful to Sara Harvell, who helped turn a nightmare into an adventure; and to Janet Little, Ruth Hillman, Mohsina Somji, and Sally Bragg, who have given me shelter and support. To my dear friends who also read drafts of this book—Natsu Hattori, Kelly Fritz, Kristen Heitman, Roberta Bivins, and Susan St. Ville—I owe special thanks. As each of these amazing women already knows: you are family.

I would also like to thank my more "traditional" family. To my parents, Rick and Sue; to my sister Jodi, brother Jon, nieces and nephew; to my cousins (especially Scott and Paul), my aunts and uncles: I love you all and *promise*, now that this book is complete, to attend more reunions. (I may even reply to e-mail messages!) I owe particular thanks to my grandmother, Veronica Skierkowski, who has always believed I was capable of more than I thought.

Finally, my love and deepest thanks to Derek Bond, who has been in my life even longer than this project, and who has remained with me despite its constant "competition" for my attentions. You're "the tear that hangs inside my soul forever."

Abbreviations

Journals
AIP	Annales de l'Institut Pasteur
AIPAN	Archives des Institutes Pasteur de l'Afrique du Nord
AIPT	Archives de l'Institut Pasteur de Tunis
BHM	Bulletin of the History of Medicine
BIP	Bulletin de l'Institut Pasteur
BSPE	Bulletin de la Société de Pathologie Exotique
CRAS	Comptes Rendus de l'Académie des Sciences
CRSB	Comptes Rendus de la Société de Biologie
JHM	Journal of the History of Medicine and Allied Sciences

Archives
AIP	Institut Pasteur de Paris, Archives, Paris, France
ASM	Archives Départementales de la Seine-Maritime, Rouen, France
HML/CLM	Harvard Medical Library in the Countway Library of Medicine, Boston, Mass., USA
RAC	Rockefeller Archives Center, Sleepy Hollow, NY, USA

Books by Nicolle
NVM	Naissance, Vie et Mort des Maladies Infectieuses (1930)
Biologie	Biologie de l'Invention (1932)

Introduction	*Introduction à la Carrière de la Médecine Expérimentale* (1932)
Destin	*Destin des Maladies Infectieuses* (1933)
Responsabilités	*Responsabilités de la Médecine*, 2 vols. (1935–36)
Nature	*La Nature: Conception et Morale Biologique* (1934)
Destinée	*La Destinée Humaine* (1935)
IPP	*l'Institut Pasteur de Paris*
IPT	*l'Institut Pasteur de Tunis*
AEEP	*l'Association pour l'Extension des Etudes Pastoriennes*
SEAN	*Société des Ecrivains de l'Afrique du Nord*

Prelude

The Substance of Shadows

> It wasn't a science—it was a crusade, this business.
> —Paul de Kruif, *Microbe Hunters*

Charles Nicolle was a Nobel Prize–winning French bacteriologist. Director of the Pasteur Institute of Tunis from 1903 until his death in 1936, he was founder and editor of the institute's *Archives* and prime mover of the (French-) Tunisian medical "cosmos" he had carefully orchestrated to revolve around that institute. He is best known for his 1909 demonstration of the louse transmission of typhus—research that helped earn him the Nobel. He also made significant contributions to the understanding of—among other diseases—relapsing fever, toxoplasmosis, trachoma, and kala-azar. On a level at once theoretical and practical, he constructed a type of acute, symptomless infection—"inapparent" infection—that informed his philosophical treatment of disease evolution and his pioneering theories of emergent diseases. France awarded him with its Osiris Prize, election as a nonresident member of the Académie des Sciences, and appointment to the Chair of Experimental Medicine at the Collège de France. In his spare time, he wrote seven novels and a number of short stories. Above all, however, Charles Nicolle was a microbiologist on a mission.

Nicolle's "mission" was defined and animated by his "Pastorian" identity. He himself described this identity: "In our country, we are often given the name *Pastorians*. It is not only a title of honor because it evokes one of the greatest human intellects, whose life exemplified discipline. It is also, on account of this discipline, a comparison with members of a religious order."[1] The Pastorians were "created" by Louis Pasteur's miraculous act: the salvation of a young boy who had been bitten by a rabid dog from otherwise certain and agonizing death, through the audacious application of his recently developed antirabies vaccine in 1885. Monetary contributions and infected pilgrims subsequently poured into Paris from around France and the globe, culminating in the opening of Pasteur's "institute" in 1888. His humble collaborators were elevated to the status of "disciples," who served the "Master," and trained new Pastorians, at the place they called the "*Maison mère*": the "Mother House." The Pastorian understanding of the microbial origins of infectious diseases blended with recent German work, giving force to a "germ theory" of disease that led the faithful to believe they were living in a revolutionary "Golden Age" of medicine. Although many clinicians at first resisted declaring their allegiance to this new medical church, a great number of eager young converts came to the Pasteur Institute to proclaim their fidelity and to be initiated into the mysteries of Pastorian microbiology. They were eager to go out as Pastorian missionaries, to proclaim the Pastorian "gospel" and save the suffering with their new mastery of disease. Charles Nicolle was one such Pastorian missionary.

It so happened that this microbe-oriented medicine—a medicine that brought the universalizing methods and ideologies of experimental science to the understanding and control of infectious disease—came into prominence just as western Europe was taking the globalization of its technologies and values (for better or for worse) to a whole new level. The West's earlier colonial forays into countries such as India and Algeria were, in scope, mere dress rehearsals for the great "Scramble for Africa" that escalated in the last quarter of the nineteenth century. France's Third Republic government, formed in the wake of the country's humiliating defeat by the Prussians in 1870–71, had its own agenda for expansion. The desire for profit and prestige motivated all Western nations engaged in the "scramble," to varying degrees. France's decision to describe its colonial endeavor as a "civilizing mission," however, underscores the particular manner in which the country embraced colonialism. It was a secular version of the older Christian "missions." As the French physician-anthropologist Lucien Bertholon, who had long worked in Tunisia, noted: "Formerly, one sought to transform the savages . . . into Christians. . . . Today, the mission is the same; only, instead of religion, it is the exportation of the principles of [17]89 that has become the *providential mission* of France."² The universal extension of French ideas of civilization and science—including the administration of French medicine and hygiene—would thus serve to raise up the world by controlling nature. At the same time, it would make that world more hospitable for French colonials to inhabit, all the while providing undeniable proof of France's continued glory.

It has been said that Louis Pasteur charged his followers to "go forth and teach all nations." Articulated—if perhaps apocryphally—in the context of France's *mission civilisatrice,* Pasteur's mandate took on the force of a double mission. "Pasteur Institutes" (and laboratories) extended around the globe, often appearing in French colonial possessions, forming, in a sense, their own "scientific empire." Charles Nicolle, who would first take the Pastorian mission to his provincial hometown in Normandy, witnessed firsthand the relative ease with which microbiology, and the "rational hygiene" it dictated, could be applied in the colonies as compared to France. In Tunisia he would find a more malleable environment for his missionary transformations. There, in accordance with what was quickly becoming a kind of overseas Pastorian "etiquette," Nicolle built up his institute, maximized his autonomy (including the orientation of all medical services around that institute), and adopted a "signature" disease: typhus fever. What he perhaps did not expect, however, was the extent to which typhus and Tunisia would shape *his* future—and even reshape his identity.

These, then, were the times, convictions, and decisions—the *context*— that gave broad shape to Nicolle's self-image and his conception of his mission. He was a *dutiful* Pastorian. Yet, like so many other citizens of the French Third Republic, he was a fierce individualist. Pastorism's respect for such individualism is one of the reasons Nicolle could embrace the "religion": "I am at once too French and too much a doctor—that is to say, too much an individualist (and, by character, too untamed [*trop sauvage*])—to regret that this [Pastorian] assimilation is only a moral one, and that a communal life, and the renunciation of personal self-interest, does not unite laboratory doctors in a kind of closed society."³ Bright, imaginative, and ambitious, Nicolle was also motivated by a private mission: to become the "next Pasteur." Again, this was not a unique aspiration—other ambitious Pastorians expressed a similar desire; however, the way Nicolle shaped this mission *was* unique. It was precisely through his awareness of his changing context—social, cultural, and scientific—that he would alter his ideas about what it meant to be the next Pasteur. As Nicolle's views came into conflict with the chosen direction of Pastorism in France, he would make choices that would redefine himself, his institute, and his conception of the best *means* to achieve his tripartite mission. Colonial distance, both geographical and cultural, would sharpen his perspective on Parisian developments and embolden his designs to change those he found objectionable.

One might well expect that the path of a "dutiful individualist" would be far from straight and narrow. In Nicolle's case, that expectation would be correct. At every turn, his dutiful life was shadowed by tensions and countervailing forces. He was a medical doctor who struggled with deafness; a husband who wrestled with traditional ideas of marriage and family; a son who sought to define himself outside the long shadows cast by his father, a provincial French doctor, and by his spiritual father, Louis Pasteur. Any simple faiths he might have held were shattered by World War I, the "Great War"—the same war that ushered him, through his typhus discoveries, onto the international medical stage. Thereafter, shadows loomed larger. Science was increasingly overshadowed by literature; reason, by imagination; Tunis, by Paris; laboratory, by nature; even "rational" typhus, by "absurd" relapsing fever. Nicolle's literary efforts employed images of light and shadow. His very disease construct, inapparent infection, shadowed disease—and acted as a constant shadow over civilization, as the means by which new diseases were "born."

Finally, the faithful missionary began to suspect that traditional means could no longer achieve desired ends. Heresy seemed necessary. Nicolle began to gather up the fragments of traditional beliefs—even of traditional Pastorian disease models and guiding policies—rearranging them and altering their contexts. After the war, he drew upon international collaborators, the rapidly changing life sciences, and his own scientific successes and literary skills, to craft a metaphor that he believed gave new meaning to the fragments of Western civilization: the "mosaic of powers." All life renewed itself through the constant rearrangement of its many pieces within a dynamic equilibrium. "Power" was not brute force, but proper *balance* among shifting alliances. Old diseases disappeared and new ones emerged; old civilizations crumbled and new ones arose from the dust. Nicolle believed his vision would salvage his multiple missions, including his private mission. And so, in the final years of his life, he took bold action, confronting the Parisian center with the reformulated Pastorian plan and model that he had created in the colonial periphery. The consequences of that action would bring about a final set of redefinitions.

This book, then, is about the intertwined identities of a man and his mission, as seen through the double lens of his chosen disease and his adopted country. The time in which he lived, the diseases he chose to investigate, the colonial life he embraced, and the trials he faced all helped direct these changing identities, shaping a unique individual who made substantive contributions to science and society. These contributions would in themselves justify a book devoted to their study. Yet, on another level, Nicolle was less unique. He was like so many other individuals in the modern West, struggling to find (or create) meaning in a rapidly changing world. In this struggle, we witness an aspiration more universal still.

Two years before he died, my undergraduate mentor, Stephen J. Rogers—perhaps one of the last true Renaissance humanists—wrote:

> There are certain subjects that concern all human beings in every age. We find that Sophocles and Shakespeare and Dante have written about love and death and happiness and sorrow. . . . But Sophocles and Shakespeare and Dante, despite all their power, cannot say loving or dying or rejoicing or grieving or believing for us. We have to say love for ourselves, and death, and being happy, and losing, and striving, and needing, and feeling for ourselves. The generation that does not say these things well for itself has failed. The person who has not said these things with some adequacy for him- or herself has missed out. But these are always the hardest things to say . . .[4]

By following Nicolle's struggle for meaning, we find, if you will, his "humanity"—with all the particularities and convictions, constraints and contradictions, that the term, in practice, implies.

Introduction

The Door of the Sadiki

> The center of my observations was the indigenous hospital in Tunis. Often, when I was at the hospital, I would walk over the typhus-ridden bodies [of patients] who had come to be admitted, but fell, extinguished, before the door. . . . The typhus patients were treated in the hospital's common rooms. Up to the door of these rooms, they spread contagion. . . . Yet, once admitted into the common room, the patient contaminated none of the patients in neighboring beds. . . . This observation guided me. I wondered what happened between the door of the hospital and the hospital room. What happened was this: the typhus patient was stripped of his clothing and undergarments, shaved, and washed. The agent of the contagion was thus something attached to the skin, to the undergarments, which the soap and water removed. It could only be the louse. It was the louse.
> —Charles Nicolle, 1928

Charles Nicolle is remembered today as the man who won the 1928 Nobel Prize in Physiology or Medicine, largely for his demonstration that the louse transmitted typhus. Outside France and Tunisia, he is principally remembered through his Nobel speech—and, from it, for the above discovery narrative. The "hospital" to which he referred was the Sadiki Hospital in Tunis, where Tunisian patients were treated. The moment when his revelatory walk took place is less clear. It may have been any time between 1903 and 1909. The best guess is 1906, but Nicolle never really specified. Also unclear is when Nicolle first came up with the "Door of the Sadiki" discovery narrative. He had published the articles demonstrating the louse's role as typhus vector in 1909, but he did not relate the discovery as a grand intuitive flash. Instead, he described it as the product of a collaborative effort between laboratory, clinic, and field, resting on multiple layers of evidence. It was only in the 1920s that Nicolle told the Sadiki story as a coherent public narrative about the "genius" of scientific discovery. It emerged in this "telescoped" form, I believe, out of an awkward convergence of personal ambition (fueled by assorted successes), colonial location (he was director of the Pasteur Institute of Tunis), and a kind of socioreligious displacement that occurred in the wake of world war and that desperately sought new definitions for old faiths. Nicolle placed his faith in the "Pastorian mission," which was itself embedded in the nineteenth-century positivistic belief in "science." The "door" was a metaphor that gave him the means to create another metaphor, the "mosaic of powers." It was this latter metaphor that shaped his own revised version of this faith and, thus, the missions that dominated his life.

Charles Nicolle was born in Rouen, a city in Normandy about 75 miles northwest of Paris, in September 1866; he died in Tunis, Tunisia, 900 miles south and slightly east of Paris, in February 1936.[1] Though he *lived* in Paris for only seven years—the years during which he prepared to become a doctor and medical researcher—it would be fair to say that his focus never strayed far from France's capital city.[2] He both loved and loathed the place and its politics; and the place and its politics defined this man who often felt placeless and abhorred politics. Paris was the heart of French culture, science,[3] and government: during Nicolle's lifetime, that government was the country's third experiment with Republicanism. Indeed, Nicolle was born four years before the rise of France's Third Republic and died four years before it ended.[4] His earliest clear memory was of looking out the window of his home over a column of Prussian soldiers: "It lengthens, falls into line, comes to a stop; black, powdery, hostile." Ten of its members presented themselves to his mother (his father, a doctor, was away seeing patients) for accommodations. "They didn't seem to be very difficult people."[5] France's defeat by Prussia in 1871 was costly. France lost Alsace and part of Lorraine, and was burdened by a war indemnity of five billion francs. It also lost face. The Prussian victory helped shape the identity and heighten the nationalist sentiments of both of the newly allied German state and the newly instituted French Third Republic.[6]

Though less than a century had passed since France first overturned its monarchy, the country had experienced the subsequent reign of three kings; rule by two emperors—Uncle and Nephew Napoleon; and two periods of republican government.[7] Comparatively, the Third Republic, if not wildly popular, enjoyed longevity. It was able to do so in part because of its successful establishment of institutions that helped ensure its perpetuation.[8] Not least of these was the extension of public schooling and the concomitant exclusion of religious teaching in these secular schools. Indeed, the tensions between the Catholic Church and the French state were a central defining force in the Third Republic. Although France's traditional links with the Church were being attacked by the Republican government (leading to an official separation of church and state by 1905), the influence of Catholic organization and values remained strong. The French still embraced the Church's centralized, hierarchical structure. France had already elevated science to a kind of religion earlier in the nineteenth century, when Auguste Comte devised his positivist philosophy.[9] The Third Republic government similarly looked to science to fill the role once played by religion.[10] Nation and science were thus offered as the new substance of society, if its structure was still informed by older religious categories.

During the early years of the Third Republic, France joined other European nations in extending what had previously been a relatively circumscribed interest in colonialism into a global project. Successful mapping expeditions in Africa combined with increased interest in colonial domination to create a perfect demonstration of the relationship between knowledge and power. In the 1870s and early 1880s, European countries, in search of new sources of raw materials and new markets for their growing industries, as well as of demonstrative proof of their own power, began laying claim to non-Western countries at a rapid pace. In short, this was no cooperative endeavor: it was a nationalistic competition. The so-called Scramble for Africa, which subsided only with the outbreak of world war, was formalized and codified at the 1885–86 Conference of Berlin.[11] At its peak, this imperialist impulse resulted in Europe's (divided) possession of nearly 85 percent of the earth's surface.[12]

The French tended to work outward from earlier colonial possessions, protectorates, and trading posts, laying claim to what would be called "French Indochina" as well as to great portions of North, West, and Central Africa.[13] Tunisia, for example, was made a French protectorate in 1881 in part to strengthen France's hold on its earlier colonial possession in North Africa, Algeria.[14] If profit motivated some to support the colonial project in its early years, the relatively dismal financial output and high cost of the colonies themselves would hardly have sustained it over the decades. Rather, nationalism—given impetus by the perceived humiliation by the Prussians, but quickly generalized beyond military defeat—was more central to the extension of French colonialism.[15] Nationalism, in France and elsewhere, was no simple force but, rather, an emerging collective identity informed by a complex of forces, each pulling with varying degrees of strength in differing directions.[16] It brought together such things as a rising appreciation (and particular formulation) of a nation's own history; a belief in its international significance; and a conviction, increasingly supported by a particular take on "biology," of its racial superiority.[17] France, still stinging from its recent military defeat, was particularly interested in demonstrating the importance of "power" beyond physical force: the power of its culture.

A revealing expression of French nationalism came in the country's justification of its colonial project as a "civilizing mission." The religious foundations of this secular mission are evident. Though many countries claimed that their imperialistic expansions offered the opportunity to spread "civilization" throughout the world, France's *mission civilisatrice*, as historian Alice Conklin has persuasively argued, went well beyond rhetorical justification, informing the very direction of the country's colonial governments. The civilizing mission acted as a kind of metaphor, allowing France to reconcile apparent opposites: its "aggressive imperialism" and "republican ideals."[18] The mission's content, she argues, changed over time; however, its central tenet, its faith in "mastery," persisted. This was "mastery" in the sense made famous more than two centuries earlier by Sir Francis Bacon: mastery of nature through knowledge, freeing humanity, Conklin continues, "from specific forms of tyranny: the tyranny of the elements over man, of disease over health. . . . Mastery in all these realms was integral to France's self-definition under the Third Republic."[19] "Mastery," by the extension of French civilization to the colonies, thus gave French colonialism the weight of a (secular) moral imperative, and its successful application in turn helped substantiate France's identity as the embodiment of true civilization.[20]

By now, it has become commonplace to argue that science, technology, and medicine were all "tools of empire," central to the effective establishment of colonies.[21] It should also be evident how medicine not only made the colonies safer for the colonizers and helped win over the trust of indigenous peoples, but also, for France, could sustain and amplify the civilizing mission. The Pasteur Institute, its so-called "filial" institutes, and even Louis Pasteur himself, at once exemplified and enacted this coupling of medicine and mission in support of French nationalism. To understand this dynamic more clearly, and to set the stage for Nicolle's work, it is necessary to say a few words about Pasteur, germ theory, and the network of Pasteur Institutes.

Indeed, Charles Nicolle would be almost incomprehensible without first understanding the research path, and the myth, of a man he met just once: Louis Pasteur.[22] Pasteur was not a physician, but a chemist. He had made his name earlier in the nineteenth century by working on optical isomerism. Ever on the lookout for opportunities to bring science to industry—and public attention to his work—Pasteur soon turned to studies of fermentation, investigating the diseases of wine and, in the wake of the Franco-Prussian War, beer. In the course of these investigations, he became convinced that the existence of the spontaneous generation of life could not be supported by scientific evidence, and that human disease was produced in a manner similar to the diseases of beer and wine. He eventually made the leap from chemical ferments to living microbes as the causal agents of disease. In so doing, he moved from chemistry to medicine, making a formal declaration of his convictions to France's Académie de Médicine in 1878.[23] Actual proof followed later. His first large public display occurred in 1881 and concerned veterinary rather than human medicine. Yet, it concerned a very *costly* animal disease: anthrax. This was his theatrical demonstration of the efficacy of his anthrax vaccine at Pouilly-le-Fort, so marvelously analyzed by Bruno Latour.[24] The vaccine itself, quite consciously named after Edward Jenner's famous vaccine against smallpox,[25] was a product of Pasteur's laboratory. It was created by the systematic reduction, or "attenuation," of the *virulence* of the microbes that caused anthrax.[26] Thereafter, attenuation and the production of vaccines from viruses—"virus-vaccines"—would be central to the Pastorian project.[27]

Pasteur employed what would become his most famous virus-vaccine four years later. This was the vaccine developed to prevent the onset of a disease that was far less common than anthrax, but that had long held sway over the public imagination because of the horror, and inevitability, of the death it produced: rabies. Pasteur and his followers had developed a series of vaccines of varying degrees of attenuation by transferring rabies from dogs to rabbits, then hanging the rabbit spines (it was known that rabies affected the nervous system) to dry for varying lengths of time. The vaccine's apparently successful human trial in July 1885 on the "young Joseph Meister"—many times bitten by a rabid animal and almost certain to die—became the stuff of legends.[28] It also became a focal point for pilgrimages and financial gifts. The money was used to create the Pasteur Institute, which opened in 1888. Pasteur's colleagues, often referred to as his "disciples," continued to work on the production of new vaccines, administered the rabies vaccine to infected pilgrims, and, given Pasteur's fragile physical state after suffering from a series of strokes, helped shape the new institute. They also trained more followers in the mysteries of the rising new medical science of bacteriology: Pasteur's disciple Emile Roux devised the institute's famous *Cours* to that end, thereby forming future generations of "Pastorians"[29] who would be ever faithful to the *Maison mère* and eager to "go forth" and spread the "gospel" of Pasteur.[30]

All this religious rhetoric is not the precious construction of postmodern historical interpretation but, rather, was woven into the very thoughts, actions, and institutions of our historical actors. Like the French Third Republic, the Pasteur Institute was profoundly shaped by Catholic forms—even while, in both cases, the religious content of those forms had been replaced by more secular beliefs.[31] Remnants of Catholic values remained, even shading into cultural and political imperatives that animated both the civilizing and the Pastorian missions. The particularly French approach to profit in medicine, for example, was central to the structure and functioning of the Pasteur Institute. During the nineteenth century, there was a strong expectation that human medicines would not be made for profit: there was even a law prohibiting the patenting of such medicines.[32] Accordingly, the Pasteur Institute developed, manufactured, and distributed vaccines, acting as its own pharmaceutical company, in a manner driven by this nonprofit understanding of medicine. Both Pasteur and Roux (who would himself eventually direct the institute) rejected personal profit from their human vaccine discoveries; researchers generally existed on meager salaries.[33]

Pasteur, however, was a savvy enough administrator to establish programs of animal vaccines and agricultural testing that helped pay the bills.[34] Moreover, he established a unique relationship between his institute and the French government. The Pasteur Institute did not follow the traditional lines of the state-centralized French university system. Instead, it was a private *foundation*—even though Pasteur expected the state to help with vaccine production costs and occasional budget balancing. The institute's private, nonprofit status meant that it was both required to serve the public and allowed to accept public donations.[35] Pasteur thus created a center of medical research that collected both state and private funds in support of its ministrations, but remained autonomous in its direction. This autonomy allowed Pasteur's institute to focus on research in addition to treatment and teaching. Yet, preserving medicine's nonprofit status presented a constant challenge to the institute's profitable maintenance.[36] The challenge would only grow after Pasteur's death. At the same time, this "charitable" self-image fitted nicely with the missionary mentality of Pastorism.

Spreading the "gospel" of bacteriology in accordance with Pasteur's wishes found a convenient vector in the extension of France's civilizing mission.[37] Europe had become freer from infectious diseases over the course of the century, leaving the "tropics" as the most promising grounds for "microbe hunters" to make new conquests (and, in so doing, an international reputation).[38] At the same time, the missionary microbiologists promised to make the "dangerous" colonies safer for colonial troops by controlling disease, as they helped colonial governments convince indigenous populations of the advantages that could be had by embracing Western domination.[39] Although many independent countries established "Pasteur" institutes and smaller laboratories, a great number of the overseas "filial" institutes were created in French colonial possessions.[40] The first was established in Saigon by Pastorian Albert Calmette—future assistant director of the Paris institute—just two years after the *Maison mère* was inaugurated.[41] In 1893, both Tunisia, a French protectorate, and Turkey, by no means a French possession, were similarly "pasteurized." Many other Pastorian laboratories and institutes followed: some sixty, altogether, by the onset of World War II.[42] Historian Anne Marie Moulin has justly dubbed the resulting network a "scientific empire."[43]

In their overseas locales, the Pastorians mirrored Pasteur's actions, setting up rabies clinics, evaluating crops and livestock, taking control of local health and hygiene concerns, and developing virus-vaccines. The Pasteur Institute of Paris (IPP) now functioned much like the Vatican, as the center of doctrine and authority. (The Pasteur Institute of Tunis was a rare exception, as it was administered directly by the French colonial government in Tunisia.) Ideally, the filial institutes would follow Pastorian doctrine, applying the "pure" research from Paris by adapting it to the local conditions of their own affiliated institutes.[44] Each of the filials even had a share of the "one true" rabies vaccine, thus mirroring Catholic churches boasting splinters of the "one true cross." Furthering the Pastorian myth and mission, directors of the overseas Pasteur Institutes commissioned busts of Pasteur—and, eventually, of each other—to be inaugurated around the world, and they delivered "homilies" on great Pastorian achievements to all who would listen.[45] In this way, the 1922 centennial of Pasteur's birth was truly the festival celebrated around the world. Moreover, as Pasteur had been buried in a gilded and mosaic-filled crypt located in part of his institute, many a director of an overseas Pasteur Institute chose his own "churchyard" as his final resting place. Charles Nicolle was buried behind what was once the entrance of his Tunis institute; his successor, Etienne Burnet, selected a quiet location in the institute's gardens.

Thus far, I have painted the Pastorian mission and its colonial extension with broad strokes that would allow one to believe that an old-fashioned diffusionist model, with medical science moving passively from metropole to periphery, applied. Such a model would suggest that the extension of Pastorism was somehow inevitable—whether by the march of "truth" or the domination of might. But the Pastorian mission did *not* extend through inevitable diffusion. Recent scholarship, on the history of colonial medicine as well as on technology transfer within and beyond colonial spheres, has been actively engaged with exploring the dynamic interrelation of the so-called "core" and "periphery."[46] Charles Nicolle provides a striking case study for such concerns. He moved from the quintessential metropoles—Paris and the Pasteur Institute of Paris—first to the French provinces (Rouen) then to a French possession (Tunisia). In these "peripheral" locations, he enjoyed great success and, particularly in Tunis, made discoveries, and constructed an institution that would find international acclaim. Study of the means by which Nicolle made his achievements offers insight into the kinds of networks and negotiations necessary for Western science to be recognized when conducted in the colonies.[47] It also highlights the constraints that colonial distance imposed upon such success: despite his many accomplishments, Nicolle always defined himself in relation to Paris. In a favorite autobiographical formulation, he referred to himself as an "ultraprovincial infraparisian."[48]

As one considers Nicolle and his work, it is important to remember that he was, as he himself observed, a "second-generation" Pastorian. He was not among Pasteur's original disciples.[49] At the same time, he *was* studying at the *Maison mère* quite soon after it opened. Pasteur, if no longer terribly active, was still alive, and Pasteur's institute was still in the process of being defined. Nicolle may have been too young to be a disciple, but he was not too young to be swept away by the excitement of being present at the establishment of this so-called Golden Age of medicine.[50] He was already a Pastorian when the myths that would come to enshroud Pasteur were being woven. When Pasteur died in 1895, the institute was formally handed over to his chosen successor, Emile Duclaux. In fact, Pasteur's poor health meant that Duclaux had been shaping the institute from its earliest days.[51] Although Duclaux had studied medicine, he was more inclined toward biology and chemistry, and the institute he directed continued to encourage a broad application of "microbiology."[52] He would also help shape how history would long perceive Pasteur and his work: a year after the "Master" died, Duclaux wrote his scientific biography. (This biography was followed, four years later, by the better known contribution of Pasteur's son-in-law, René Vallery-Radot.)[53] Just as significantly, Duclaux would contribute to Pasteur's myth in his 1898 textbook of bacteriology by attributing to him the doctrine of specificity.[54]

The doctrine of specificity, which rested on the notion that one specific microbe caused one specific disease, has often been held up as the heart of the bacteriological "revolution." Clearly, Duclaux had come to see it as such and thus sought to fold it into the Pastorian myth. In fact, the codification of causal specificity was the product of German, not French, investigations: the German physician Robert Koch, following his teacher Joseph Henle, outlined a series of conditions that had to be met to demonstrate the causal relationship of a particular microbe to a distinct disease. His formulations came to be called "Koch's Postulates," but this did not deter the periodic recurrence of priority disputes between the researchers of such clearly divided nations as were France and Germany.[55] Recently, historical studies have raised questions about whether there was a "bacteriological revolution"—and just how fair it is to attribute this apparent revolution to a singular "germ theory" or to attach it to too strict a conception of specificity.[56] Beneath the ambiguities of historical reality, however, lay a belief in specificity that was a central tenet of those who then had faith in bacteriology. If specificity was in fact a "straw man," it did have a very real impact on the disease concepts, research choices, and larger conceptual questions of individuals such as Nicolle.[57]

After Nicolle completed his training in Paris, he returned to Rouen, where he attempted to actualize his newly minted Pastorian mission. In its details, this mission was informed by Pasteur's life and work: it would encourage the extension of microbiology to all possible spheres of existence, ensuring the health of humans, animals, industries, and environments. Nicolle faced resistance in the form of the Rouen medical establishment. Subsequently, he took the same model to Tunis, where he faced far less resistance and enjoyed greater success. Shortly after Nicolle arrived in Tunisia, however, Duclaux died, leaving Emile Roux to direct the IPP. Roux's reign in Paris was largely coextensive with Nicolle's in Tunis.[58] Roux, a physician by training, lacked Pasteur's dramatic flair, preferring instead an almost monastic existence. These inclinations were evident in his administrative style. Under Roux's direction, the IPP moved along paths that Nicolle thought to be increasingly narrow and, consequently, damaging to the future of the Pastorian mission. In response, Nicolle began to revise certain key elements of his own mission. His critique of Paris, and the revised mission it informed, were not limited to administrative decisions. They extended even to the Pastorian conception of infectious disease, questioning in particular its understanding of specificity. Ultimately, sheltered by colonial distance and personal success, Nicolle devised a series of plans to force change upon Roux and Paris—largely from the shores of Tunisia.

Neither Nicolle's decision to act, nor the substance of his missionary revisions, was *wholly* determined by his experiences as director of the Pasteur Institute of Tunis. There was a deeply personal element in the process as well. In all public forums until he was nearly fifty years old, Nicolle had been a dutiful son, husband, and Pastorian. In *private* communications, a more critical persona is evident. Still, these more subversive inclinations did not often come to the surface, nor did they preclude Nicolle from enjoying a few certainties. His deepest faith was reserved for "science": reason informed by careful observation, whose proper application would bring about the progress and perhaps perfection of human civilization.[59] He was, after all, a child of the French Third Republic. Suddenly, however, the line between private and public, the sustaining faith in select certainties, *ruptured*. (Nicolle would become particularly fond of this word.) It was 1914, and the Great War shattered his beliefs. Science and technology, the leading lights of Western civilization, had led to the degradation, rather than the perfection, of humanity. "Scientific reason" had had its critics before World War I. The war brought their concerns outside the fairly narrow circle of the philosophical elite and into the thinking of a far broader populace: a populace that included Nicolle.[60] Nicolle's close friend, medical doctor and cultural critic Georges Duhamel, illustrated the horrors that the expansion of science, technology, and even the successful practice of medicine, had allowed, in his prize-winning novel, *Civilization, 1914–17*.[61]

The years of war and "postwar"—the latter of which, history would redefine as "interwar"—were difficult ones for Western culture in general, and for its medical researchers in particular. They were years when old certainties were challenged, even down to the meaning of existence itself. They were marked by a growing awareness of the enormous *complexity* of existence, which applied to societies and psyches as well as to medicine and science. Perhaps it was most difficult for men of Nicolle's generation, who were born, trained, and even became professionally established in a time of certainty, only to be forced in the prime of their well-established lives (Nicolle was forty-seven when World War I began) into an era of doubt.[62] Nicolle himself spent the rest of his life trying to reconstruct "science" (particularly biological science) so as to strip it of violence and open it to dynamic change. Only through such redemptive redefinition of science, he believed, could the Pastorian mission—and thus civilization—be saved.

Even before the war began, the fragmentation of life-oriented science was underway. As Western countries were using colonies as social laboratories, biologists were increasingly turning to their own laboratories for new insights into sciences that were once principally grounded in observation and description.[63]

This experimental approach gave rise to rapidly proliferating biological subdisciplines, at once diverging and claiming territory from each other.[64] By the 1920s, the old field of natural history had been tilled and appeared to be fertile; however, the nature of the fruit it might bear was not yet evident. It had been twenty years since Gregor Mendel's seminal work on heredity had been rediscovered, and since Hugo de Vries proposed *mutation* as the force creating the variations in living organisms that nature eventually "selected." Evolutionary questions had been given further immediacy by Wilhelm Roux's experimental work on embryo development.[65] Yet, it remained unclear how heredity and variation functioned, and how, precisely, "evolution" worked.[66] In its darker manifestations, biology also served to legitimate so-called "scientific" racism, which had existed long before the war but hardened in the interwar period. Indeed, it took on such popularity that it even altered the content of France's civilizing mission.[67]

By the time World War I ended, bacteriology's "Golden Age" was (arguably) forty years old. There had been much time, and many opportunities, both national and international, to test its assumptions and methods. Indeed, the war itself had acted as a kind of litmus test for bacteriology's progress. Claims for its successes—for example, the rarity of typhus on the Western Front[68]—could be countered by abundant evidence of its limitations and even its failures.[69] When put into action, early bacteriological thinking was found to be overly simplistic. Human host, microbial parasite, and the host/parasite relationship, were far more complex in nature than in textbook formulations. There were, for example, an increasing number of so-called "filterable viruses" being discovered. These were entities that caused disease but, unlike "normal" microbes, passed through standard filters, were too small to be seen under standard microscopes, and could not be cultivated outside a host. Were they simply tiny microbes? How could they be controlled?[70] Similarly, vaccination—the word was applied by Pastorians to cover both preventive and curative inoculations—was going through a period of reconceptualization. The early days of relatively straightforward "virus-vaccine" production were gone. Vaccines for many of the diseases that could be prevented or cured with the older methods of attenuation and antitoxin production had been developed. What remained were the more difficult cases, such as diseases caused by filterable viruses. These difficulties were exacerbated by a growing appreciation that the body's immune response was far more difficult to account for than early appeals to phagocytes and lock-and-key antigen–antibody models had suggested.[71]

Indeed, it was increasingly suspected that the very concept of specificity was too rigid. Sometimes, one microbe produced two diseases; sometimes, two microbes produced one disease. The role of asymptomatic or "hidden" carriers in the conservation and distribution of infectious disease was well known and appreciated.[72] Nicolle himself extended this complicating formulation with his concept of acute, symptomless disease: "'inapparent' infection."[73] Moreover, bacteria were not fixed entities. If interwar research did not press the issue as far as did earlier transformist theories,[74] it had offered striking evidence that bacteria *changed*. Even the emergence of new disease species through bacterial mutation seemed plausible.[75] Problems and questions multiplied.

Tangible progress toward providing answers to these questions came only later. These answers began to take shape in the 1930s. (This was also the time that evolutionary theorists' widely acclaimed "synthesis" was accepted.) In medicine, the possibilities of vaccine production were greatly widened with the development of yolk sack cultivation. Insight into the nature of filterable viruses came in 1935, when Wendell Stanley crystallized the virus of tobacco mosaic disease. Curative medicines moved beyond things such as antitoxins and convalescent sera (and Ehrlich's salvarsan) with the discovery of sulfa drugs that same year. This was, of course, followed by the appreciation and usable production of penicillin during World War II.[76] The new "Golden Age" of biomedicine emerged fully in the 1940s and 1950s, which boasted the rise of microbial genetics and the widespread distribution of the new "miracle cures." In short, the biomedical sciences became powerful, laboratory-based disciplines, and medicine again showed its miraculous powers, only *after* Nicolle had ended his years of active research—indeed, largely after he had died.

One may take issue with the idea that golden ages exist. Nicolle himself did.[77] I appeal to the formulation only to emphasize that Nicolle experienced his professional formation during a period of heightened certainty, and then carried that certainty into a world that was far more complex than early expectations had suggested. The perception of certainty—and it is the *perception* that gives the concept of a Golden Age some analytic substance—was partially eclipsed during the years when Nicolle was director of the Pasteur Institute of Tunis. The subsequent era of perceived certainty in medical research cast a long shadow over the history of bacteriology—so long, in fact, that it reached back almost to the discipline's formative days. Despite the fact that historians have long decried the writing of history by and for "winners," they have largely neglected this shadowy period of medical history.[78] The case of Charles Nicolle hints at what its closer study might reveal.

Nicolle approached the escalating uncertainty of his time in a manner that may not always have produced answers that would eventually be accepted as "correct." Yet, the approach itself is revealing of both the man and his time, as are the answers he devised. He combined his long-standing interest in natural history with a broad review of biology's latest developments to help him better understand the relations between varieties of typhus and relapsing fever. To this, he added his continued efforts to perfect virus-vaccines, his understanding of inapparent infection, and his careful review of changes in immunological and (to a lesser extent) epidemiological theory, and constructed his own theory of the "birth, life, and death," or "destiny," of infectious diseases.[79] He applied it not only to the rise of individual epidemics, but to the evolution of disease *species*.[80] If many bacteriologists had come to suspect that old concepts of specificity no longer explained the available evidence, it was Nicolle who was among the first to give coherent shape to a new understanding of "emergent" diseases, articulated within what in other countries would be called an "ecological" framework.[81]

Further, Nicolle would combine a number of cultural currents, including the French effort to define power outside brute force, in his redefinition of specificity. This redefinition rested on a metaphor, the "mosaic of powers," that maintained balance between allied individuals through perpetual "equilibrium." He would extend this metaphor to ideas about creativity; he would use it to explain the enduring force of both morality and Plato's old triumvirate of "beauty, goodness, and truth"; he would appeal to it to dictate the proper (biological) nature of society and to indicate the path by which "civilization" might be preserved. In all this, he never strayed far from his Pastorian mission: he used the mosaic to redefine the very heart of Pastorian ideas about disease and cure—"virulence" and vaccines. It was this vision of infectious disease that he added to his administrative critique of the Pasteur Institute of Paris to formulate his own approach to the Pastorian mission's salvation. All this was done—perhaps could only be done—at a colonial distance from Paris. Nicolle knew this, too: "I am a captive who complains of his prison, but who perhaps could not live outside of it."[82]

Today, we again live in a world of medical uncertainty. As Nicolle himself predicted, new diseases have emerged, and international efforts to produce effective vaccines and cures to control them have met with only limited success. Infectious diseases once "conquered" have adapted to medicine's arsenal, with no pill or no shot left to curb their spread.[83] It seems timely to produce a study of a medical researcher, one of the leaders in his field, who spent his life attempting to find a way out of ambiguity.[84]

Nicolle would not live to see the efforts he and his colleagues made achieve the goals they had set for them. This, too—if by the chance timing of his death—was a central component of Nicolle's identity. He spent much of his professional career in a kind of "no-man's-land" between eras of certainty. In many ways, his struggle to re-create certainty defined him. It guided his early efforts to recreate Pastorism in Tunisia as it guided his later efforts to redefine Pastorism so as to save the Pastorian mission from the ravages of an uncertain and rapidly changing world. Wrapped within this struggle were smaller but no less constant struggles with isolation, tradition, religion, and science. Nicolle was looking for a sense of place, of connectedness, in a fragmented world. He did so in a way that was unique to his situation, and that made him unique. Yet, in this way, he was like so many other French citizens, both at home and in the colonies, seeking meaning in an era no longer quite "modern," but not yet post-modern. Mutual isolation rarely creates community. Where, after all, is the "*patrie de nomade*"?[85]

Part One

Thesis
Embracing Missions

1

Staring at the Sea

Nicolle and the Pasteur Institute of Tunis

> The heaviness of the warm air hung over the sea. The fishermen's lanterns made furrows in the gulf's steamy haze, like living reflections of the fires lit in the sky. And my thoughts, in search of their chimerical and nomadic prey, glided among these moving lights, and went astray on the dark and distant horizon.
>
> Every now and then a rustling of life—the noise of their nets falling upon the water, or the tardy silhouettes of silent passers-by—ruptured the spell I was under, and my reason, awakened, ran up in haste, as would a dog with the slightest encouragement. . . .
>
> And I dreamed of Apuleius, before the sleeping sea of Carthage, by the light of a lamp made of clay.
> —Charles Nicolle, "La Naissance des Muses," 1915

Outre-Mer

For historical reasons, Charles Nicolle was captivated by the town of Carthage in his newly adopted country of Tunisia. Its faded glory, its cultural heritage, came to inform his ideas about civilization and to animate his works of fiction. For more visually aesthetic reasons, though, he loved the village of Sidi Bou

Saïd. "Sidi Bou" lay (as it does today) about 20 kilometers northeast of Tunis, on a hill overlooking the sea.[1] There, drinking mint tea at a café, Nicolle would hold court, discussing the composition of the country's many ancient mosaics with archeologist friend Père Delattre, lamenting the perils of war with novelist friend Georges Duhamel, or composing articles on bacteriological research with his collaborators at the Pasteur Institute of Tunis. The sea was always in view. Nicolle was fond of the sea, not only as an object of visual beauty but also as a highly personal metaphor, a symbol of both treachery and salvation.[2] Geographically, it acted at once as barrier and gateway between Europe and its "less civilized" neighbors. The Mediterranean Sea had been Nicolle's means of escape from what he considered the narrow-minded conservatism of his native Normandy; yet, at the same time, it was a most immediate source of his isolation from France. The eminently logical Nicolle was perched atop a sea of ambiguity, even of outright contradiction.

It was late in 1902 that Charles Nicolle had crossed the sea to take up his life as a "Tunisian" Pastorian.[3] He was thirty-six years old and brought with him his wife, two young children, and a host of assumptions and aspirations. Like many Pastorians then being sent overseas to proliferating colonial institutes, he was motivated by a deep sense of mission.[4] This mission had as its goal the almost biblical propagation of Pasteur's words and deeds, embodied by the formation of Pasteur Institutes that ritualistically repeated the actions of the "Master." The directors of these institutes would work to place themselves at the center of their adopted country's health and hygiene; they would, following Pasteur, produce Pastorian products: vaccines, laboratory tests, and original research. This Pastorian mission was never far removed from France's "civilizing mission." Microbiology would make the world safe for French cultural expansion, which, in turn, would preserve civilization itself. For Nicolle, this dual mission was sustained by a third, more private, mission: to become the "next Pasteur."[5] Nicolle embraced these intertwined missions enthusiastically. He was ambitious, talented, and well prepared to face the challenges ahead by the lessons he had learned in his first attempt to preach the gospel of Pasteur, something he had done with only limited success in his native Rouen.

Rouen

Nicolle was born on September 21, 1866, in Rouen, France.[6] The moral climate of this damp, beautiful Normandy town was conservative: only a decade earlier, Gustav Flaubert had captured the setting masterfully in *Madame Bovary*.

Nicolle's family was perfectly at home there. Like Flaubert's characters, the Nicolles were self-consciously bourgeois, looking to solidify their place in society. Father Eugène, himself from a family of artisans and shopkeepers, practiced medicine, while mother Avice tended to the housework and the moral work of teaching her three sons to be righteous and (with only partial success) devoutly Catholic.[7] Eugène and Avice had high expectations for their sons, particularly their two eldest: Maurice (b. 1862) was to become a famous medical researcher and Charles a provincial doctor, destined to take over his father's practice. Youngest son Marcel (b. 1871) was freer to pursue his own inclinations, which leaned toward art and the humanities.

Charles, however, did not fit perfectly into his parents' plans for him. A solitary and imaginative child who longed for adventure, he found Rouen "such a desert, such a tomb"—and dealt with it by turning inward. Writing of himself in the third person, he later recalled that "to save himself from boredom . . . he had his imagination and his reading. . . . At home, he lived, during his free time, a life within himself."[8] He found in literature the furniture for his interior life. His earliest literary memories were of Jean de La Fontaine's fables, which presented grim morality tales in the guise of children's stories. Like children throughout France, Nicolle memorized many of these fables. Later, he would weave their images and lessons into his philosophy of nature. Moving from La Fontaine to the novels of Jules Verne, Nicolle used fictional adventure to escape the confines of provincial life. With brother Maurice, he wrote plays that they performed for their family. At school, he excelled in history and rhetoric,[9] although for a long time, he had no great desire to succeed in his studies as an end in itself.[10] Even when he did wish to do well, he could never quite master foreign languages, calculus—or handwriting.[11]

The tangible world did offer the young Charles opportunities for more direct enjoyment. Two repeated childhood events retained an almost sacred status in Nicolle's memories. Both featured his father. The first was his family's annual seaside summer vacation. Charles, his brothers, and his mother would head off together for several weeks; Eugène Nicolle, unable to leave his patients for long, would join them for a few days each year. For those "two or three days," his father's presence would "animate" their lives and their surroundings. Yet, this "great joy" was "brief." His father would soon vanish, as would the "enchantment" he had brought with him. Long after his father's death, Nicolle continued to find great solace in summers at the sea.[12] The second event took place on those rare evenings when Eugène had a few spare moments before falling asleep. Charles and Maurice would sit near his bedside, "notebooks in hand," as their father recounted to them his lectures in natural history. For, in addition to his medical practice, Eugène Nicolle was Chair of Natural History at Rouen's École Préparatoire des Sciences et des Lettres. He even taught his young sons some comparative anatomy. Here, too, Nicolle would remember how his father's words brought the world around them to life.[13] Nature found its way into Nicolle's imagination through literature, natural history, and his father's magical, if elusive, presence.

Circumstances—again involving his father—intervened to pull Charles out of his interior world and into the reality his parents had shaped for him. Early in 1884, Eugène Nicolle died. Charles, not yet eighteen, complied with his father's dying wish and wholly embraced the medical future Eugène had envisioned for him. He focused on excelling academically for the duration of his studies at the Lycée Corneille, and in his baccalaureate examinations. Having successfully completed his qualifying requirements, Charles then entered medical school. As Maurice was already studying in Paris, Charles stayed in Rouen, where he could help his mother with his younger brother. After finishing his first two years of study at the local École de Médecine, Nicolle joined his older brother in Paris, where he continued his medical studies.[14] Impressively, he succeeded at the competitive Internat des Hôpitaux de Paris on the first try and was named laboratory *préparateur* at the Faculté de Médecine.[15] Charles Nicolle appeared to be well on his way to fulfilling his father's vision.

As he learned how to auscultate patients, however, Nicolle discovered something deeply and personally disturbing. One of his ears was able to hear those diagnostically important internal sounds far better than the other. Initially, he dealt with his growing deafness by favoring his good ear. Soon, however, Nicolle acknowledged his limitations and modified his medical course: "Prudently, I learned the least risky specialty, skin diseases, and set to work in the laboratory."[16] It was not quite the approach to medicine his father had had in mind but, rather, a digression necessitated by forces even stronger than the posthumous will of Eugène Nicolle.

At the time, "skin diseases" and "the laboratory" intersected most obviously in the study of sexually transmitted diseases. And "the laboratory" where one went to study disease in France ca. 1890 was Pasteur's. (Maurice Nicolle was already there.) Indeed, it was the year after Nicolle's father died that Pasteur conducted his mythic vaccination of "The Young Joseph Meister" against a seemingly inevitable, and inevitably deadly, case of rabies. Nicolle was in Paris as the world's gratitude for Pasteur's miraculous interventions took material shape in the construction of the Pasteur Institute. Soon after the Institute officially opened, Pasteur's right-hand medical man, Emile Roux, assembled his famous *Cours* for instructing an influx of eager students in the ways of Pastorian knowing.[17] It was a heady time for "medical science," filled with promise. In the light of such spectacle and success, it is perhaps unsurprising that Pasteur attracted acolytes dreaming of missions, rather than simply technicians seeking to solve medical problems. Nicolle seized the opportunity to overcome his clinically limiting infirmity by immersing himself in the Pastorian lab.

Examined in a different light, however, the decision of the brothers Nicolle to follow Pasteur is less transparent. Eugène Nicolle's influence on his sons remains evident to this day. He was, as we have seen, a well-established provincial clinician who also taught natural history.[18] Yet, had he survived, both roles might have brought him into conflict with Pastorian medicine. The early tensions between Pastorians and traditional clinicians are well known.[19] And natural history was increasingly being defined as a "descriptive" biological science, *in opposition to* experimental approaches.[20] More striking still, Eugène Nicolle had been a student of the naturalist Félix-Archimède Pouchet, a man who had made his name in biomedical history through a very public dispute with none other than Louis Pasteur. Pouchet was Chair of Natural History at Rouen's École Préparatoire.[21] Starting in 1859, Pouchet began challenging Pasteur's experiments on spontaneous generation. While carefully attempting to distance his interpretation of the concept from "heretical," materialistic transformism, Pouchet argued in support of spontaneous generation.[22] The Académie des Sciences assembled a panel of experts to judge the disputed evidence. The debate between Pasteur and Pouchet had officially ended two years before Nicolle was born. Pasteur was declared the victor; spontaneous generation and Pouchet alike seemed discredited. It was Pouchet's institutional position that Eugène Nicolle would later come to hold, teaching the course in natural history at the École Préparatoire.[23] The Nicolles were thus at one remove from battle with Pasteur.

The decision of both Maurice and Charles to embrace Pasteur's mission in the wake of their own father's death is, at least on the surface, somewhat ironic. The fact that Charles Nicolle turned Pasteur into a veritable spiritual father and life-model is positively intriguing. Assessing the significance of this move would be difficult indeed.[24] One may safely suggest, however, that Nicolle, who delighted in reconciling apparent contradictions, attempted throughout his career to bring together his father's interests and Pasteur's. Nicolle believed that bacteriology was best viewed as *micro*-biology, and his approach to infectious disease would come to be fundamentally shaped by his understanding of natural history.[25]

At the Pasteur Institute, Nicolle worked principally with two of Pasteur's most cherished colleagues: Emile Roux and Elie Metchnikoff. It would be difficult to find two men more different in character. Roux might best be described as a secular monk of science. Cautious, guarded, and logical, he remained convinced throughout his life that true commitment to the Pastorian mission necessitated unquestioning devotion coupled with contempt for material rewards.[26] Metchnikoff, in contrast, might well have been a character out of a Dostoevsky novel. He was passionate, romantic, and imaginative.[27] Roux was trained as a clinician; Metchnikoff received his training in zoology and embryology. In 1904, Metchnikoff was appointed *sous-directeur* of the Pasteur Institute, and Roux was named director. Of the two, it was Metchnikoff who was deeply—and, for a Pastorian, uncommonly[28]—influenced by evolutionary theory, bringing it to bear on his famous phagocytic theory of immunity.[29] In a sense, then, Nicolle's very teachers at the Institut Pasteur de Paris (IPP) brought his father's interests in natural history and clinical medicine directly into the context of Pastorian approaches to disease. Throughout his life, Nicolle continued to be influenced by his two mentors: Roux, in practice; Metchnikoff, in (disease) theory.[30]

Nicolle completed his thesis, "Le Chancre Mou et son Germe le Streptobacille de Ducrey," in 1893, and he immediately set to work on his life's mission. Coincidentally, that same year, the Director of Agriculture in France's North African protectorate, Tunisia, was requesting that the Pastorians establish a laboratory in Tunis. At that time, however, Nicolle's sights were set on a more immediate mission. He hoped to return to Rouen, in order to establish a true Center of Medical and Microbiological Research at the city's École de Médecine.[31] In other words, he would attempt to extend the Pastorian gospel to the provinces. Toward that end, he was appointed professor *suppléant* of Pathology and Clinical Medicine at the Rouen École in November—a nine year position, with a regular salary, that could be made permanent at its conclusion.[32] In March 1894, he was also named *Médecin-Adjoint* to the hospitals of Rouen.

By April, when Nicolle returned to the city of his birth, everything seemed to be in order for his mission's eventual success. This promising situation persisted throughout the year. When Nicolle arrived in Rouen, a small bacteriology laboratory already existed at the École. Founded by Robert Leudet and François Hue with their own funds, it was housed in a room annexed to the anatomy lab. Leudet and Hue extended laboratory privileges to their new Pastorian colleague.[33] The laboratory's existence, and Nicolle's affiliation with it, rapidly took on larger significance that autumn, when a deadly childhood disease threatened to become epidemic. The epidemic would in turn catapult Nicolle into a position of leadership—and a recent Pastorian discovery provided the impetus for this ascendancy.

During the time Nicolle was studying under him, Emile Roux was conducting research on diphtheria, a deadly childhood disease that produced a characteristic "false membrane" in its young victims' throats, suffocating them.[34] Roux worked first with Alexandre Yersin to confirm the identity of the disease's causal bacillus. The pair then demonstrated that the bacillus released a toxin that produced diphtheria's symptoms.[35] Subsequently, in Germany, Emil Behring found that immunized animals produced an *anti*toxin. Seizing upon this discovery, Roux set to work on producing the antitoxin in large quantities. With Louis Martin—the man who would eventually succeed him as director of the IPP—Roux developed a viable antitoxin and successfully tested it on hundreds of children at the Hôpital des Enfants-Malades.[36] The Pastorians' findings were presented at an international congress in the summer of 1894. Despite the German connection in its development, diphtheria antitoxin took its place next to the rabies vaccine as evidence of the Pastorians' potential power over disease.[37]

In September 1894, as Nicolle was vacationing in Italy, early predictions were being made of an impending diphtheria epidemic. Nicolle's colleagues sent for him, and he returned promptly to Rouen, prepared to confront the grave threat. He knew well that a successful campaign against diphtheria would establish the truth of Pastorian medicine for many unbelievers. In the meantime, the École de Médecine had arranged a special service for the production and distribution of diphtheria antitoxin. It was to be supported financially by public subscription and implemented by the bacteriology lab. Nicolle, who was charged with heading up the laboratory arrangements, left immediately for Paris. There, he sought permission from Roux himself to use his methods of antitoxin production in Rouen. Roux assured him that the Pasteur Institute "will not monopolize the production of serum" and conferred upon his former student his blessings and a quantity of active diphtheria toxin.[38] Nicolle returned to Rouen, where his laboratory began to produce antitoxin, and the École and city officials collected funds to support the production process. In the calm before the epidemic struck, Nicolle educated local physicians about the bacteriological approach to diphtheria control. When the epidemic took hold in early January, the Rouen medical community was prepared with a supply of serum[39] and a functioning diagnostic laboratory. In the end, Nicolle judged their campaign a stunning success.[40] And success had its advantages: in addition to helping to save a number of young lives, Nicolle had emerged as leader of an expanded laboratory and as a recognized force for medical reform in Rouen.

By this time, Nicolle was nearly thirty and still unmarried. His father had directed his career choice; his mother's preferences were now satisfied with his marriage to Alice Avice, a young woman from a "good" family. Maurice Huet, one of Nicolle's biographers (and thoughtful on all matters), is unable to suppress his distaste for Mme. Alice Nicolle, whom he considers to have been far beneath her husband in intellect, etiquette, sociability—indeed, everything except playing the piano.[41] (Many others agreed with this assessment.) Later, Nicolle himself would criticize medical systems that forced talented young men of limited means to marry women of place and purse to secure a successful career. More immediately, however, Alice and Charles Nicolle embraced the traditional duties of married couples, producing two children: Marcelle (b. 1896) and Pierre (b. 1898).[42] The family's personal troubles lay in the future. By 1895—the year of his marriage—Nicolle could feel a sense of accomplishment. He had realized his parents' wishes, had brought the Pastorian mission to the provinces, and appeared to have his life well and dutifully ordered.

These positive appearances would have sustained scrutiny on a number of levels: even if some did not quite take on the status Nicolle had envisioned for them. His laboratory, now in a new location, assumed an increasing number of medically useful, Pastorian-oriented functions. The laboratory staff produced and distributed vaccines, conducted medical analyses, and analyzed the city's water supply. And it was, now, "his" lab. Nicolle had been appointed director of the laboratory and given the official title of *chef de service*. With institutional functions, medical appointments, and personal reputation in place, Nicolle added yet another element essential to the successful extension of the Pastorian mission. In 1896, he began to teach his own *Cours,* "the analogue of the universally known course taught by Dr. Roux at the Pasteur Institute."[43] The *Cours* was, in fact, two courses. He offered the *"petit"* session twice a year; between the two small sessions, he presented his annual *"grand"* course of forty lectures. The former attracted around ten students per session; the latter, about twenty.[44]

The year 1896 brought Nicolle still more opportunities. A technological advance announced that summer enabled him to perfect his laboratory's routine procedures. Moreover, it prompted him to extend the lab's functions in a direction that would complete its Pastorian pedigree: into original research. In June, Fernand Widal published details of the typhoid diagnostic test that would soon bear his name.[45] To perform the test, one added a quantity of known typhoid bacillus to a sample of the patient's blood serum. If typhoid antibodies were present in the serum, the meeting of bacillus and antibody would cause the cells to clot, or agglutinate.[46] By July, Nicolle had not only begun using the Widal test, but had developed a modification thereof.[47] He published his findings in the area's most notable medical journal, the *Normandie Médicale,* which had added him to its editorial committee that same year.[48] By 1898, Nicolle had expanded his agglutination studies with original research that merited publication not only in the IP's *Annales,* but also in the *Comptes Rendus* of the Society of Biology.[49] Before leaving Rouen, he extended his studies still further with investigations of the connections between agglutination and bacterial motility and, within a single bacterial species, on the variation of agglutanitive properties between "races" and on changes that occurred when that species was placed in different environments.[50] In still other original investigations, Nicolle continued his thesis research, successfully producing *chancre mou* in a monkey.[51] Both projects displayed research priorities he would take with him to North Africa.

Five years after his return to Rouen, Nicolle took stock of his laboratory's accomplishments in a special review article. He noted the many tests performed within its walls; he reminded his readers—with statistical evidence—of the tangible benefits its antitoxin production had brought to Rouen's families.[52] Moreover, Nicolle's microbiology classes, which were rooted in the laboratory, had served to raise Rouen's medical status in the world outside Normandy: "Before this course was organized," he observed, "no foreign doctors came to study at the École de Médecine of Rouen." That, he boasted, was now changing. Clearly, Nicolle and his laboratory had greatly benefited the city and its citizens. Yet, there was still more the Pastorian pairing could contribute:

> We believe that this rapid review will suffice to demonstrate that, with a little energy, *it is possible to work in a provincial laboratory.* With a less faulty installation, however, it would have been easier to do this, and such will become necessary: with the current state of our knowledge, *medical science, veterinary science, hygiene, agriculture, and industry have the right to demand much* from microbiological laboratories.[53]

Wrapped within this dense paragraph are a number of interconnected elements. Central among them is a model: Nicolle's understanding of the Pastorian model of laboratory function. *Medical* microbiology, which Nicolle believed he had successfully established in Rouen, was only one part of that model. Other parts, less fully developed, extended to plants, animals, human populations, and human productions: indeed, all life might benefit from the expert application of Pastorian microbiology. It was Pasteur's life's work, systematized and generalized. Yet, Nicolle was discovering just how difficult it was to apply in a provincial French city.[54] Resistance abounded; his frustration grew.

None of Nicolle's successes in Rouen had been unqualified. The campaign against diphtheria had provided him with funding, an expanded lab, and evident medical accomplishments. Yet, it also proved the start of a larger power struggle that would persist throughout his professional tenure in his native town. Troubles became apparent when subvention funds for the 1894–95 effort exceeded immediate need.[55] Nicolle had hoped to use the additional amount to turn the small serum production lab into a state of the art facility. Leaders of the École, however, had other plans for the money. It might, for example, be used to build a new facility for *all* the medical school's laboratories, including histology, physiology, and bacteriology. In the end, none of the plans came to fruition. Nicolle's lab did move to another building, but it was far from the well-funded, modern facility he hoped for.[56] Moreover, although he remained the lab's designated leader, he was not given the title of "Director" that he'd sought. He remained, instead, *chef* of the laboratory.[57] Funding continued to be a problem. His 1899 review article was, on one level, an elaborate appeal for financial contributions.[58]

Nicolle's troubles did not, of course, simply arise from an anonymous medical school "will." Raoul Brunon, who was appointed director of the École de Médecine late in 1895, was Nicolle's chief nemesis.[59] Later, Brunon would be described by one of Nicolle's admirers as "an aggressive redhead" who sought to "become omnipotent," displaying "a burgeoning and dangerous rivalry" with Nicolle that was most evident in his opposition to Pastorian reforms.[60] By all accounts, Nicolle and Brunon quickly surrounded themselves with opposing medical "clans" that roughly conformed to the "conservative/clinical" versus "progressive/bacteriological" categories that have so intrigued historians of germ theories.[61] Nicolle certainly believed in the truth of these oppositional categories; he argued that "there was a consensus among Brunon and others to harm the laboratory"[62] and blamed Brunon for blocking plans for its expansion. It appears that Nicolle and his supporting "clan" had been brought onto the editorial board of the *Normandie Médicale* to work alongside their opponents, in an effort to force some return of harmony. There is little to suggest that the appeasement had any long-term effect. Indeed, the frustrated Nicolle even took to the pen on several occasions, to support his perspective. He wrote the partially polemical laboratory review article; he composed a short story about his travails.[63] And, when all else failed, he and his "clan" broke ranks with their medical confreres and established their own journal, the *Revue Médicale de Normandie*, in 1900.

What was principally at issue in the Great Rouen Medical Feud? Was it *simply* a reactionary rejection of the laboratory by a privileged and powerful clinical old guard? Probably not. Both Brunon and his predecessor at the École seem to have had at least a basic understanding of the laboratory's potential contributions to medicine. It will be recalled that they hoped to spread the diphtheria subvention between a *number* of labs. At more immediate issue, it seems, was the place of the *microbiology* lab. The directors of the École de Médecine were attempting to fit an assortment of laboratories with apparent medical applications into the structure of medical education. This was, after all, the country of Lavoisier and Claude Bernard as well as of Louis Pasteur.[64] Nicolle, on the other hand, saw all the living world from the perspective of his microbiological lab. Medical bacteriology was but one component of a larger project—a conviction reflected in his 1899 Report's charge to society to demand more from its microbiologists. Nicolle was a convert to the Pastorian cause and behaved in ways consistent with a true believer.[65]

Here, then, was the main problem: Nicolle's mission was microbiology-centered and extended far beyond the medical school; Brunon's mission was to direct medical education. Both men certainly had their personal agendas and a fair share of hubris. But, fundamentally, the tension seems to have arisen from their contrasting vision of the place of the bacteriology lab: of *Nicolle's* bacteriology lab. That lab, it should be remembered, may have been started out of the private initiative (and financing) of École faculty: yet, it remained an École lab. The model Nicolle had imported into Rouen had been shaped by the legacy of Pasteur and the reality of his institute—an institution that had carefully preserved its autonomy by casting itself as a *private* establishment, supported by *public* (and, to some extent, government) contributions.[66] One could hardly hope for a bacteriology laboratory to achieve, within the confines of a medical school, the grandeur and scope of Pasteur's institute. Nicolle himself seems ultimately to have realized this restriction. In Tunis, he would work tirelessly to assure his institute's autonomy—eventually, from the Pasteur Institute of Paris itself.

Even if his battle with Brunon was not simply an expression of clinical medicine's opposition to the laboratory, Nicolle soon found that, when he was himself the clinician, Rouen's medical establishment opposed his plans. In 1900, he was appointed *chef de service* at the Hospice Général de Rouen.[67] In accordance with his training and his growing deafness, he was placed in charge of the venereal and dermatological wards. It was his approach to treating prostitutes that brought him more controversy.[68] In accordance with the laws of the day, prostitutes in Rouen who were diagnosed with a venereal disease were hospitalized in one of the Hospice Général's wards—wards Nicolle was assigned to oversee. The often-unwilling patients were kept there for the duration of their treatment. Conditions on the wards made their hospital stay resemble a prison sentence, and the women occasionally displayed their discontent by rioting.

Before Nicolle arrived, the instigators of such riots were sent to cold, humid prison cells known as the *loges*. Upon taking up his new position that July, Nicolle banned this practice. All was calm for several months, when another riot took place. The hospital administration, arguing that the absence of punishment encouraged such behavior, held Nicolle personally responsible. Still, Nicolle would not change his position: the women were patients to be treated, not prisoners to be punished. Eugène Nicolle, who had lectured extensively on public hygiene, would have approved. Calm eventually returned. Then, in April 1902, one of Nicolle's patients was sent to the *loges* in his absence. Incensed, he hand-delivered his strongly worded letter of response to the hospital's director. When the letter failed to persuade its recipient, Nicolle threatened to retrieve the imprisoned woman and escort her out of the hospital personally, to ensure that no one dragged her back to the *loges*. The director relented but expressed displeasure with Nicolle's methods.[69]

At about the same time that Nicolle was facing conservative disapproval as a clinician, two of his other positions were being reevaluated. Brunon was at the center of both processes; in his hands, these "processes" became challenges. The first challenge came to Nicolle's status as *chef* of the serological lab. Brunon sought to change the duration of the appointment—originally unlimited—to three years, a move that would allow him to replace Nicolle more easily in the future. The Administrative Council of the lab, however, did not approve the change, and Nicolle's position remained safe.[70] Review of his appointment as *professeur suppléant* at the École was another matter. The initial nine-year appointment period was coming to an end and was up for extension. Nicolle depended on the position not just for status in the Rouen medical community but also for a fixed, reliable source of income. Unfortunately for Nicolle, Brunon had the power to veto tenure and, in this case, used it. There was no appeal.

If there was a last straw that broke Nicolle's faith in his ability to accomplish his missions in provincial France, this was it.[71] Fortunately, Nicolle had been quietly working on an alternative plan. Late in 1902, he put that plan into action: he resigned from his assorted obligations, packed up laboratory and life, and left Rouen.[72] For decades, he would speak of his hometown with a mixture of fondness and contempt.[73]

The Shore

> The moment came when the agonizing peril of deafness bore down upon me. Like a ship whose captain is unable to fill its cracks, I took in water. I was

sinking. My impending drowning became my salvation. I decided to abandon everything before everything abandoned me. Courageously, I cast myself into the sea and swam to the shore that has since been the site of my suffering and my success.

—Nicolle, "Lettre aux Sourds," 1929

In December 1902, Nicolle dove headfirst into an uncertain sea. At least this is how he described his move to Tunis, nearly thirty years after the fact, to readers of his "Letter to the Deaf." He hoped to inspire these readers with a stylized retelling of his own life story.[74] In the famous "sinking ship" passage, Nicolle cast his deafness as a horrific storm that was destroying the life—here, the clinical life—he had so carefully constructed for himself. Fighting against it only heightened its power to wreak havoc. Finally, he embraced the storm: casting aside the vestiges of his former life, he followed the course of his deafness to the shore of his new homes—Tunis, and its nascent Pasteur Institute. Implied in his rejection of the "sinking ship/clinical life" is a kind of surrender to laboratory life. And, in Tunis, Nicolle did embrace the laboratory wholeheartedly. Yet, he always kept the sea, with its untamed life and its ambiguous connotations, close by. Further, he even brought along a few planks of timber from his otherwise sunken clinical ship. All these he would integrate into his methodological approaches and (at least in theory) standards of evidence for "treating" disease.

Taken out of context, this metaphor-driven life narrative might encourage the assumption that Nicolle erased from later accounts the pesky personal animosities that had also driven him from Rouen. He did not. He continued the story: "I went to Tunis. . . . In this new country, my initiatives did not meet with the difficulties and hostile stinginess of the provinces. One was more alone there, but also more one's own master."[75] It is an enticing assertion for historians hoping to evaluate the "resistance" provided in the metropole, provinces, and—in Nicolle's apt formulation—"ultraprovinces" like Tunisia, to the seemingly inevitable progress of the "empire" of laboratory medicine. Yet, as we have already seen with Nicolle's experience in Rouen, one must not to rush to embrace stark assertions simply because they neatly substantiate one's historical assumptions. Resistance levels certainly varied, but they did not *necessarily* vary to the extent that some—Nicolle included—would have us believe.[76] By the time he arrived in Tunis, Nicolle met with an array of extant medical structures that constrained his actions. He would spend years gathering up select pieces of those structures—emphasizing or amplifying some, erasing others. Eventually, he would create a kind of mosaic from these pieces that appeared to demonstrate that all health and hygiene in Tunisia somehow began and ended with his institute. It was not an uncommon strategy for colonial Pastorians: selective obliteration and appropriation of the past was one of the ways they established their medical religion.[77] Nicolle was just uncommonly successful in applying it.[78]

The missionary fervor that had compelled Nicolle to return to Rouen in the 1890s also took hold of other Pastorian microbiologists. Conveniently, if not wholly coincidentally, they had before them a wide array of potential destinations, all open to Pastorian conversion. Alongside the many self-governing nations requesting samples of rabies vaccine and permission to establish laboratories bearing the Master's name were a growing number of countries with far less autonomy and far more obligation to France. Germ theory had found its footing just as the West was scrambling to lay claim to the rest of the globe.[79] Moreover, since "the rest of the globe" tended to harbor dangerous and unruly diseases—often a hindrance to colonial designs—Pastorian medicine increasingly accompanied Western troops and entrepreneurs to their overseas destinations. Colonial doctors began enrolling in the IPP's *Cours,* and Pastorian researchers themselves went out to start up laboratories and institutes around the world.[80]

Albert Calmette, who would eventually be named assistant director of the IPP and lay claim to the "C" in the tuberculosis vaccine "BCG," established the first overseas Pasteur Institute in Saigon in 1891.[81] (Alexandre Yersin would join him there before starting up his own Pastorian lab in Nhatrang in 1895.) A year after the Saigon institute was established, a member of the Algiers Faculty of Medicine suggested that his city, too, would benefit from the presence of a Pastorian laboratory. Two years later, the institution that would become the Institut Pasteur d'Alger (IPA) was founded.[82] In 1893—the same year Tunisia's Director of Agriculture was requesting a laboratory for Tunis— Maurice Nicolle himself was sent to Constantinople to fulfill the Sultan's wish for a local Pasteur Institute.[83] Pastorian labs and institutes appeared in Madagascar, Brazzaville, and Morocco; in Lille and in Athens—indeed, all around the world. The Pasteur Institute of Tunis was founded as a humble laboratory in 1893 and was directed by Pasteur's own nephew, Adrien Loir.[84]

The foundation and even future direction of the Pastorian lab in Tunis were intimately linked to Tunisia's status as a French protectorate. Underpinning the structure of that protectorate status was Tunisia's unstable nineteenth-century development—an instability rooted in the country's rulers' responses to changes in Western society and exacerbated by a series of internal hardships.[85] Tunisia had long been part of the Ottoman Empire and its leader, the Bey, technically answered to the Sultan. By the early nineteenth century, the Bey had more autonomy in governing Tunisia. The Napoleonic Wars and the French invasion of Algeria served to bring Europe's military and industrial progress to Tunisia's immediate attention. Husayn Bey reformed the Tunisian military (on the French model) in 1831.[86] His successor, Ahmad Bey, expanded upon this military project and, at the same time, took on further Westernizing projects. In these endeavors, he appears to have been motivated at once by personal interest, concerns for parity with his country's modernizing neighbors to the north, and "suggestions" from European advisors that he undertake enormous and expensive projects. While his successor, Muhammad Bey, set aside the military project, his tenure was brief (1855–59), and his own successor, Muhammed al-Sadiq Bey, returned to it energetically. Drought, crop failure, and epidemics of cholera and typhus in the 1860s caused the country's already precarious financial state to decline further, until it was officially declared bankrupt in 1869.[87]

Meanwhile, increasing numbers of Europeans were coming to Tunisia.[88] Tunisia was *relatively* salubrious, temperate, and, for Europeans, close.[89] Even before the Protectorate was established, lively French and Italian communities were thriving. During the acquisitive excitement of the "Scramble for Africa," the small country, sporting an expat community, excellent location, and sizable debts (allowing for persuasive negotiation), was an obvious prize. These assets also promised to buffer French interests in Algeria and, for some, to offer entrepreneurial advantages. In April 1881, the French Expeditionary Force invaded Tunisia. Shortly thereafter, the Bey signed the Treaty of Bardo, establishing the country as a protectorate of France.[90] Technically, "protectorate" status was less invasive than "colonial": the Tunisian government was to remain intact, with power preserved; the French would simply establish some of their own administrative structures and claim rights over certain local interests. The 1883 Convention of La Marsa, however, transformed the protectorate, in all but name, into a de facto colony.[91] The Bey, now Ali Bey, retained his place at the head of the Tunisian government, but the French ran the country and headed up its *directions*, or government departments. The Department of Education was established in 1883, Agriculture, Commerce, and Colonization in 1890.[92] Three years later, the director of the latter was asking Louis Pasteur for his expert assistance.

The Pastorians found a foothold in Tunisia not as a consequence of a human epidemic, but because of a business opportunity that arose out of a plague on

French grapes. In the early years of the Protectorate, French entrepreneurs had bought up Tunisian properties, including farms, in hopes of making a profit from the land.[93] Meanwhile, an outbreak of phylloxora in France threatened its grape (and therefore wine) supply. Perhaps, with proper cultivation, quality grapes could be grown in the Protectorate that would supplement the scanty French crop—and profit the new landholders. Microbiological study could help achieve this goal. Pasteur had, after all, established his early reputation by analyzing the diseases of wine and of beer.[94] Thus it was that the director of Tunisia's Department of Agriculture contacted the IPP. The Parisian institute responded to Agriculture's inquiries with a laboratory that opened—without the official title of "institute"—on September 7, 1893. Adrien Loir was appointed its director, ensuring the Pastorian pedigree. Loir's laboratory studied the diseases of wine, as it had been established to do; but it also moved into medical analysis proper.[95]

Loir soon became interested in medicine more broadly. Here, he entered into a Tunisian medical universe whose adaptation to European ideas was well under way. Historian Nancy Gallagher has described the shift in Tunisian medical power over the course of the nineteenth century. At the beginning of the century, any European doctor who wanted to practice in Tunisia had to find favor with the local medical elite. European and Tunisian medicine, she argues, were not terribly different at the time, given their common roots in Hippocratic and Arabic medicine. Yet, they were quickly diverging, as industrialization and professionalization were transforming European medicine. Moving along the same path followed in reconfigurations of the country's military and society in the nineteenth century, Tunisian medicine came increasingly to be patterned after European medicine. In 1835, the Bey even established an advisory Sanitary Council.[96] During the country's bout of epidemics in the 1860s, the Sanitary Council seized the opportunity to expand its status from advisory to active, increasingly implementing hygienic and medical reforms.[97] The protectorate government subsequently took over the Sanitary Council and created the Maritime Sanitary Police, which divided the country into sanitary districts and established quarantines to stop pilgrims, who were passing through Tunisia on their way to Mecca, from spreading disease.[98] More generally, however, the country's protectorate status formalized the century-long shift in medical power. Following an 1888 decree, all medical practice was regulated by the new government. Doctors now had to be credentialed in European fashion, meaning principally in Europe, given that Tunisia had no medical school.[99] The first license for a Tunisian doctor was not granted until 1897. By the onset of World War I, only three more Tunisians were officially licensed to practice medicine.[100] Empiricists of long experience were permitted to continue practicing, though labeled in a way so as to discourage patient confidence: as *médecins tolérés*.

The licensing of doctors was but one move toward a more European approach to medicine taken in the final decades of the nineteenth century. Another was the establishment of hospitals. Granted, hospitals were not foreign to the Arab medical tradition. But, as historian Mohamed Zitouna points out, hospitals had long disappeared from Tunisia. At mid-century, the Hôpital Saint Louis, a tiny charitable establishment, took in foreigners. Only in 1879 was a hospital established for Tunisians. This was the Hôpital Aziza Othmana, better known as the Sadiki Hospital. Built in the Medina and surrounded by souks, the Sadiki was more hospice than hospital, soon burdened with chronically ill patients and a poor reputation.[101] When the French Expeditionary Force invaded Tunisia, the military established a small ambulance[102] to attend to soldiers and opened its full hospital, the Hôpital de Belvédère, in 1886. In 1891, the Italians opened an Italian hospital; in 1894, the Jewish hospital opened its doors. Only in 1897 was the Hôpital Civil Français de Tunis created by beylical decree. (In 1944, the French civil hospital would be renamed the Hôpital Charles Nicolle.)[103] Moreover, shortly after the Pastorian laboratory was created in Tunis, the French military opened its own bacteriological laboratory. The Institut Pasteur de Tunis (IPT) under Nicolle would come to have close relations with the military lab.

Loir was in Tunis from 1893 to 1901. Nicolle's subsequent dismissive accounts of this period have greatly influenced historical perception of his predecessor's contributions. Fortunately, historians have recently returned to Loir and reevaluated his work.[104] The medical context Loir entered was indeed undergoing Westernization. Unfortunately, as we have seen, the establishment of the Protectorate essentially translated "Westernization," as "dominated by European practitioners." Tunisians were marginalized, and Loir hoped to temper this trend. One opportunity came out of the nationalistic bickering that dominated relations between Europeans in Tunis. The Europeans, like their hospitals, tended to separate along national lines, and were wholly unable to work together. In an effort to carve out some common cultural ground, the Institut de Carthage was formed in 1893.[105] Some two hundred members, drawn from the city's competing cultures, assembled to discuss history and geography, physical and natural sciences, and arts and letters.[106] Medical members—including Loir—presented their work in the "physical and natural sciences" section. They could also publish their papers in the institute's journal, the *Revue Tunisienne*. By 1898, however, eight of the city's leading doctors had determined the need for a separate medical section of the institute. Loir, one of the eight, was the new section's first secretary. By 1901, the group had decided to sever ties with the mother institution and to form an autonomous medical society, the Tunisian Society of Medical Sciences (*Société des Sciences Médicale*).[107] Its members would continually provide the clinical evidence the Pastorians needed for their research. Nicolle, like Loir, would serve as its president.[108]

While Loir was still in Tunisia, the medical group, consciously seeking heterogeneity, invited Béchir Dinguizli to join it. Dinguizli was Tunisia's first local doctor to be licensed under the Protectorate's restrictive regulations. Loir himself had encouraged him to study medicine in France, and Dinguizli responded by not only completing his studies in Bordeaux but also dedicating his thesis to Loir.[109] Indeed, it was Loir's hope that a cadre of professional Tunisians could be formed—individuals who would be sent to France to study law or medicine and would then return home to practice. The French *colons* opposed Loir's plans with predictable if occasionally revealing arguments,[110] and Dinguizli remained his one immediate success. Loir did, however, also add Tunisian technicians to his laboratory staff.[111]

Meanwhile, the Tunisian government and the Pasteur Institute of Paris agreed that Tunisia's need for bacteriological services could not be met by the small laboratory on the rue du Contrôle Civil, and so elevated it to the official rank of "institute" on February 14, 1900. As the Institut Pasteur de Tunis it would broaden the old laboratory's functions and enlarge its structure: it was now expected to oversee original research and could charge for many of its products and analyses.[112] The institute itself would remain under control of the Department of Agriculture, and its director's salary would be paid from Tunisian government funds. Loir was appointed to this position but held it for only a year; in 1901, he left both institute and country.[113] Starting in June, veterinarian Edouard Ducloux was acting director.[114] The IPT now had a research mandate, a budget for reconstruction—and no one fit to oversee either.

Colonial Constructions

Just about the time Loir was returning to Paris from Tunis, Maurice Nicolle was returning from Constantinople. A solution to the Tunisian power vacuum seemed evident: might the elder Nicolle be interested in trading in the frustrations of directing a Pastorian facility in an autonomous country for the more pliable environment of France's North African protectorate? He was not, but he knew someone who might be. His brother Charles was similarly frustrated with resistance to his Pastorian mission in Rouen. Moreover, he had experience directing a microbiology lab and was conducting original research. The IPP asked Charles if he was interested in the position. Yet, despite his problems in Rouen, Nicolle hesitated.[115] He did not wish to move from one limited position to another; and the IPT, wedged as it was between the IPP and the Tunisian government, appeared from a distance to be similarly constrained. The Tunisian government wanted power over Pastorian appointments; the Pastorians balked. Eventually, the two institutional bodies found common ground in colonial interests and scientific aspirations.[116] Albert Calmette, now back in France and acting frequently as the IPP's colonial ambassador, wrote to Tunisia's central authority, *Résident Général* Stephen Pichon, about these shared concerns:

> I am honored that you have asked me to organize the Pasteur Institute of Tunis along the main lines that are needed in the interests of the influence of French science in Tunisia . . . . An establishment organized on this basis will doubtlessly come to offer very important services to the Regency and will effectively serve to diffuse French influence among the indigenous population.[117]

Back in Rouen, Nicolle's problems were mounting, and Calmette's negotiations had made the Tunisian solution more promising. Nicolle accepted appointment as director of the IPT in November 1902. He and his family sailed for Tunisia in December. By January 1903, his new position was official.

Nicolle arrived in his new country with a clear vision of his mission's requirements: "For now," he wrote to his mother, "we must be cautious: if we start from a solid foundation, we will be able to rest easy for the future and will have no financial worries. I think that we will be entirely successful in this endeavor."[118] His optimism was short-lived. Soon after he arrived in Tunisia, Nicolle discovered that the Institute's foundation was, quite literally, far from "solid." Ignoring an agreement reached with Calmette, the Tunisian government had approved a plan for the IPT's reconstruction that was designed in Nicolle's absence. The selected land was in the Jardin d'Essais de l'Ecole d'Agriculture, just north of the city limits. The "garden" location was not as idyllic as it sounded. The land had only recently been reclaimed from a lake, making it essentially swampland. Nicolle protested that it was "unstable" and wholly unsuitable for sustaining a modern medical research institution. When the Tunisian administration dismissed his arguments, Nicolle, in response, threatened to take the next steamer back to France.[119] Eventually, it was agreed that he could make changes, but those changes took months to approve. His request for a different plot of land in the Jardin, on a hill behind the land he had rejected, was finally accepted in April. Additionally, the cost of construction became an issue. M. Guy, architect for the Department of Public Works, had been assigned the task of designing the institute according to Nicolle's specifications.[120] The projected costs had doubled. Lacking the money to cover this increase, Nicolle acknowledged that his additions of a personal residence and veterinary services to the original plans had driven up the costs. He feared he would have to cut back.[121] A timely visit from the French Minister of Agriculture resulted in the extension of the institute's credit.[122] Still, even this extension was insufficient to enable Nicolle to realize the whole of his design.[123] Finally, in August 1903, eight months after his arrival in Tunis, Nicolle's final plans for the IPT were approved and construction commenced.

In the meantime, Nicolle had discovered the key to virtual autonomy and professional success in Tunisia. Technically, the IPT still fell under the aegis of the Department of Agriculture and its most current director, M. Hugnon. For all practical purposes, the true lines of power lay elsewhere: "we have here the good fortune of being under an absolute master," he noted conspiratorially in one of his letters. "The *Résident Général* need only say the word, and that word immediately becomes deed."[124] Consequently, Nicolle began focusing his persuasive powers on Stephen Pichon and encouraged his colleagues in Paris—where Pichon appears to have spent much of his time—to do the same.[125] Given the lengthy approval process to which his plans were subjected, it is evident that Nicolle and the Parisian Pastorians enjoyed only mixed success in their efforts. Still, considering Nicolle's many achievements, it is clear that he ultimately won the favor—or at least earned the respect—of Pichon, and of most of his successors.

Despite the Tunisian power struggles and perpetual negotiations, construction moved ahead. The new institute comprised two main buildings, a staff residence, an incinerator, and a shed. The main building contained offices, research and fermentation laboratories, a photographic darkroom, the (isolated) rabies clinic, a library, and, upstairs, the Nicolle family apartment.[126] A second building, located behind the main building and a small garden, housed animals for experimentation and vaccine research. Although the inner institute displayed the structures of Western medical research, its outer design reflected traditional Tunisian architecture. Surrounded in part by a wall and in part by a "*grille artistique*," its buildings boasted arched doorways and windows. Such outward adaptation to surrounding culture was a hallmark of the Pasteur Institute's overseas extensions, and Nicolle drew attention to this aesthetic aspect of his institute's design.[127]

The new institute began operations in October 1904. Its small staff consisted of Charles Comte, *chef de laboratoire*; Gaston Catouillard, *préparateur*;

J. Chaltiel, *aide-préparateur*; a "*garçon de laboratoire français*"; a "*chaouch indigène*"— Habib; and Mektouf, a "*garçon de service indigène.*"[128] (The last two staff members were the Tunisians that Loir had brought in.) Finally, months after it had begun functioning, the IPT was officially inaugurated. The festivities, such as they were, took place on May 3, 1905. Tensions between the Tunisian government and the IPP over their joint venture were evident. Although the Director of Agriculture had formally invited Roux or another Parisian representative to the inauguration, Pichon strongly discouraged this. In a letter to Nicolle explaining the IPP's absence from the celebration, Roux dismissed Pichon as proof that "the politician remains the politician, incapable of raising himself up from his parliamentary depravity."[129] The inauguration itself seemed to Nicolle a parody of orchestrated and superfluous bureaucracy. He was given a detailed schedule of events that articulated each step and accounted for each moment. The gravity of administrative planning was made more absurd in practice, when a visiting dignitary fell asleep during the ceremonies. Nicolle's accounts of this event were publicly respectful but privately ironic.[130]

Nicolle's early constructions extended beyond laboratory buildings and into origin myths. He had long thought himself at once ordered and imaginative. He was a passionate advocate of the Pastorian mission, with real-life experience in the difficulties of realizing that mission. He was personally ambitious. And, if he had largely abandoned the Catholic faith in which he had been raised (he would embrace it again only at the very end of his life), he was steeped in its symbols, traditions, and organization. All these qualities prepared him well for his work in Tunis. He drew upon several of them in his campaign to construct the institute he had envisioned. Yet, he knew that his successes on this level were not sufficient to make the IPT his own. A pesky bit of prehistory stood between him and his hopes of claiming the "creation" of scientific medicine in Tunisia. Thus, along with working on the physical construction and staffing of his institute, Nicolle began constructing a narrative of the IPT's origins that effectively negated Loir's contributions. In short, he was creating an origin myth.

Traces of that myth are scattered through Nicolle's early correspondence. Dismissing the history of the Pastorian institution in Tunis, 1893–1902, as "a delicious chapter to add to the Human Comedy"[131] in one letter, Nicolle described his initial reaction to his new surroundings in another:

> M. Ducloux, a veterinarian who is to be assistant director, acted as my guide, introducing me to everyone and everything. He impressed me: his temperament is well suited to my own. Moreover, the old Pasteur Institute owes him

a great debt. Only through his influence did it escape the potentially devastating effects of my predecessor, who not only committed blunders, but also proved worthless as a microbiologist.[132]

Ducloux was not a Pastorian, had only been the interim director, and was, after all, a veterinarian: he hardly posed a threat to Nicolle's position in the IPT's grand narrative. It was Loir who needed to be discredited. Nicolle was certain to have the sympathy of friends and family in Rouen when he wrote such critiques of Loir. Private letters, however, did nothing to change the very public fact that Loir not only had been director for the Institute's first year, but had been the guiding force for Pastorian efforts in Tunisia for nearly a decade.

Nicolle turned to his own public format to tell his official version of the institution's history, in the guise of simple fact. In the opening article of his new house journal, the *Archives de l'Institut Pasteur de Tunis (AIPT)*, he interspersed descriptions of the institute's services with attacks on Loir's competence.[133] As a prelude to statistics on the effectiveness of rabies treatment at the Pasteur Institute, for example, Nicolle pointed an italicized finger at the inadequacies of Loir's direction: "*the statistics that I publish here today annul all other statistics previously published*, as the earlier figures contained several errors."[134] Describing the institute's vaccine services, he made a similarly double-edged apology: "We lack information on this service's functions until 1901. . . . In 1901, M. Ducloux reorganized the service, which has since functioned quite regularly."[135] He also underscored the poor statistical record of fermentation services and the complete disregard of teaching that characterized the pre-Nicolle institute.[136] In short, Nicolle wove the physical and conceptual threads of the IPT's history together in a way that left him as its sole designer.

This mythic position, once devised, became central to Nicolle's autobiographical narrative. Thirty years later, arguing for the broad acceptance of his model of bacteriological research, Nicolle could summon this now well-established origin myth as evidence of his model's success:

> The Pasteur Institute of Tunis had a very modest beginning. Upon my arrival I found it in a state of ruin, as the result of difficult circumstances. In a few short years, I successfully got it on its feet by regaining the confidence of the medical corps and by creating resources for it.[137]

Loir's failure underscored Nicolle's success. Nicolle could be at once true founder and sole savior of the Pasteur Institute of Tunis. His accomplishments, set against so bleak a background, became all the more impressive. Obscured by his narrative, however, was the fact that the relevant administrative bodies had decided to expand the institute before Nicolle was even selected as its director. Also made invisible were Loir's many efforts to improve the health and the medical structures of Tunisia.

Creating a Medical Cosmos in Tunis

It took more than careful constructions of laboratory facilities and origin myths to create a fitting overseas "House of Pasteur." Echoing the work of religious missionaries who established churches abroad, the Pastorians performed definite functions for their adopted community—functions that also served to spread their influence and their doctrine. This in turn helped them fulfill their mission. In the case of the overseas Pasteur institutes, this mission, though centrally focused on Pasteur and bacteriology, was rarely far removed from the more famous "civilizing mission."[138] These functions mirrored Pasteur's own work, although they were adapted to local circumstance where necessary.[139]

In his first report of its functions, and in many a subsequent report, Nicolle was careful to mention the ways in which his institute was a true house of Pasteur. The same article that had opened both the *AIPT* and his lifelong campaign to discredit Loir also underscored the many ways in which the IPT was a *Pastorian* place. Naturally, Nicolle devoted a lengthy section to rabies work. The institute also prepared and/or distributed other vaccines and antitoxins. In 1903, the government had passed a law requiring that all individuals moving to Tunisia be vaccinated against smallpox; the IPT produced the vaccines. From the start, Nicolle was careful about which of his services he charged for, and, depending on the recipient, how much he charged. His institute provided medical analysis for private physicians and public hospitals, including free service for the Hôpital Civil Français and the Hôpital Sadiki.[140] It also continued to fulfill its original function, offering fermentation analysis for vintners. Attending to the public's health, Nicolle conducted a study of the pollution of the Lake of Tunis (1905) and, from the first full day of his directorship, commenced drinking water analysis for the city.[141] At the same time, Nicolle and his colleagues engaged in a series of public lectures dedicated to improving the public's health.[142]

Occasionally, conducting the standard business of being a Pastorian institute demanded adaptation of methods to local conditions. Nicolle (in a way Bruno Latour himself might admire) boasted of the adjustments he had made. Tunisia's heat in particular demanded flexibility.[143] Vaccines transported during summer months were often attenuated or even sterilized by the sweltering temperatures. The institute worked with the Department of Health and Public Hygiene to develop a cylindrical clay vase that could be filled with cool water to surround the fragile materials, thereby insulating them. The heat also caused another problem that positively begged for a Pastorian solution. It was ruining the yeast used to produce bread. As Nicolle described the problem,

> Currently, French bakeries in Tunisia must depend on Europe to buy [yeast], and often in the summer—especially in the interior villages—the leaven is spoiled, preserves poorly, gives mediocre results, and conveys an unpleasant taste to the bread. The Tunisian production of a high quality, affordable yeast will appreciably ameliorate the current condition. This result does not appear impossible to achieve.[144]

And so they set to work developing a local variety of yeast that could achieve the results produced by French yeast in France. In this way, the IPT addressed the problem of adapting both bread and wine production to a local climate in which the necessary ferments did not naturally tend to thrive. This work met both the Pastorian predilection for solving fermentation problems and a fundamental need of French civilization. How could Tunis ever be an acceptable dwelling place for French colonists without those two life staples, bread and wine? Moreover, who could miss the religious resonances? The limits that the Tunisian elements imposed on French expansion might be overcome by microbiological adaptation.

Aided by his provision of vaccines and bacteriological analyses, Nicolle established good enough relations with local doctors, practicing both privately and in hospitals, to have access to a constant supply of clinical material—patients—for his various studies. Indeed, he seems to have negotiated a careful clinical alliance. He and the IPT were the heart of Tunisian laboratory research, while the still-active Tunisian Society of Medical Sciences attended principally to clinical cases. The Society welcomed Nicolle, even electing him president in 1909—a fortuitous year to boast Charles Nicolle as president. His typhus studies at the Sadiki Hospital were of central importance both to the reputation of Nicolle and Tunisian medicine and to potential future typhus sufferers around the world.[145] Yet, Nicolle managed to gain more from his medical relations than just patient access and general notoriety. He also found in them the men who would work with him at the IPT.

Over the years, Nicolle brought many of his Normandy colleagues to Tunis, to play important roles in his institute. He had, for instance, brought Gaston

Catouillard from Rouen to Tunis almost immediately. Yet, his two most important collaborators during the institute's early years were both affiliated with the Sadiki Hospital. When last we left the Sadiki, it was in poor condition, a hospital more in name than in function. Efforts were undertaken to improve it in 1900, but it was only in 1902, with the appointment of Dr. Brunswic-le-Bihan, that a real change became evident. Brunswic, a surgeon who had been born and educated in Paris, came to Tunisia in 1899 for health reasons. He settled in Nabeul, where he established an infirmary/dispensary and an excellent reputation. When named medical director at the Sadiki in 1902, he rapidly implemented an impressive set of reforms.[146] To assist him in his efforts, Brunswic summoned a promising doctor with whom he had studied in Paris: Charles Comte.[147] Nicolle, too, saw Comte's promise; in 1904, he hired Comte away from Brunswic to act as the IPT's first *chef de laboratoire*. Two years later, Brunswic recruited another promising practitioner from France: Ernest Conseil, who, despite his intention to become a surgeon, wrote his thesis on typhus while at the Sadiki.[148] This may well have been influenced by the interests of his former medical school teacher back in Rouen: Charles Nicolle. In 1907, however, Conseil contracted osteomyelitis after suffering a cut on his finger during a procedure, incapacitating his arm—and thus his surgical career—permanently. Nicolle was impressed by Conseil's typhus work and empathized with the way fate had altered his career options. Comte and Conseil became Nicolle's closest collaborators on typhus, and Nicolle would soon secure a permanent post for Conseil.[149]

When it came to his relations with the Tunisian government, Nicolle made every effort to maximize his institute's influence and thereby its autonomy. He used the country's assorted epidemics to help him gain this authority. He had noted immediately, as we have seen, that true power rested not with the Department of Agriculture and Commerce, to which Nicolle directly answered until 1921, but with the *Résident Général* himself.[150] His relatively successful relationship with the changing cast that filled this position is reflected not only in the expanding number of products and services he provided (often for a fee) to the government, but also in the steady growth of the IPT's influence over Tunisia's public health.

When malaria broke out in 1906, the Director of Agriculture turned to the local Pasteur Institute. What did its director recommend? Nicolle asserted that the central position of any effective "campaign" against malaria (here he adopted the ubiquitous battle rhetoric of tropical medicine) should be played by the IPT. Moreover, in the public report on his response, he carefully connected the institute's services in this matter to the continued success of France's colonial mission in Tunisia:

This study underscored the considerable damage that malaria did to the work of colonization and the subsequent need to organize the campaign against this disease by using the latest prophylactic methods. M. Bartholome, recently appointed Director of Agriculture, Commerce, and Colonization, did not hesitate to adopt the Pasteur Institute's plan and created a special service.[151]

Nicolle appointed Dr. Albert Husson, a colonial physician, to direct this service at the institute and to lecture doctors throughout Tunisia—in French and in Arabic—on malaria prophylaxis.[152] The Pastorians, with Nicolle at their head, were accepted as authorities on more effective ways to prevent disease. The Tunisian government valued the promise of disease control this specialized knowledge held; Nicolle prized the promise of authority and concomitant flexibility that a good governmental alliance offered.

Plague struck the following year.[153] The dreaded Black Death mobilized Pastorian disease control efforts.[154] After Nicolle personally established the presence of the plague bacillus in Tunisia, he appointed Conseil head of the new Pasteur Institute antiplague service.[155] Conseil examined hundreds, sometimes thousands, of rats each year for evidence of plague. Disease control provided Nicolle not only with subjects for research, but also with opportunities for administrative extension. In another example of Pastorian influence, a 1907 cholera epidemic led to the construction of a sanitary station in La Goulette, to examine ships' passengers before they entered Tunis. Station director F.-J. Guégan, sketching the station's function in an *AIPT* article, concluded by thanking Nicolle and his collaborators, "who were never sparing of either time or labor, and who graciously placed all their knowledge at our disposal."[156]

Nicolle did not stop at disease-specific services and general assistance with epidemics. He also, gradually, moved Pastorians (and Pastorian sympathizers) into key government positions in public health. We have seen how the Tunisian government proper had, since the first half of the nineteenth century, embraced the importance of European-style public health boards. These became further integrated into Tunisian society with the establishment of the Protectorate. By 1908, the recent rash of epidemics in Tunis helped convince the government to split the position of Directeur de la Santé et de l'Hygiène Publique into two parts. With Nicolle's influence, Ernest Conseil was named director of the Bureau of Hygiene of Tunis.[157] The government expanded the new Bureau and its official power. A *brigadier* and two police agents were assigned to seek out infractions and punish offenders; city police were instructed to assist. Conseil assembled detailed annual municipal health reports that presented statistics on births, deaths, and diseases, by nationality.[158]

The thorough Conseil acted as both government representative and Pastorian tentacle. Through him, Nicolle could extend his control over public health, thereby furthering a Pastorian-centered model of health administration and authority. Western hygiene could make the colonies safe for Western habitation, trade, and culture by making them more like Europe. Conseil stated his young Bureau's goals in 1911: "The primary concern of the Bureau of Hygiene thus continues to be the popularization of hygiene's essential ideas. The great sanitary efforts we are making will thus give Tunis a mortality rate comparable to European cities."[159] Moreover, in an early annual report, Conseil called for continued assistance in this hygienic endeavor from civil doctors, whose collaboration had been "particularly helpful" to the new Bureau.[160] Nicolle's collaborator was clearly faithful to his teacher's goals. Two years later, the "pasteurization" of Tunisian public health was extended, as Comte himself was named the Tunisian government's "Doctor of Epidemics." Nicolle commented: "This nomination will not deprive the Pasteur Institute of a precious collaborator. Comte will retain, in addition to his new functions, his position as director of the Pasteur Institute's antimalaria service."[161]

Nicolle was successfully creating a Tunisian medical cosmos that revolved around his institute. Yet, there was another essential component to the making of a true House of Pasteur: research, with the laboratory at its center.[162]

Research, Inside and Out

Attending to the epidemics of the moment was quite important to Nicolle. Such efforts were not only part of the practical mandate of the institute, but also central to the Pastorian mission: overseas Pastorians were to adapt bacteriology to the pathological conditions indigenous to their adopted homes.[163] This mission also helped Nicolle make a number of original disease discoveries, most of them in his early years in Tunis.

In 1907, studying small rodents resembling guinea pigs—*gondi*—native to southern Tunisia, Nicolle identified a microscopic organism that killed the creatures. Initially he thought it to be a new variety of leishmaniasis, but he soon realized it was a separate organism. He called it "toxoplasma" and named the disease "toxoplasmosis."[164] At about the same time, Nicolle began to work on kala-azar, a form of leishmaniasis that is "characterized by fever, hepatosplenomegaly, lymphadenopathy, anemia with leukopenia, and progressive emaciation and weakness"; postinfection lesions of the skin are common.[165] Untreated, kala-azar is often fatal. Nicolle first differentiated the

Tunisian form from the previously identified Indian variety: unlike Indian kala-azar, Tunisian kala-azar primarily struck children under the age of six. The two forms also had slightly different symptomatic expressions. Having determined this, Nicolle turned to the question of transmission, which he studied through epidemiological observation. In Tunisia, the disease was proportionally most common among poor Italians. The French were second, Muslims third; the Jewish community, however, was almost free of the disease. Attempting to make sense of this, Nicolle identified the dog as the disease's likely reservoir. For proof, he returned to the laboratory. Culturing the organism from the dog entailed a technical innovation that later would come into widespread use. Starting with a culture medium designed by Novy and McNeal, Nicolle adjusted the composition to fit his particular needs. This medium became known as "NNN," with Nicolle's name contributing the final initial. The newly adapted medium in hand, Nicolle confirmed the presence of leishmaniasis-causing organisms in dogs.[166]

To this point, we have seen how Nicolle built institutional networks in Tunisia that also served to elevate his own power, and how he backed up that power with original research on several of the country's diseases. Yet, beyond an apparently singular link between the IPT and Albert Calmette, it is unclear how developments in Tunisia became known outside the country. In fact, by the first decade of the twentieth century, the Parisian Pastorians had created pathways for exchange between the colonial "filials" and the better known institutions of Western medicine.[167] In addition to Calmette's reign over colonial diplomacy, these pathways were overseen by Emile Roux (now director of the IPP) and parasitologist Félix Mesnil. Roux acted as a veritable mentor-at-a-distance, writing Nicolle, for example, with abundant suggestions for future experiments that arose out of his research projects. He was also the principal link to France's prestigious Académie des Sciences. When a colonial Pastorian made a discovery of sufficient merit, it was Roux who would ensure that the discovery was noted at a meeting of the Académie and published in its journal. He also made certain that Pastorians overseas were considered for the Académie's assorted prizes: though he tended to deliver news of such awards in an offhand way that suggested he saw prizes themselves as merely a necessary evil. In 1909, he informed Nicolle that the Académie had awarded him its Montyon Prize in a postscript to his letter.[168]

It was Félix Mesnil, however, who acted as the central conduit for the exchange of personnel, prestige, and information between metropole and periphery.[169] A contemporary of Nicolle, Mesnil had worked on cellular immunity and comparative pathology in Metchnikoff's lab and acted for a time as

Pasteur's secretary, then went on to conduct important work on sleeping sickness with Alphonse Laveran. In 1899, he was put in charge of the parasitology section of Roux's *Cours* and used the position to appropriate the most promising students—many of whom were colonial doctors—for the overseas Pasteur Institutes. In addition to this important recruiting role, Mesnil helped create new pathways of information exchange. He was one of the founding editors of the *Bulletin de l'Institut Pasteur*, established in 1903 to facilitate the dissemination of microbiological developments in summary form. (The journal complemented and extended the more formal functions of the IP's *Annals*.[170]) Responding still more directly to colonial needs, he helped found the Société de Pathologie Exotique in 1907 and its *Bulletin* the following year.[171] Mesnil's journals filled important niches in the division of labor of microbiological publications, and, with them, the overseas Pastorians had an array of journals to which they might contribute their work. Mesnil and Nicolle frequently exchanged letters in which Mesnil advised his friend where to send his various articles, making sure he did not neglect, for example, the Society of Biology. Mesnil thereby helped ensure that colonial names were made familiar to the metropolitan centers of medical authority.[172]

Nicolle was keenly aware of this network of information exchange and did his part to contribute to it. His experience in Rouen, first with the *Normandie Médicale*, then with his own *Revue Médicale*, had taught him the importance of editorial control. Tunisia did have its own medical journal, which was attached to the Société des Sciences Médicales.[173] Principally a clinical journal, and not a publication he could easily control, it was not sufficient for Nicolle's designs. In 1906, he started his own journal, the *Archives de l'Institut Pasteur de Tunis*.[174] Later, he would describe his motivations for starting the journal in colonial terms, noting that, in the metropole, one could simply cross the hallway, or attend a conference, to elicit a critique of one's ideas. In the periphery, however, other means were necessary—means such as one's own journal.[175] Whether or not he had such considerations in mind in 1906, Nicolle did create in his journal a forum that allowed him to make his work, and that of his collaborators, known broadly and in full detail. Frequently, he would publish in his own *Archives* greatly expanded versions of his papers that had appeared in the Academy of Science's *Comptes Rendus* (where contributions were generally limited to three pages) or the IP's *Annales*. Although the journal helped bring Nicolle and the IPT to international attention, it is clear, at the same time, that the *AIPT* came to be increasingly popular among medical researchers and libraries throughout the world as Nicolle's reputation grew.[176] Here, it was the Parisian journals that directed international attention to Tunis.

Within five years of crossing the Mediterranean Sea and "becoming Tunisian," Nicolle had successfully established his institute as worthy of bearing the name "Pasteur." He had also established himself as a worthy participant in the de facto bacteriological conquest of the colonial world: he was a "microbe hunter," a master of disease (and organization). At least rhetorically, he linked his work with the successful extension of France's civilizing mission. His conviction that microbiology, properly undertaken, was essential to the civilizing mission, and thereby to the survival of civilization itself, deepened over time, until it became the very heart of his understanding of both humanity and disease. Yet, to Nicolle, too close an identification with his fellow colonial-microbiological colleagues was dangerous: despite Mesnil's best efforts, it was rare that they ever received even a fraction of the recognition so abundantly lavished on their colleagues back in the metropole. Even at this early stage in his direction of the IPT, it is clear that Nicolle was ambitious, both for himself and for his institute. The faithful Pastorian wanted to be the intellectual son of Pasteur, an accomplishment that would take far more than the successes he had achieved thus far. Most of the colonial IPs had adopted an emblematic disease. Nicolle selected his signature disease carefully. He sought a disease that would be recognized by the Western world as significant but that was also, in a sense, distinctly "Tunisian." He found this locally grown yet internationally significant disease in typhus.

2

THE THRESHOLD OF CIVILIZATION

Typhus in Tunisia (1903–11)

> Human knowledge and human power meet in one; for where the cause is not known the effect cannot be produced. Nature to be commanded must be obeyed, and that which in contemplation is as the cause is in operation as the rule.
> —Sir Francis Bacon, *New Organon* I.3, 1620

> In this historic place, typhus fever is thus [both] a very old plague and a permanent threat to man and to civilization.
> —Charles Nicolle, 1911

"The *history of typhus*," wrote August Hirsch in his classic nineteenth-century *Handbook of Geographical and Historical Pathology*, "is written in those dark pages of the world's story which tell of the grievous visitations of mankind by war, famine, and misery of every kind."[1] Besides its association with poor conditions in temperate climates, typhus fever remained mysterious even after enthusiastic applications of the germ theory had clarified the inner workings of many other diseases. By the time Nicolle adopted the disease for special attention in the first decade of the twentieth century, it had been more clearly differentiated from typhoid fever (with which it was often confused) and, for the most part, had been banished from western Europe. It did, however, continue to exist in both endemic and epidemic forms in countries near Europe's borders.

One region that typhus continued to menace was North Africa. The epidemics in Tunisia in the 1860s had made history, as we have seen, for helping to ensure the country's bankruptcy. Still, such occurrences were subsequently rare. Typhus was endemic in neighboring Algeria but not, it seemed, in Tunisia. Indeed, in 1894, Lucien Bertholon, best known for his anthropological studies of North Africa (and for his position as head doctor to prisons in Tunisia), published a statistical study of disease distribution among French colonists in Tunisia. Although several diseases were described as presenting challenges, *typhus* did not even merit a mention: it was not regarded as a problem in Tunisia. Indeed, Bertholon judged the country to be relatively healthy—"*une terre de colonisation par excellence.*"[2] Even the IPT's own Adrien Loir, in his subsequent listing of diseases fatal to the inhabitants of Tunis, made no mention of typhus.[3]

In short, before Nicolle came to it, typhus was thought to be a disease occasionally *in* Tunisia, but not a disease *of* Tunisia. His "selection" of typhus as his institute's "signature" disease thus raises a number of questions. Why did Nicolle neglect closer study of, for example, typhoid, which he had investigated so carefully in Rouen, and which was more obviously a disease "of" Tunisia? Why did the other diseases he studied in Tunisia fall short of his aspirations (and on what levels?)? Why did he instead choose typhus? How did typhus become a disease of Tunisia—and how, and to what end(s), did Nicolle redefine understanding of the disease, both locally and internationally? Before we can begin to answer these questions, we must look more closely at Nicolle's conception of Pastorian "medical science" and at the many mysteries and complications that hindered efforts to explain typhus in scientific terms as Nicolle began to investigate the disease more closely.

Pastorian Medicine à la Nicolle

Nearly three centuries before Charles Nicolle made public his initial discoveries about typhus fever, Francis Bacon gave his charge to the scientific revolution.[4] Knowledge and power would coincide, he argued, when knowledge was derived *inductively*. Gradually ascending from careful observation of particulars, one eventually gained solid understanding of nature's laws. With knowledge of these laws, one could in turn control nature: "Nature to be commanded must be obeyed." This was the *scientific* method of knowing.[5] Science was a universalizing process, and the laws it revealed were, by definition, applicable to all nature. Yet, for three centuries (and more), it had been wholly unclear how such seemingly universal scientific analysis could be applied fruitfully to the unruly particularities of human bodies.

Germ theory, particularly as postulated by Jakob Henle and his student, Robert Koch, was perceived by its supporters to be a successful marriage of science and medicine. Dutifully applied, it would allow doctors to determine the *cause* of infectious diseases and, eventually, to control such diseases. Louis Pasteur and his followers tended to be less impressed by such strict rules and methods; and time, with experience, substantiated their caution. By the first decade of the twentieth century, the German ideal of specificity, in which one microbe caused one disease, was being challenged by the discovery of a number of instances to the contrary.[6] This did not mean, however, that German bacteriologists, or even French microbiologists, were ready to abandon the dream of discerning the universal laws determining human sickness and health. Instead, they acknowledged that things were more complex than they first seemed—and pressed forward with more elaborate models of disease causation and immunity.

The Pastorians, as Moulin has shown, found yet another path toward universalizing scientific medicine.[7] They housed microbiological technique within the trappings of Catholic social structure, then set those enshrined techniques in motion with the force of France's civilizing mission. Once this socio-microbiological package arrived at its destination—and there were dozens of international destinations—it took root in the local soil, where, nourished by science's universalizing tendencies, it grew into a true *"filial"* Pasteur Institute. These institutes, as we have seen with the IPT, featured local external architecture that housed within it the more global contents of scientific medicine. The Pastorian preference for coupling the local and the universal is seen also in the institutes' preferred model of relations between clinic, laboratory, and hygiene, and in their specific research choices.

In Rouen, Nicolle had been guided by the way Pasteur carved out a place for microbiology that was autonomous from clinical medicine and hygiene, but that also drew upon those disciplines as needed for its own advancement. Nicolle's frustrating experiences with clinical medicine in Rouen, however, taught him valuable lessons about achieving autonomy as they solidified the model of "scientific medicine" he brought with him to Tunis. In his second year in Tunisia, Nicolle provided a striking portrait of this model, in the course of participating in a dispute at the Société des Sciences Médicales about professional control of medical practice in the Protectorate.

French doctors in Tunisia, like their colleagues in other French possessions, were divided about how best to approach medical practice in the colonies. At opposite ends of a well-shaded spectrum lay capitalism and socialism: Should French doctors concentrate their efforts on fellow Europeans, or should a universal system of medicine and hygiene be available to all (and paid for by the wealthiest)?[8] By the early twentieth century, it was evident that doctors neglected local health problems at their own risk. Still, many questions remained about proper distribution of limited resources. If one supported an all-inclusive medical system, one needed far more licensed medical practitioners than were available in Tunisia.[9] One also needed practitioners whom locals would trust. To that end, Brunswic-le-Bihan, then engaged in the daunting task of overhauling the struggling Sadiki Hospital, proposed the creation of a new school. Affiliated with the Sadiki, it would train young Tunisians to act as "medical auxiliaries" to licensed doctors. These auxiliary practitioners would also help other Tunisians feel more comfortable receiving care at the indigenous hospital. The school was approved by the Tunisian government in October 1903.[10]

In the spring of 1904, the new school's validity was challenged by several members of the Société des Sciences Médicales. Indeed, the doctors were indignant: it had taken years to weed empiricism out of Tunisian medicine, and now Brunswic's school was allowing it to reenter through official channels. Clearly concerned that such empiricism threatened to strangle the ideal of medical "professionalism" they had so carefully cultivated, the protesters ignored certain practical facts in order to press their claims. Hospital staff, particularly at the Sadiki, were stretched thin; the number of Tunisian *médecins tolérés* was declining rapidly; and only one Tunisian doctor had been officially licensed since Dinguizli.[11] Nonetheless, these protesting members urged the Société to challenge the school's continued existence. They met opposition from a vocal minority, whose concerns necessitated the addition of an "extraordinary" meeting to discuss the Société's right to take such action.[12] This minority's leading voice was that of Charles Nicolle. His objections had to do with his understanding of fair play, both personally and professionally. It was an understanding that, though tinged with a certain amount of self interest, was principally driven by his concern for preserving "scientific medicine."

The personal component of Nicolle's challenge concerned the propriety of engaging in such a debate when the prime mover of the opposition, Brunswic-le-Bihan, was absent.[13] Nicolle had several viable motives for making this argument. One was personal respect: earlier that year, Nicolle and Brunswic had coauthored a provocative article for the Presse Médicale. More literary than scientific, the piece effectively condemned the preferred Tunisian method of hanging prisoners, simply by detailing one such execution.[14]

Another plausible motive combined personal and professional interest in preserving the smooth functioning of the parts that, together, made up scientific medical practice in Tunis: Nicolle would long rely on Brunswic's hospital for "clinical materials" to support his research. Yet, the core of his challenge was informed by his conception of scientific medicine and his understanding of the Société's self-definition as it intersected with that conception: "remember, Messieurs, that our bylaws forbid us to engage in politics: that we are a *scientific, and, above all, an international society*. In the interest of our Society, we must be extremely prudent and wise when we enter any realm that borders on the political."[15] "Medical science" thus effectively excluded both politics and the concerns of clinical professionalism. (Throughout his career, Nicolle would, at least publicly, hold both spheres at arm's length).[16] Yet, he denied that he was being dismissive of clinical medicine's professional designs: "I would not dream of denying that doctors have the right to defend their professional interests," he responded to his critics at the Société's extraordinary session. "What I refuse to admit is that the Société des Sciences Médicales of Tunis may do so without violating its statutes. This is not the role [of the Société], but of medical individuals, syndicates, and professional associations."[17]

The majority of members present rejected Nicolle's cautions and went forward with protests in the Société's name.[18] In the end, such efforts proved futile, and the protesters' arguments, at least in this case, were largely superfluous.[19] Five years later, Nicolle would act as the Société's president. If he had aspirations of bringing the institution into closer alignment with its scientific statutes, he lacked the time to do so. A typhus epidemic in 1909 demanded most of his attention. Indeed, in his outgoing presidential speech that October, Nicolle apologized for being "the most unfaithful of presidents" and asked his colleagues to "forgive my many involuntary absences." The speech was delivered by the Société's general secretary: for "professional reasons," Nicolle could not be present at the meeting.[20]

Although Nicolle's conception of scientific medicine transcended the particularities of medical practice and politics, it was by no means an autonomous entity. In the Pastorian tradition, it contained within itself the categories of laboratory, clinic, and hygiene, all in proper (or laboratory-centered,) alignment.[21] In 1911, Nicolle participated in the creation of a useful institutional amalgamation of these elements. It took the form of a new medical journal, *La Tunisie Médicale*, whose editorial committee—influential doctors at "the principal Civil and Military Hospitals (The French Civil Hospital, where the reactions of Europeans to the African climate are effectively studied; the Sadiki Hospital, rich with indigenous documentation) and the Directors of the principal biological and medico-demographic services (Pasteur Institute; Bureau of Hygiene)"—reflected this ideal.[22]

Functionally, the new journal also reflected Pastorian concerns with coupling local and global scientific interests. Its pages were open to contributions from "all our confreres in the Regency," and its primary goal was to act as a "useful instrument for work and a place to bring together the scientific activity of the country."[23] Grounded in the "local interests" of "Tunisian pathology," the journal would encourage consideration of the ways in which these local discoveries were of "general interest" to "science."[24] The particularities of Tunisia itself would link the local and the global: the country, located on a small "plot of African soil," was a "crossroads of diverse races," all of which exhibited "distinctive predispositions and reactions" to local conditions. Such diverse local findings might well have international significance. Moreover, they might—and here we find an increasingly central theme in Nicolle's model of medical functions—be *profitable* to the Tunisian government. The Regency had largely "relied, for aid and medicine, on the dowry of the metropole." It "is just, and it is time," for Tunisia to take advantage of its unique resources, both for its own benefit and for "the public treasury of medical sciences."[25] (This "public treasury" would, of course, benefit the institutions represented on the journal's editorial board.) The very first issue of the journal boasted articles reflecting its integrative ideals about medical science, written by editorial board members: Ernest Conseil, on the treatment of syphilis by "606"; Brunswic-le-Bihan, on abdominal wounds—and Charles Nicolle, on "New Findings on Typhus Fever."[26]

The Mysteries of Typhus

Typhus fever is perhaps best remembered in the United States—when it is remembered at all—through the lively popular history written in the 1930s by Nicolle's good friend, Harvard bacteriologist Hans Zinsser. Zinsser described typhus as an acute fever

> which does not always behave in a conventional manner. In its typical course . . . the onset may vary from extreme abruptness to a more gradual one. As a result the initial stages resemble closely those of severe influenza. The temperature rises rapidly, often to from 103 to 104 Fahrenheit, with chills, great depression, weakness, pains in the head and limbs. The eruption appears on the fourth or fifth day after the onset. . . . It is at first composed of pink spots which disappear on pressure, but soon become purplish, more deeply

brownish red, and finally fade into a brown color. These are the "petechia" and "peticuli" of the older descriptions.[27]

The stupor that so often accompanied the disease also inspired its name.[28] Treatment in Nicolle's day tended to be palliative: mortality rates during epidemics could reach upwards of 40 percent.

To get a sense of the dangers presented to researchers studying typhus in the early twentieth century, one need look no further than the causal microorganism itself. *Rickettsia prowazeki* was named after two men who noted the presence of the very tiny microbe that was *eventually* agreed to cause typhus.[29] Henry Ricketts, an American conducting research on typhus in Mexico City, contracted the disease and died in 1910; Bohemia-born bacteriologist Stanislas von Prowazek, working on typhus during World War I, died of it in 1915. Still more immediately to our story—though with somewhat more positive outcomes—both Nicolle and Zinsser, as well as most of their collaborators on typhus, contracted the disease in the course of their research.[30] Even Lucien Bertholon, herald of Tunisian salubrity, was stricken.[31]

If typhus remained a mysterious disease, its mysteries were of the tragic, rather than romantic, variety. It tended to haunt people in confined spaces, such as jail cells and overcrowded dwellings; it struck when these marginalized men and women were at their weakest.[32] As August Hirsch noted:

> It is always and everywhere the wretched conditions of living, which spring from poverty and are fostered by ignorance, laziness, and helplessness, in which typhus takes root and finds nourishment; and it is above all in *the want of cleanliness, and in the overcrowding of dwellings, that are ventilated badly or not at all and are tainted with corrupt effluvia of every kind*.[33]

War was an infamous breeding ground for typhus. Soldiers were often crowded together, hungry, cold, and exhausted. Typhus seemed drawn to them. Zinsser recounted the details of several major historical battles whose outcomes, he argued, were dictated more by the presence of typhus than by the strategies of generals or the power of their weapons.[34] Moreover, when typhus struck with epidemic force, it spread rapidly, overcoming even those who were better fed and better off.

Writing in the early 1880s, Hirsch also observed that nineteenth-century Europe enjoyed a historically unprecedented absence of epidemic typhus. From 1815, "whole regions of the continent of Europe have remained almost entirely exempt from typhus." Instead, "the disease appears to be now confined to particular spots."[35] These were not *tropical* spots, but "mostly . . . temperate and cold zones."[36] More specifically, typhus continued to erupt in Ireland, Russia, "Upper Silesia" (Poland), Mexico—and North Africa.[37] What did these places, "whatever be their differences in climate, and in terrestrial and national characters," have in common? "There is a remarkable agreement among them in respect of certain *blots in their social well-being*."[38] The typhus epidemic in Algiers and Tunis in 1868 served as an example of this rule.[39]

In short, by the later nineteenth century it was evident that the presence or absence of typhus was somehow connected to cleanliness and constitution. It was not evident *how* the disease was connected to these conditions. Nor was it evident how typhus spread when epidemic or where, precisely, it went when it was not epidemic. Yet, given the disease's rapid epidemic extension and the fact that typhus persisted in countries bordering western Europe and the United States, healthier countries could not afford to ignore the disease altogether. Researchers in these more fortunate countries, however (for reasons that will be clarified later), were unable to study typhus in their laboratories. Instead, they had to rely on colleagues working on the peripheries of the West for a better understanding of the elusive and menacing disease.

Between 1860, when the first volume of Hirsch's magisterial study of pathology was published, and 1881, when his revised volume on acute infectious disease appeared, Pasteur and Koch had conducted the research that was warming doctors to the possibility that "germs" caused many of these diseases.[40] Except for the addition of a few epidemic appearances, however, there wasn't much more to say about typhus in the second edition than there had been in the first. The disease's continuing tendency to avoid much of Europe was an important, but mainly fortuitous, development. Indeed, the century's greatest contribution to the *understanding* of typhus had occurred nearly twenty-five years before Hirsch's first volume appeared. As part of efforts to classify fevers (with the help of anatomical-pathological correlation), "*typhus*" had been diagnostically differentiated from "*typhoid*" in the 1830s.[41] Still, typhus itself remained quite difficult to diagnose. Later in the century, Widal's agglutination test for typhoid would help doctors determine a diagnosis of typhus by eliminating typhoid as a possibility. Yet, typhus remained hard to diagnose with any certainty: in 1898, the American master diagnostician Nathan Brill used the Widal test to demonstrate that a mysterious but mild disease thought by most doctors to be a form of typhoid was not, in fact, typhoid.[42] Only in 1912 was that disease shown instead to be a mild form of *typhus*.[43]

Back in North Africa, when Bertholon asserted Tunisia's healthiness, he made a large exception: typhoid fever continued to be a widespread, and often deadly, problem.[44]

The Persistence of Typhus Mysteries

The heart of germ theory was the germ. The so-called "Koch's Postulates" for demonstrating disease causality were straightforward and germ-centered. One must find the suspect microbe in patients suffering from a particular disease— and not in individuals without the disease. One must then cultivate that microbe on an artificial medium (potato cultures were initially quite popular, then agar), then inoculate a susceptible animal with the resultant pure culture. If the microbe is indeed the etiological agent of the disease, an inoculated animal will exhibit that disease. To complete the causal circle, one then needed to find the organism in the sick animal. When Nicolle began to work seriously on typhus, around 1906, not one of these steps seemed possible for the disease. No microbe had been found that caused it; no cultures containing any causal typhus agent could be grown. Typhus appeared to resist the progress of scientific medicine at every turn. Then again, by 1906, a number of qualifications had been attached to the famous postulates. Of most immediate importance for understanding typhus was the work being done on the so-called "filterable viruses."[45]

The term *"filterable virus"* was devised to refer to a growing class of causal agents that passed through porcelain filters. In 1884, Charles Chamberland, one of Pasteur's original "disciples," addressed the difficulties often encountered in obtaining a "pure" culture of any etiological agent by borrowing a method from water filtration. He devised a porcelain filter that helped researchers remove fluids from a sample, leaving only the larger elements— including microbes—for analysis. The "Chamberland Filter" was rapidly adopted, and a variety of other such filters were soon developed. In the 1890s, however, two researchers independently determined that the causal agent of tobacco mosaic disease passed *through* the filter with the liquid. In a move indicating how central filtration had become to research on microbes, the phenomenon was found to be significant and its manifestations were called "filterable viruses"—as opposed to normal "viruses," as microbes generically continued to be called.[46] Soon, other diseases, including fowl plague and rabies, were added to the category.[47] In 1903, the first article in the first volume of the *Bulletin de l'Institut Pasteur* was a review of findings on filterable viruses. It was written by Emile Roux himself.[48]

When Nicolle began his typhus research, "filterable virus" had become a well known and continually expanding category. It was unclear, however, what these agents were and how they functioned. Indeed, they were wholly defined by negatives: they were not stopped by standard microbiological filters, they were not seen with a light microscope, and they appeared not to be cultivable on artificial media.[49] They were wholly resistant to postulate-oriented demonstration. The agent of typhus was possibly a filterable virus.

Had typhus simply resisted cultivation on artificial media and eluded microscopic sight, it still might have received more thorough study before 1906. But the disease had another complicating characteristic: no animal had been found to exhibit typhus symptoms, either in nature or in the lab. Humans alone appeared to be susceptible. Human experimentation had by no means faded from the laboratory landscape, but the often-fatal outcome of typhus infection made intentionally cultivated cases difficult to justify.[50] Without a susceptible animal to inoculate, samples of the typhus "virus" could not be maintained for study between epidemics. Even during epidemics, laboratory investigation proved to be of limited value. No diagnostic test had been developed to help clinicians identify patients with the disease, and pathological examinations turned up little more of any promise.[51]

In 1906, typhus had a complex status in the West. Although it no longer visited western Europe (or the United States) with epidemics, it continued to dwell in the West's immediate periphery. The disease's ability to extend beyond its normal confines during epidemic outbreaks made typhus a constant threat. As the mystery of its nineteenth-century redistribution persisted, no one was certain how to stop the disease, once it became epidemic, from striking the West. Moreover, its absence from the West meant its absence from laboratories in the West: no cultures, no inoculated animals, could take experimental typhus from periphery to center. The West, however, had extended itself far beyond its traditional continental confines, sprouting up in colonies around the globe. Typhus continued to menace some of the most proximate Western possessions; there, colonial microbiologists could study the disease directly. Moreover, wherever typhus continued to exist locally, it would draw the considered attentions of the more geographically conventional West. It perfectly combined the qualities of local specificity and international interest. This made typhus an enticing disease for the Tunisian Pastorians. Its relatively frequent epidemic appearances in the first decade of the twentieth century gave Nicolle and his collaborators pathological materials to study directly. But, despite its local visitations, was it fair to claim typhus as a "Tunisian" disease?

Typhus in Tunisia

> It is thus natural and necessary that the study of typhus was undertaken in a country such as our own, which has been so cruelly afflicted with the disease, and it is precisely the goal and the utility of Pasteur Institutes to study the pathological conditions specific to [*la pathologie spéciale*] the countries where those institutes were created.
>
> —Charles Nicolle, 1911

Shortly after Nicolle arrived in Tunis, he had his first, unforgettable encounter with typhus. In 1903, an epidemic struck the country. Hoping to determine how the disease could be moved from field to laboratory for closer analysis, Nicolle planned a trip with two medical colleagues. The trio was to go to a town about fifty miles south of Tunis, where they would examine typhus patients.[52] Just before they were to depart, Nicolle fell ill and could not make the trip. His two colleagues set out alone. Both contracted typhus and died. Later, in his Nobel Prize speech, Nicolle recalled this early escape: "Without this incident, my first contact with typhus would doubtlessly have been my last."[53] The disease appeared, though in limited form, in both 1904 and 1905; 1906 brought a true typhus epidemic. During the 1906 epidemic, Nicolle and his collaborators continued their efforts to study the disease in the laboratory, while his newly adopted colleague, Ernest Conseil, studied its epidemiological characteristics in the field. It was Conseil's work that allowed Nicolle to claim typhus as a disease *of* Tunisia. Laboratory progress had to wait for the next epidemic outbreak.

The collaboration of Nicolle and Conseil was so close that Nicolle would later confess he wasn't always certain where Conseil's work ended and his own began.[54] That collaboration started in earnest with Conseil's 1907 study of typhus in Tunisia. Published in Nicolle's *Archives de l'Institut Pasteur de Tunis,* it was the first original study of typhus to appear in the young journal. The article's simple descriptive title, "Typhus Fever in Tunisia," was accurate but incomplete. While Conseil carefully detailed the disease's nature and distribution in his newly adopted country, he also had another motive for writing. He sought to prove that typhus was *endemic* to Tunisia—in short, that typhus fever was a local disease.

In the article's opening, Conseil noted that typhus was long known to exist in North Africa and that, "since the conquest of Algeria, hardly a year has passed" in which military doctors in Algeria had not seen it take epidemic form. Despite the abundance of evidence for Algeria, there were few accounts of typhus in Tunisia beyond its occasional epidemic appearances. "However," Conseil mused rhetorically, "the frequency of relations and the identity of etiological conditions allow one to think that [in Tunisia], as in Algeria, each springtime brings with it small, localized epidemics." Indeed, upon closer inspection of more recent evidence, it was possible "to affirm the endemicity of typhus in Tunisia."[55] The article proceeded to substantiate this assertion. In essence, Conseil demonstrated the local endemic existence of typhus by pulling it out of obscure corners where it had hitherto been overlooked: dank jails; dark bodies; and shadowy diagnostics.

Having just completed his thesis on typhus at the Sadiki, Conseil was well acquainted with all of the occasions on which typhus was known to have claimed victims in recent years. Many of these cases had been noted but never written up and published. There were, he explained, "several cases" of typhus in the "Tunisian prisons and Israelite Hospital" in 1901 and 1902. The year 1903, of course, produced the recorded and more extensive epidemic appearance of the disease. Between 1903 and the 1906 epidemic, typhus had struck, if only marginally, each spring, "localized in indigenous prisons." It was spring again when typhus arrived in 1906.[56] This record, Conseil concluded, "not only shows the endemicity of typhus in Tunisia; if one examines it more closely, one is struck by the regularity of its appearance." Each year, typhus emerged with the start of spring weather and disappeared when the summer's heat became intense. It was odd, Conseil noted, that this disease of confined spaces tended to manifest itself in North Africa just as people were moving out of winter enclosures to take up "lives in the outdoors."[57] He left the observation without explanation, turning instead to the particular "biological characteristics" of local typhus cases.

Conseil argued that the extent of Tunisia's typhus problem had gone unnoticed because most (Arab) Tunisians who contracted the disease went undiagnosed. Western doctors in North Africa had long known that typhus was particularly difficult to diagnose in the local population. When locals contracted the disease in its endemic form, it was quite mild and appeared not to be highly contagious. During epidemics, which tended to break out when conditions were particularly poor, Tunisians often displayed typhus in its more deadly form. In both cases, however, they did not clearly display all the symptoms associated with typhus in Europeans. Conseil noted that Arab-Tunisians exhibited typhus in a "*forme fruste*"—literally, a "rough" or "unsophisticated" (not quite civilized?) expression of the disease.[58] (Even if the term was generally used among French doctors, it seems an unsettling word choice for the circumstances.) Of course, the presence of typhus was more easily confirmed when Tunisian patients transmitted it to nearby Europeans, who then expressed "all the classic symptoms of typhus."[59] Failing that, diagnosis was tricky. In the disease's local, rough form, its characteristic rose-colored spots tended to be "transient, even wholly absent." The problem of finding these petechia was complicated by their tendency to be camouflaged by "the brown skin of the patients" and still further obscured by the frequency with which that skin was mottled by "all species of parasites."[60] Finally, to reclaim typhus from "typhoid" misdiagnoses, Conseil, with Nicolle, conducted serodiagnostic tests "systematically on all of our patients."[61] By the time typhus was again epidemic in Tunis, Conseil argued explicitly that many cases had been misdiagnosed over the years as typhoid.[62] Reclaimed from the dark places that had previously hidden it, typhus was most assuredly a disease *of* Tunisia.

The year 1909 saw the typhus epidemic that made Nicolle—and his Institute—famous. It started in January with three small foyers, all at some distance from Tunis.[63] By mid-March, typhus was in Tunis, where a soldier "who frequented Moorish cafes" and a prisoner fell ill.[64] Spreading slowly at first, it picked up steam in April; May saw the epidemic's peak, with 360 cases in Tunis alone. By this time, patients with typhus were being sent to a lazaret in la Rabta, just outside Tunis (largely because their numbers were too great for the Sadiki).[65] "The European sick," Conseil noted, were "far less numerous" and were therefore treated by "their respective national hospitals."[66] The epidemic continued into June, striking over 200 people in Tunis that month. Finally, in July, it subsided. In the end, typhus had stricken some 4,000 individuals in Tunisia, 836 of whom were in Tunis.[67] The mortality rate in the city, where more precise statistics were available, was 32.6 percent.[68]

Conseil was now Director of Hygiene for the City of Tunis. The position did not, however, limit him to the administration of prevention and cleanup: as Nicolle's right-hand man in the field, Conseil was first and foremost the city's epidemiologist. Moreover, he gathered much of his statistical insight from the data supplied to him by his clinical colleagues throughout the country.[69] In this way, Conseil's work embodied the combined forces of "hygiene" (broadly defined) and "clinical medicine" that Nicolle was so fond of attaching to the lab within his idealized conception of scientific medicine. The typhus epidemic offered Nicolle and Conseil an opportunity to demonstrate how that conception might work in practice, and they seized it. Within this model formulation, it was the multilayered epidemiological evidence gathered by Conseil that guided Nicolle and his colleagues to the most likely explanation for typhus's mysterious transmission. The laboratory gave demonstrative weight to the hypothesis, resulting in *knowledge* that contained within itself the *power* to control the disease.[70] Later, Nicolle would find still more lessons he could teach with the story of the typhus studies undertaken in Tunisia.

Within his epidemiological study of the 1909 typhus epidemic, Conseil drew attention to a number of apparently significant observations. Typhus, as he had taken great pains to demonstrate in 1907, was "endemic in Tunisia."[71] Early each spring, the disease would appear first, often in its "benign" or "rough" form, among poor men in the countryside. The spring of 1909 brought particularly miserable conditions, with drought and famine. A bit later, typhus arrived in Tunis itself, where it was particularly prevalent in "Moorish" cafes and temporary lodging places. Examining the victims, Conseil noted that 90 percent of the patients were men—most of them *single* men, between the ages of 20 and 40. Closer examination of the victims' professions revealed that more than 60 percent could be classified as "the wretched": the unemployed, beggars, day laborers, agricultural workers—often, the "miserable souls" who had descended on Tunis from the countryside.[72] Typhus was far rarer in families, even in the countryside where endemic foyers of the disease were evident. Moreover, "when a case appears in the street, it almost always remains an isolated case. Typhus," Conseil observed, "is not spread in ordinary times by simple contact; one needs another element, one that creates foyers in the *zaouïas* and cafes."[73]

What about the men and women in Tunis who contracted the disease but did not frequent such establishments? Conseil found that most of them had jobs that brought them into contact with such individuals: "doctors and male nurses . . . but only those who approached the sick before they entered into the hospital; . . . police officers . . . in charge of transporting the sick; railroad employees . . . small shopkeepers, grocers, café workers . . . whose clientele were the wretched; bath keepers . . . prostitutes; in short, all those who had direct relations with the sick" and their garments.[74] An "interesting example" of this phenomenon had been "furnished by the hospitals." At the Sadiki, typhus patients were not initially isolated from other patients. Still, none of the other patients contracted typhus. However, "the nurses who admitted the patients at the hospital's entrance and several patients in rooms near the entrance were afflicted."[75]

Conseil assembled this evidence in support of a probable description of the 1909 epidemic's trajectory, one that strongly suggested a particular causal explanation for that trajectory. Poor men in the countryside were the perpetual reservoirs of typhus in Tunisia. The mildness of their infections tended to hide the disease from clinical sight. (Besides, there were very few Western doctors in the countryside.) In the spring, when the nomads left their shelters to find work, they carried the disease, and the agent of its transmission, with them. Most years, they remained localized. In 1909, however, conditions were particularly bad: famine gave rise to "an exodus of the unemployed," and Tunis quickly became "the refuge of all the miserable souls that famine had chased out of the countryside."[76] More specifically, they congregated in "the Moorish cafes, the *zaouïas* and the inns" that were transformed by their presence into "veritable foyers" of typhus.[77] From these foyers, however, the disease did not spread generally, as did truly contagious diseases such as smallpox. It tended to strike only those in direct, close contact with the sick and their effects. The "peculiar fashion" in which the disease moved suggested that typhus was transmitted by an insect.[78] Other epidemiological observations pointed to one insect above all others. Over in the laboratories of the IPT, Nicolle and his colleagues were working to make it possible for the laboratory to substantiate the hypothesis that epidemiological study had helped formulate.

Behind the Curtain

During the 1906 typhus epidemic, Nicolle and his collaborators attempted to reproduce the disease in laboratory animals. They failed.[79] In 1909, Nicolle decided to inoculate monkeys; he hoped that their closer physiological proximity to humans would make them more likely candidates for expressing this human disease. Nicolle had previously used monkeys to study other diseases (such as *chancre mou*) in the lab.[80] Monkeys, however, were tricky to procure. Fortunately, since 1908, Nicolle had had an inside source for monkey acquisition—the dashing Alfred Conor. Conor, who had been Nicolle's student in Rouen, was now a military doctor and had recently received an appointment at the military bacteriology lab in Marseille. Among his duties was the distribution of lab animals to researchers in other laboratories. Nicolle addressed many a letter to his former student that year, requesting monkeys for experiments. By the time he needed the animals for his typhus experiments, however, he no longer had Conor to fill his orders: Conor, who was also a talented bacteriologist, had moved to Tunis in the spring of 1909. There, in addition to his post in the bacteriology lab of the military hospital in Tunis, Conor was ordained assistant director of the Pasteur Institute of Tunis. He arrived just in time to see typhus become epidemic.

Although his preferred animal provider was no longer in Marseille, Nicolle was able to conduct preliminary experiments on monkeys already in his possession.[81] He inoculated Chinese monkeys (*bonnet Chinois*, or *Macacus sinicus*) with blood taken from typhus patients. Again, he failed: "*Two attempts to transmit typhus by the direct inoculation of infected blood into the Chinese monkey gave negative results.*"[82] He needed something closer still to humans in physiology: a chimpanzee. Chimps, however, not only were more difficult to procure than monkeys; they were far more expensive. The Tunisian government, which continued to supply the institute's budget, was (as Conseil would later note) already being quite lenient about all the expenses the local Pastorians were incurring in their typhus research.[83] Nicolle turned to Paris. Proving he could make sacrifices when the cause was sufficiently noble (or potentially prestigious), the fiscally conservative Emile Roux arranged for a chimpanzee to be sent to Tunis, and even paid for it with funds from his own budget.[84] In possession of a chimp and with the epidemic rapidly waning, Nicolle repeated his inoculation experiments. The blood sample came, as statistical probability would suggest, from a thirty-five-year-old Tunisian male who had been admitted to the Sadiki in mid May.[85] Nicolle inoculated the chimp with this blood and waited. Twenty-four days later, the chimp began to exhibit symptoms of typhus: fever, then skin eruptions, prostration, and so on. An experimental animal now was available. Yet, Nicolle was well aware that the cost of chimps would make them impractical for any longer term study, particularly because preserving typhus for experimental purposes would depend on the regular passage of the "virus" between lab animals. Nicolle turned again to his Chinese monkeys. Drawing blood from the sick chimp, he inoculated a monkey. Thirteen days later, the monkey had typhus.

Late that June, after receiving Nicolle's letter describing his results, Roux responded with evident excitement: "I received your dispatches and am delighted with the excellent results. . . . Send me a note on your experiments and I will present it to the Academy of Sciences." He even offered to send another chimp to Tunis.[86] Roux presented Nicolle's note to the Academy on 12 July. In it, Nicolle heralded the dawn of a new era in the understanding of typhus fever: "the experimental study [of typhus], which had previously seemed impossible, has become possible with its successful inoculation into the monkey."[87] Nicolle had set the stage for a subsequent announcement that would reveal the mysterious culprit responsible for typhus's transmission. Experiments in support of this impending revelation were already in progress at his Institute.

At some time in the 1920s, Nicolle began recounting his discovery of the means of typhus transmission as an epiphany: the "Door of the Sadiki" narrative. He located his intuition at the Sadiki Hospital, at the door separating the unwashed from the washed (admitted) typhus sufferers. Whereas previously he "would walk over the bodies of typhus sufferers awaiting admittance," he suddenly found in them the key to typhus transmission. Before crossing the threshold, patients transmitted the disease to doctors, nurses, and even those who undressed them and cleaned their garments. Once the patients were clean, however, they did not transmit typhus to other patients. Why was this so? The answer, he claimed, came in a flash: "The agent of disease was . . . something attached to the skin, to the undergarments, which water and soap removed. This could only be the louse. It was the louse."[88]

At the time of his discovery, however, Nicolle did not describe it as a sudden, intuitive flash. Instead, he presented it as the rational outcome of thorough epidemiological observation and informed laboratory analysis. Field observations of the disease offered evidence supporting or eliminating certain options; these options were eventually narrowed to a single suspect, which was then tested in the laboratory: "What observation allowed us to divine, our experiments definitively demonstrated."[89] The very structure of his next note to the Academy of Sciences reflected this formulation. Presented on September 6, it was, unlike the July note, a coauthored piece, signed by Nicolle, Comte, and Conseil.[90] It opened with epidemiological evidence supporting the hypothesis that insects parasitic on the human body were the vectors of typhus. The Sadiki phenomenon was one of several observations listed. Cumulatively, this evidence pointed to the louse as the most likely suspect for typhus transmission. Nicolle's previous success with animal inoculation allowed him and his collaborators to test the hypothesis. Using a Chinese monkey inoculated with infected chimpanzee blood, they allowed "29 lice" to feed on it; then, over the next few days, they transferred the lice to other Chinese monkeys.[91] Eventually, monkeys in the latter group developed typhus. One died. Nicolle had his rational, multilayered proof of louse transmission.

Typhus was not the first disease to be linked to louse transmission. In 1907, Britain's F. Percival Mackie, studying an outbreak of relapsing fever in Bombay, argued on the basis of epidemiological evidence that the disease was being transmitted by the louse.[92] It had only recently been discovered that the *tick* was the vector of relapsing fever.[93] Mackie's work increased the possibility that two separate varieties of the disease existed. Over in Algeria at about this same time, an outbreak of relapsing fever had drawn the attention of Pastorian Edmond Sergent and his colleague, Henri Foley.[94] Also suspecting the louse but not yet having eliminated other insects, the pair sent potentially infected specimens up to Paris. There, the insects were crushed, mixed in a physiological solution, and injected into monkeys. Only the monkeys inoculated with the louse mixture became infected. Sergent and Foley wrote a preliminary report on their findings for the first volume of the *Bulletin de la Société de Pathologie Exotique* and expanded upon their work in a 1910 publication.[95] In both articles, they dismissed Mackie's work as being "mere" epidemiology supported by a bit of faulty lab work, thereby allowing them to claim priority for *demonstrating* the louse transmission of relapsing fever. Subsequently, Sergent and his followers argued that their 1908 work inspired Nicolle to suspect the louse for typhus transmission.[96] Nicolle, though privately annoyed, did not address Sergent's charges in any public forum and simply continued to tell his own—changing—discovery story.

The one point on which Nicolle did confront Sergent in print—though without naming him directly—concerned their respective definitions of "demonstration." Sergent had claimed that the successful inoculation of a monkey with crushed lice *proved* the louse's role in transmitting relapsing fever.[97] Nicolle, on the other hand, only considered the louse's role to be "demonstrated" when he successfully transmitted typhus between monkeys by the louse *bite*. In other words, Nicolle required that the conditions of "nature" be reproduced in the laboratory before laboratory evidence could be asserted to carry demonstrative claims beyond mere possibility. Another component of his strict conception of scientific medicine, Nicolle's standards of evidence—standards that often at once irritated and awed his own collaborators—illuminate why he placed such emphasis on the epidemiologically derived nature of the hypotheses he tested in the laboratory.[98] Later, even after he lost faith in the exclusive power of Enlightenment-variety inductive logic, he continued to espouse this model of demonstration. Before World War I, however, that logic, with its promises of power, remained Nicolle's guiding light. It was in these terms that he worked out the significance of his typhus discoveries.

Knowledge Is Power

For Nicolle, then, discovery of the louse transmission of typhus was the result of epidemiological observation and experimental demonstration that brought together in triumphant practice the three component parts—clinic, hygiene, and laboratory—of Pastorian scientific medicine. It was given further weight by the attention he and his collaborators paid to determining the path of "nature" and having that path (at least in idealized presentation) guide work in both field and lab. In short, it produced reliable knowledge of how nature—in this case, typhus fever—actually worked. It even provided the key to typhus's mysterious proclivity for association with human misery:

> In all the great epidemics of typhus, certain auxiliary causes have been noted: filth, misery, severe weather, gatherings of men, and overcrowding. All these conditions were found during the epidemic we observed, and our recent knowledge of the vector explains why this is so. Famine, by creating an exodus of paupers, encourages the dissemination of the disease. Harsh weather forces workmen into unemployment, and they take refuge in the numerous Moorish cafes, where they contaminate others. Large gatherings and overcrowding equally facilitate the transmission of the insect-inoculator.[99]

Their rational, inductive path to enlightenment brought them to knowledge with heuristic powers—powers that acted, in turn, to substantiate that knowledge.

The power of their new knowledge of typhus fever was not only explanatory (and potentially predictive); it was also prescriptive. Soon after Nicolle sent Roux his initial evidence for louse transmission, Roux, full of ideas for vaccine development, could not help but note pragmatically, "the true means of combating the disease is cleanliness. The disappearance of lice will bring about the end of typhus."[100] Nicolle, Comte, and Conseil drew attention to this very formulation at the end of their September 1909 paper.[101] As Nicolle would later remind his readers, "we demonstrated the role of the body louse in the transmission of the disease, and the rules of proplylaxis were fixed."[102]

Having painstakingly demonstrated the endemicity of typhus in Tunisia, the Pastorians sought to control the disease by louse eradication and, as a secondary but supporting goal, by improving habits of cleanliness among the local population. Success in this endeavor would not only be of practical value, but would also go a long way to demonstrating the truth, and the significance, of their discovery. By "Pastorians" here, I include, for the practical components of the eradication plan, the adopted but unofficial Pastorian Ernest Conseil. Prophylaxis was the responsibility twinned with epidemiology under the broad rubric "Hygiene" that Conseil controlled for the city of Tunis. To carry out his program of typhus eradication, Conseil relied, as he had for epidemiological fact-gathering, on the country's medical practitioners. He also, as a result of new legislation, was able to rely more fully on government assistance to enact his plans.

In his report on the 1909 typhus epidemic, Conseil underscored the prophylactic conclusions he and the Pastorians had drawn from their investigations: that typhus was "only contagious through the convergence of certain circumstances—the sick and the parasite—against which it is now easy to fight."[103] "Easy" in terms of the rational deduction of disinfection, it was not so easy in terms of finding all typhus patients and destroying their lice. Indeed, the doctors of Tunis, "long convinced of the possibility of typhus contagion by parasites," had practiced, "as much as was possible, disinfection by sulfur." Yet, the inns, the cafés, and other locations frequented by the poor and lousy were many; their owners would often hide the sick, for fear of their businesses being closed for disinfection.[104] The 1909 epidemic had raged, despite doctors' best efforts to stop it. In the countryside, where the "reservoirs" of typhus were preserved and persisted, the task of eradication was more difficult still: "one rarely had available the means to undertake sufficient disinfection." Often, for lack of resources (apparently both chemical and manual), the huts (*gourbis*) and all their contents were simply burned to the ground, and more huts were then erected. The efficacy of this "radical measure," Conseil argued, was "illusory." On the one hand, the locals still "carried with them" to their new huts "the most dangerous elements of contagion: the parasites." On the other, it "terrorized the natives, who hid patients and even decided not to care for them, rather than risk exposure to such a disaster."[105] The lesson was clear: "the destruction by fire of *gourbis* in the countryside should not be employed."[106]

In that same article, Conseil lamented the "absence of the civil state" in the Tunisian countryside, which made it difficult to track the diseases and shifting dwellings of the nomads.[107] Efforts to remedy this absence were soon in place. In January 1910, the government divided Tunisia into *cordonnes médicales* and assigned a *médecin de colonisation* to each of them. This new cadre of medical assistance in the countryside was specifically instructed to watch for cases of benign typhus and control them with the rational hygienic measures that followed from Pastorian experiments.[108] Once again, Pastorian control over Tunisian health and hygiene was permanently extended in response to an immediate epidemic emergency.[109]

Many clinicians not only embraced the new Pastorian-informed dictates of the Director of Hygiene and the Tunisian state, but even went so far—in true Pastorian spirit—of adapting them to local circumstances. A striking example of this active communal spirit was provided in 1912 by A. Poirson. A doctor at the Hôpital-Dispensaire de Medjez-el-Bab in Goubellat, Poirson wrote an article, published in the *AIPT,* about his successful control of a small epidemic that had started there in January. He had achieved this happy result by "applying the thesis of M. Nicolle. . . . The colonial doctor," Poirson explained, "has neither the time nor the means to do pure science; but, if the results of his practice confirm experimental, scientific principles, those valuable results should at least be discussed."[110] He went on to describe his efforts.

Following Pastorian suggestions, Poirson had disinfected the hospital, but he knew he also needed to attend to homes. The sulfur he had used for the hospital, however, would be difficult to apply to the huts that dominated the area. Poirson thus adapted Pastorian prescription to fit local conditions. First, he found that boiling water served his purposes. Then, he assembled "locals that I knew to be the most intelligent" and explained to them how the louse transmitted typhus. To kill the lice, he told them, they needed only boil their clothing in water. They followed this practice in four of the neighborhoods (*douars*), and typhus cases declined. Shortly thereafter, three other neighborhoods were found to be contaminated. Within three weeks, and with no additional efforts on Poirson's part, all three foyers had been extinguished. How did this happen? Taking evident delight in the story, Poirson recounted how the people he had first taught about typhus, living near the new foyers, took it upon themselves to go to their neighbors and "explain how we had proceeded" to contain the disease. They "told them the story of the louse." Shortly thereafter, the residents of the contaminated *gourbis*, of their own accord, abandoned their lodgings and set up new ones, about two hundred meters away, cleaning their effects in the process.[111] The epidemic's containment had at once helped "substantiate the theory of Nicolle" and made "great progress" in teaching hygiene to the local population. It is no wonder Nicolle included the article in his *Archives*.

With Tunisia a proven endemic reservoir of typhus and louse eradication the focus of Pastorian-dictated rational hygiene, Nicolle and his followers soon turned their attentions to the *success* of their typhus control efforts, as demonstrated by a general decline in the number of annual typhus cases.[112] Initially, that decline was noticeable, but perhaps not as great as they might have hoped. In Tunis, the 856 cases of 1909 were reduced to 148 in 1910, then rose slightly to 180 in 1911. Conseil gave the relatively modest decrease a positive spin, noting that their louse-oriented control efforts allowed them to *contain* those persistent typhus reservoirs among the poor of the countryside and their extensions to the poor cafés and inns of the city.[113] Control of these reservoirs, he argued, had to be the focus of hygienic efforts: "Prophylactic measures must especially be directed against these persistent reservoirs [of typhus], even before the epidemic spreads. Knowing about these reservoirs and their habitual winter locations will facilitate the application of rigorous measures that will make them disappear."[114] Typhus numbers were subsequently kind to the Tunisian Pastorians. There were a mere twenty-two cases in Tunis in 1912; six in 1913, and just three—"all 3 imported," Nicolle and Conseil emphasized—in 1914.[115] Scientific medicine—and, specifically, scientific medicine produced in *Tunisia*—had demonstrated its power to control disease.

Within this story of success, it is important to note how Conseil shifted his understanding of typhus reservoirs after 1910, and to what effect. We have seen that, in his accounts of the 1909 epidemic, he had concentrated on single, poor, and generally itinerant males as the vectors of the vectors of typhus.

By 1911, the filthy bachelor/clean family (/woman) divide had been replaced by a clearer country/city divide:

> In Tunis, cases of familial contagion were very rare (pockets only). . . . The presence of the cutaneous parasites is indeed exceptional in the houses of the cities where a more civilized population has embraced bodily cleanliness. The *fondouks*, the *zaouïas*, where workmen and paupers, covered in parasites, take refuge, are the usual centers of contagion. . . . In the countryside, where all are covered with parasites, family contagion is the rule and [typhus] *indiscriminately strikes men, women and children.*[116]

By implication, the relative healthiness of Tunis brought it closer to "civilized countries," where "typhus has almost completely disappeared because the hygienic habits and the cleanliness of its people have rendered the necessary vehicle of the disease, the louse, rare."[117] Dwellers in the countryside, who had yet to be purified by the practices of Western civilization, were the dangerous reservoirs of disease.[118]

This reservoir shift was not simply the product of Conseil's (and Nicolle's) desire to claim progress in the Westernization of Tunis proper. As doctors continued to gather information on typhus distribution in Tunisia, Nicolle and his colleagues "were struck by the scarcity of cases in children." This meant either "that typhus was truly rare in infants, or that it manifested itself in them in a form so benign that these cases passed unnoticed. It is this last opinion," Nicolle asserted, "that is the true one."[119] With the encouragement of the Tunisian government, more colonial doctors had gone into the countryside to look for typhus among the nomadic populations. Their experience appears to have shattered Conseil's earlier conception of family life, even in the countryside, as relatively hygienic. Typhus appeared among the women and the children of the countryside, just as it did among the men. And, just as it did among the men, typhus appeared in a milder form in these women, and particularly in their infants, than it did in city-dwellers.[120] The women and children, however, did not tend to travel to cities with the men. Employing this revised reservoir formulation, Pastorian knowledge had already brought Tunis closer to Europe. In future, such civilizing effects might—with increased "medical surveillance"—even extend throughout the countryside.[121] Indeed, Conseil was hopeful that their "new etiological knowledge" would soon permit them to see "the disappearance of typhus in North Africa, just as it has been seen in Europe, through the practices of hygiene and bodily cleanliness."[122]

In 1909, Conseil's fieldwork had fed Nicolle's laboratory studies of typhus; subsequently, the pair worked in tandem not only to instruct their colonial colleagues on the practical difficulties of controlling typhus in North Africa, but also to inform more distant colleagues of the significance of their work. Nicolle picked up on Conseil's analytic categories and statistical studies, then used his own particular rhetorical skills to package them for effective exportation. Setting the stage with the props of Tunisia's glorious ancient history, Nicolle increased the drama of typhus's epidemic appearances on that stage: "ever since the days written of by the bishop of Carthage, typhus has not ceased to strike North Africa with cruelty."[123] Typhus in Tunisia was therefore of historic stature. It was also, as it had been in the West, attached to human tragedy: "The varying intensity of these epidemics has been determined by the extent of well-known etiological factors: famine, overcrowding, emigration and population displacement; still," he emphasized, "there has been no year when the disease was wholly absent" from Tunisia. Nicolle heightened the dramatic tension with reference to typhus's persistent reservoirs: "Silent and unsuspected during the autumn and the winter, typhus reappears each spring in the form of small foyers which can be born and die on the spot; in other cases presents a moderate diffusion and which, some years, spreads rapidly through much or all of the land." In sum, "typhus fever is thus, in this historic area, [at once] a very old plague and a permanent threat to man and to civilization."[124]

How, if typhus had been banished from Europe, did it remain a "permanent threat to ... civilization"? In fact, it had not quite been banished: "Its retreat from civilized countries has not completely extinguished it."[125] Outside of Europe, lousy populations remained, in which many benign typhus cases, undetected by medicine, persisted. Indeed, patients with such "silent infections" could not even be detected by animal inoculation with their blood.[126] Following Nicolle's words, one can almost imagine these typhus-ridden patients hovering, ghostlike, at the edges of civilization, awaiting the moment when guards would be dropped and they could drink up the liquid that would give them substance. "There exist at the door of better-favored countries," he warned his readers, "enough permanent foyers to constitute a serious menace, should the conditions of hygiene worsen even temporarily."[127] As long as typhus was endemic in Tunisia, Tunisians remained a threat to French health: should the conditions of French hygiene fail. However, "when the social conditions and values of North Africans are modified by the progress of civilization and by general well-being, typhus fever will be here, as it is in France, but a curiosity, on its way to becoming a disease of history."[128] The Pastorians in Tunisia were, it seems, the vectors of Western civilization, whose successful inoculation of the local population would at once improve the health of North Africans as it ensured the continued health of the West.

Was it a fortuitous coincidence that Nicolle and his institute came to be identified with a disease that was of such pressing concern for both North Africa and the West? It is possible, but doubtful. Each overseas Pasteur Institute was, as we have seen, expected not just to attend to local pathological conditions, but also to specialize in the study of one particular local condition. Each institute was to adopt an emblematic disease. As Nicolle himself observed, "it would be hard to justify studying diseases that strike Europe here" in Tunisia, "as the laboratories of France—and, first among these, the Pasteur Institute of Paris," were "so well placed and well equipped" to study such diseases themselves.[129] By 1909, Nicolle had done original work on a number of diseases that were distinctly *local*. Explicitly comparing these diseases to typhus, he noted that typhus "is not a rare affliction like Kala Azar, or a benign one such as the Oriental Sore, but one of the gravest and most ancient diseases, justly regarded as one of the great plagues of humanity." Despite the disease's important status, "not a fact was known about it before we undertook its study."[130] Moreover, as we have seen, typhus, because it was absent from Europe, could *not* be studied in European laboratories, even while it remained of great concern to Western nations. Indeed, as Nicolle pointed out on several occasions, his recent typhus discoveries had been confirmed by two teams of American researchers studying the disease in Mexico. On many levels, typhus was a savvy choice of signature disease for a man intent on overcoming the anonymity that so often enshrouded his colonial colleagues and establishing himself, and his institute, among the elite of medical research internationally. He was a model Pastorian, extending France's civilizing mission in measurable fashion in a model medical research institution, practicing model scientific medicine.

Inside the Institute

A central component of Nicolle's institutional model-building was staff selection. Alfred Conor's 1909 arrival in Tunis was not the chance result of a fortuitous military reassignment but, rather, the planned outcome of Nicolle's painstaking efforts to secure his former student for the IPT. By mid-January 1909, Nicolle was promoting his institute to Conor and his wife; by month's end, he had spoken with "Doctor Roux, Director of the Pasteur Institute of Paris," as well as "The Director of Agriculture, Commerce, and Colonization [of Tunisia], on whom the Pasteur Institute of Tunis depends," about his desire to bring Conor to Tunisia. Nicolle was now in a position to make Conor a solid offer: "A new place will be created" at the IPT, "intermediary between mine and that of the *chef du laboratoire*—I would be pleased if you would occupy that place."[131] As part of this project, Nicolle had negotiated with the army to give Conor a position at the Military Hospital of Tunis (Belvédère), a move that would conveniently put him in place to take up the post of assistant director of the IPT. Conor arrived in Tunis that spring and immediately set to work on a variety of diseases, including typhus. He also brought an addition to the IPT that Nicolle came to cherish even more than he did Alfred's bacteriological expertise: his wife, Marthe.

Nicolle had known Marthe even before he met Alfred. She was the daughter of Georges Bugnot, one of Nicolle's medical colleagues in Rouen. Born in 1883, Marthe was a child of ten when Nicolle, "without attaching any interest to the girl I was," first met her.[132] At the time, Nicolle was swept up in medical politics, grand ambitions, and the literary life of Rouen; only later did he notice young Marthe. It was during a medical examination, Marthe later recalled, that she, still a child, began discussing her newly discovered love of literature with Dr. Nicolle. Intrigued, Nicolle lent her a copy of Huysmans's *En Route,* which she found "a revelation."[133] A long and life-changing friendship thus began with a shared passion. Then, in 1903, Marthe married Alfred Conor. As she became proficient in the administration and function of laboratory research, she continued her literary explorations. Nicolle would rely on her for both talents.

A year after the Conors arrived in Tunis, another important change took place in the IPT's staffing. Charles Comte, who had worked closely with Nicolle on typhus, left the institute, ostensibly to take up the post of Tunisia's official "Doctor of Epidemics." (Later developments suggest that Nicolle and Comte actively sought distance from each other.[134]) Meanwhile, Ludovic Blaizot had been sent to Tunis by his mentors at the Faculté de Médecine in Paris, Raphaël Blanchard and Emile Brumpt, to study spirochetes in hens. Blaizot's background in zoology and parasitology, combined with his expertise in the new dark-field microscopy, prepared him well for his mission. Indeed, he did so well in Tunis that Nicolle named him *chef de laboratoire* from the start of 1911.[135] Nicolle took full advantage of the fields of expertise his new collaborators brought with them.

Most immediately, Nicolle was eager to continue his investigations of typhus fever. Many important questions about the disease remained unanswered. A central question, at least for a Pastorian intent on following in the footsteps of the Master, concerned vaccine preparation. Nicolle's correspondence with Roux demonstrates the interest both men had in developing preventive and curative inoculations for typhus. Indeed, Nicolle was testing the curative powers of serum taken from convalescent patients at the same time he was conducting laboratory tests of the disease's louse transmission.[136] Although animal transmission allowed Nicolle to conserve typhus for study between epidemics, reliance on chimps and monkeys for that conservation was a financial burden.[137] Thus, with Conor and Conseil, Nicolle began to search for a susceptible animal that was cheaper and easier to breed than were monkeys. The Pastorians had been using guinea pigs for transmitting and studying other diseases, but the rodents seemed to be resistant to typhus. A small-animal thermometer, specially developed by Nicolle, showed otherwise. Using his new instrument, Nicolle found that guinea pigs, while expressing no other symptoms of typhus, did display a characteristic febrile curve when infected.[138] Moreover, their blood, when drawn during this period, successfully transmitted typhus to other guinea pigs. The trio announced their pragmatic discovery to the Académie des Sciences in 1911.[139] It was an important breakthrough that facilitated laboratory research on typhus. Nicolle used the guinea pigs in his efforts to develop a typhus vaccine.[140]

Indeed, vaccine research was being conducted at the IPT on a variety of infectious diseases in addition to typhus. Here, Nicolle was specifically concerned with the problem of attenuation. Attenuation had defined the Pastorian school's approach to vaccine development.[141] Yet, how could one be certain that the attenuated virulence was fixed? How could one produce a vaccine that was effective, reliable, and safe? Two options were available to aspiring vaccine fabricators: use live, attenuated microbes, or use the serum left after bacteria had been killed. Vaccines produced by attenuating living microbes in an artificial medium were most effective in conferring a lasting immunity to disease, but they could be dangerous: they could sometimes produce a full-blown case of disease. On the other hand, the use of dead cultures or the sera of cured animals, though safer, conferred only weak immunity. Inoculations often had to be repeated.[142]

In their attempt to solve this vaccine production dilemma, Nicolle, with Conor and Blaizot, examined various methods by which microbes had been killed to produce vaccines. All were at once too "brutal" and too weak: in sterilizing microbes, they radically diminished vaccinating properties. Nicolle experimented with other agents and discovered that sodium fluoride both killed microbes quickly and prevented their autolysis. In 1913, the Tunis-based Pastorians tested vaccines made with sodium fluoride, which appeared to be as effective as living, and as safe as killed, vaccines. Applying this discovery, they developed fluoride-based vaccines against gonorrhea, staphylococcal infections, and cholera, testing these first on each other, then on volunteers. Their new processing method produced vaccines that were stable enough to be shipped abroad for further tests. By 1914 Nicolle could cite testimonials for his vaccine from doctors throughout the world. These international reports illustrated not only the procedure's efficacy but also its mobility: supplies could be ordered from Tunis and shipped to locations lacking serum producing facilities. Once again, the Pasteur Institute of Tunis had created an opportunity to attract international attention its way.

Model Pastorian?

By 1914, Charles Nicolle had achieved a good deal of autonomy and notoriety. He had followed the formula of overseas Pasteur Institutes, which led him in search of an original research project of local significance. With the help of Conseil's careful epidemiological studies, Nicolle could claim typhus, which still threatened western Europe, as a local pathology. He solved the problems of its animal transmission and louse vector in the laboratory, presenting these solutions not as the result of intuitive flashes of genius but as the product of rational epidemiological analysis and carefully constructed experimental investigation, made possible by close collaborations with local government, colonial doctors, and the Paris institute. Laboratory discoveries were then translated into a rational program of hygiene. These hygienic measures were again collaboratively enacted, resulting, within a few short years, in the "extinction" of a number of countryside typhus reservoirs and the lessening of Tunisia's epidemic threat to the West. Indeed, through the civilizing force of hygiene—through the *power* of *knowledge*—Tunisia was *approximating* western Europe. Moreover, in achieving this goal, the IPT and Tunisia's colonial doctors increasingly attracted Western attention. Institutionally, Nicolle had even found in Alfred Conor a candidate to groom as his eventual replacement. To all appearances, Charles Nicolle was an ideal Pastorian.

The deceptive nature of appearances is, of course, a cliché. So, too, is pointing out that sayings become clichés precisely because they contain a solid grain of truth. For Nicolle, all the pieces that made up his ideal Pastorian appearance were authentic enough. Yet, they were not the whole story. Pieces of himself that he had kept private would soon become public. The fame won by his typhus work—and by his presentation thereof—would gradually alienate him from many of his colleagues. His potentially profitable vaccine work led him far from Pastorian nonprofit ideals, further alienating him from his chosen society. Changes with both Conors disrupted Nicolle's institutional and his familial homes alike. Physical isolation, as manifested by both his ever-growing deafness and his ever-fixed distance from Paris, pulled at the edges of his carefully constructed personal and professional identities. Then, the war itself, which enhanced his (and the IPT's) international status, upended the few things he had until then privately held as truths. Afterwards, the power of reason, the accepted means for achieving his missions, and even the future of the Pasteur Institute of Paris, all came into question.

Part Two

Rupture
Things Fall Apart

3

Light & Shadow

Lousy War and Fractured Peace (1911–19)

> Your Father was human—very human, with all that that implies of brightness and shadow, . . . he only dimly resembled the quasi-monolithic image that biographers have sketched to date.
> —Marthe Conor to Pierre Nicolle, 1963

> The consciousness of life is higher than life. Science will give us wisdom, wisdom will reveal the laws, and the knowledge of the laws of happiness is higher than happiness.
> —Dostoevsky, "Dream of a Ridiculous Man"

In the bright light of medical science's triumph over typhus in Tunisia, Ernest Conseil was haunted by a growing shadow of doubt.[1] It was not that he had reservations about the transmission discovery per se: even if some medical researchers remained unpersuaded by evidence of the louse's unique role in spreading typhus, the insect was, Conseil believed, the disease's vector.[2] It was the *way* the louse transmitted typhus that concerned him. Nicolle had announced with great fanfare that lice spread typhus by *biting* their victims. Indeed, he had waited to make his announcement about the path of typhus spread until he had successfully transmitted the disease between monkeys through louse bites. Nicolle had put great stock in this formulation for at least two reasons. First, as we have seen, he believed the bite experiment to be the final, crucial step in demonstrating the course taken by "nature" itself in spreading typhus. Second, he used it to substantiate a specific program of "rational hygiene" against the disease. Secure in the knowledge that typhus was propagated in nature only by the louse's bite—not by its droppings or, as he would soon assert, by hereditary transmission to offspring—Nicolle could confidently focus on killing living lice to control the disease. It is therefore understandable that, when Conseil approached him with his concerns, Nicolle was skeptical.

In the spring of 1914, a new collaborator arrived at the IPT. Georges Blanc had, like Ludovic Blaizot, worked in Blanchard's parasitology lab at the Paris Faculty of Medicine; like Blaizot, Blanc, too, was interested in spirochetes.[3] His arrival in Tunisia corresponded with the "importation" of three typhus cases into Tunis, and Nicolle set him to work with Conseil to relieve the latter's nagging doubts about the route the disease took in moving from louse to human.[4] Blanc soon came to believe, with Conseil, that typhus was transmitted when the prospective patient *scratched* a louse bite, thereby inoculating the body with infected droppings. Indeed, they believed they had demonstrated that typhus was *principally* transmitted by scratching. Nicolle reportedly dismissed the idea as "*trop bête*."[5] In an early wartime review on the medical dangers presented by lice, Nicolle simply avoided the question, noting without comment on the insect's means of typhus transmission that "the sick person, having been cleansed of lice, is no longer contagious."[6] By 1915—writing with both Blanc and Conseil—Nicolle was willing to concede that typhus inoculation took place by scratching "as well as by the bite."[7] Years later, Nicolle would take credit for discovering that the louse transmitted typhus by *both* routes.

It is strange that neither Blanc nor Conseil protested Nicolle's later proprietary claims. The most plausible explanation for their silent acceptance is the power of direct, master–student relations within the Pasteur Institutes. Conseil was Nicolle's willing right hand; Blanc, Nicolle's protégé. Marcel Baltazard, who later recounted these events while remaining silent about the credit issue, was in turn Blanc's protégé. Pastorian stories, particularly as publicly told, remained faithful to such "familial" loyalties.[8] Harder to explain, however, is Nicolle's opposition to the louse transmission of typhus by the "beastly" route of scratching the insects' droppings into the skin when, by 1912, he—with Conseil and Blaizot—had determined that the louse-borne form of relapsing fever was transmitted by a still more absurd route. Indeed, Nicolle's ongoing work on relapsing fever reflected his typhus work much in the manner of a fun-house mirror. Ultimately, these diseases' twinned images came to have a profound influence on Nicolle's thinking, on several levels. To this end, they were aided by a series of experiences, individuals, and events, that would act at once to fragment Nicolle's carefully constructed, rational universe and to bring to the surface certain long-neglected aspects of his character. His efforts to deal with the fallout would occupy the rest of his life. They would also lead him to reconceptualize his missions—not his goals, but the means by which they might best be fulfilled.

Reminders

We have now seen Nicolle the Researcher, Nicolle the Administrator, and Nicolle the Family Man. In so doing, we have left Nicolle the Romantic as a child back in Rouen. It would seem that, when he bent to his father's wishes for his career and his mother's wishes for his marriage, he left behind all those "childish" things: writing plays, reliving human history, studying natural history, forging his own path within his otherwise traditional world. In private letters—particularly those addressed to his old friends from Rouen—we find evidence that the "other" Nicolle did indeed survive. Here, even the dutiful façade thins, revealing a man at once far more self-aware and cynical than his public image would suggest, and far more idealistic. In the years immediately after his initial typhus success, Nicolle received a number of "visitors" in Tunisia—the Conors, Blaizot, and Blanc; and also relapsing fever—that served to remind him of passions past. Initially, Nicolle tried to contain the emerging contradictions within clearly defined categories: *absurd* disease; *collaborator's* wife; *scientific* reason versus *literary* imagination. Then the world went to war, furthering Nicolle's success, and further confusing his efforts to contain the categories splintering around him.

When Ludovic Blaizot arrived in Tunis in 1910, he was twenty-eight years old. He brought with him expertise in zoology and in the new study of dark-field microscopy, and experience teaching parasitology (under Emile Brumpt) to colonial doctors training in Paris. Though sent to Tunisia to study spirochetes in hens—and to improve his own health—Blaizot soon found a more formal place among the Pastorians there.[9] Indeed, he was quite enthusiastic about his new surroundings; he commented to Brumpt that the IPT might well be superior to the IPP on many levels. (He was particularly impressed by the way Nicolle had organized the institute's services.)[10] As newly appointed *chef de laboratoire* at the IPT, Blaizot set to work on an outbreak of louse-borne relapsing fever that struck parts of Tunisia in May 1911. He and frequent Pastorian collaborator E.-G. Gobert established that the initial cases of the disease had been imported into Tunisia from Libya.[11] Although the epidemic was contained by the end of June, its occurrence brought relapsing fever to Nicolle's immediate attention. The disease was—or at least appeared to be—louse-borne, something the Tunis Pastorians felt well qualified to investigate more closely. Moreover, Blaizot's assorted fields of expertise promised to give them more power still to master the remaining mysteries of relapsing fever.

"Relapsing fever" was named for its most distinctive feature: its tendency to recur, or relapse, in an apparently improving patient. Initial symptoms are flulike and can become more severe, especially when fever escalates. Having expressed these symptoms for one to several days, the patient improves, generally for several days, after which time the symptoms recur, the patient relapses, and the cycle begins again. Recurrences eventually end and the patient, having survived to that point, recovers permanently. By the time Nicolle and Blaizot began working on it, relapsing fever was known to be caused by a type of spirochete that had recently been dubbed *Borrelia*, in honor of French bacteriologist Amédée Borrel.[12] Moreover, as we have seen, it was known to take on two distinctive forms, each with its own vector and its own species of *Borrelia*. The tick-borne form tended to be at once the more severe and the more endemic of the two.[13] The second form, suspected even before Mackie and Sergent published their louse theories, was milder but tended to be epidemic in its appearances.[14] Like typhus, it had long been associated with misery and war. When Nicolle and Blaizot came to the disease in 1911, some credited Mackie with having demonstrated the louse transmission of relapsing fever's second form; others credited Sergent and Foley, who had no doubt they were due all credit for the discovery. Nicolle, however, had serious reservations about both claims.[15]

Edmond Sergent was born to French parents in Algeria in 1879. He started his medical studies in Algiers and then, in 1899, went to Paris, where he followed the IPP's famous *Cours*. A year later, he was appointed *préparateur* to the course and expanded his knowledge of the microbiological world under both Félix Mesnil and Amédée Borrel. Soon thereafter, the IPP sent the promising young Sergent back to Algeria, to study malaria. The country already had a small laboratory bearing Pasteur's name, created through the interventions of the medical school.[16] When, in 1908, the (French) governor of Algeria requested that the IPP oversee the transformation of the facility into a true Pasteur Institute, Emile Roux agreed. In that familial manner so characteristic of Pasteur's institutes, Albert Calmette, founder of the first overseas IP, was sent to coordinate the process. On December 31, 1909, the new Pasteur Institute of Algeria (IPA) was given official existence. Calmette soon handed directorial control to Edmond Sergent.[17] It was as director of the IPA that Sergent continued his investigations into relapsing fever. Relations with the director of the IP to his immediate east vacillated between cooperative and combative; they were always highly competitive.

Sergent and collaborator Henri Foley had begun their systematic investigations on relapsing fever when an epidemic struck Algeria late in 1907.[18] At the time, Sergent, though stationed in North Africa, was *chef de laboratoire* at the IPP. Facilities at the IP's Algerian outpost were still quite basic; it is therefore understandable that Sergent sent all his insect-suspects up to Paris for analysis. The successful transmission of relapsing fever by crushed louse bits in 1908 had encouraged him to lay claim to the demonstration not only of the path the disease traveled in nature, but also of the louse as a potential disease vector more generally. In 1910, he and Foley sought to substantiate their claims by providing evidence of relapsing fever's louse transmission through actual louse bites: much as Nicolle had done a year earlier for typhus fever. As louse-borne relapsing fever was a far milder disease than typhus, Sergent and Foley used *humans* as their experimental animals. Controlled efforts to transmit the disease by louse bites consistently failed. Finally, they met with what they saw as success when they transferred a patient's louse-infested blanket to two healthy women, who then contracted the disease.[19] Unsettled by the difficulties they had had in proving transmission by louse bite, however, the pair suggested that, perhaps, lice kept under experimental conditions were somehow impaired in their inoculating abilities, compared with their more naturally maintained kin.[20]

Nicolle and his colleagues, who had faced no such difficulties with lice in their typhus work, precisely (and regularly) held up their expertise with lice in support of their own insights into relapsing fever. (They even noted, à la Pasteur, that this earlier work "prepared" them for understanding the disease.[21]) By 1912, Nicolle felt qualified to offer a critique of his predecessors' evidence for louse transmission and to present his own explanation of their difficulties in demonstrating their theory. Dismissing Mackie's work much as Sergent had done, Nicolle also dismissed Sergent's investigations even as he praised them. The "only truly important studies of the question," noted Nicolle, "were made by our colleagues in Algeria." However, he continued, Sergent and Foley had never really *shown* that the louse could transmit relapsing fever by its bite, as they asserted happened in nature. In short, "none of the research to date has provided a single demonstrative fact" concerning the insect transmission of the disease.[22] (One can only imagine Sergent's reaction to this claim.) The reason others had failed to transmit relapsing fever by louse bite, Nicolle argued, was that the louse did not transmit relapsing fever by its bite.

How does one substantiate a negative claim? Nicolle did so through what can only be described as "extreme experimentation." By the time he was conducting his experiments, it had been determined that Salvarsan (arsphenamine) effectively treated patients with relapsing fever.[23] Thus he, like Sergent and Foley, felt at qualified liberty to conduct human experiments.[24] Volunteers came forth, including some from the IPT staff, who were willing to be subjected to numerous bites from contaminated lice. Four of the five volunteers were unnamed; they received hundreds, sometimes thousands, of bites. The fifth volunteer, the only one named, was identified as "Habib ben Abdesselem, *chaouch* of the Pasteur Institute," who was bitten 6,515 times. This was the same Habib whom Adrien Loir had brought to his institute and Nicolle later decided to retain. By all accounts, Habib and Nicolle were devoted to each other, if in a highly paternalistic fashion. Yet, in a memoir Nicolle later wrote on Habib, it is clear that the loyal *chaouch* had little choice in "volunteering" to be bitten by the lice. Habib had a drinking problem that had frequently hindered his ability to work. Having tried many times, and in assorted ways, to persuade him to curb his alcohol consumption, Nicolle finally lost patience when Habib again came to work drunk. He fired him. Eventually, Habib's family intervened on his behalf, and Nicolle took him back. There were, however, a couple of conditions attached to this reinstatement. He had to remain sober—and he had to volunteer for a few louse bites.[25] In the end, Habib provided some 9,000 louse-meals.[26] At no time did he, or did the other, more voluntary, volunteers, contract relapsing fever. Nicolle felt justified in claiming he had demonstrated the negative.[27]

This negative proof raised the question of how, precisely, the louse conveyed its pathogenic microbes to human hosts. Not only was its bite innocuous; so too were its droppings. Nicolle called upon Blaizot's expertise with the dark-field, or "ultra"-microscope, to shed light on the mystery. The ultramicroscope had been developed in 1903 to study things (such as enzymes) that were too small to be seen under standard microscopic magnification. To use the ultramicroscope, one suspended the tiny objects of interest in liquid, setting this mixture against a black background and illuminating it with a light source perpendicular, rather than parallel, to the microscope's optical axis. Light scattered around the suspended objects, producing bright spots against a dark background, which were captured on a photographic plate. The ultramicroscope was soon turned on the invisible, "filterable" viruses; subsequently, filterable viruses were also called "ultra"-viruses, or ultramicrobes.

It had long been known that the spirochetes of relapsing fever seemed, under standard microscopic magnification, to disappear from human blood between symptomatic recurrences of the disease. British microbiologist William Boog Leishman used an ultramicroscope to examine what happened to the spirochetes that "disappeared" from the blood of humans suffering from tick-borne relapsing fever. He argued that the spirochetes did not wholly disappear but, instead, became tiny but abundant granules that later reformed as visible spirochetes.[28] Nicolle and Blaizot turned to the ultramicroscope early in their relapsing fever studies; they hoped that a clearer understanding of spirochete development in the louse would suggest the means by which the microbes moved from lice to humans. They found that the spirochetes ingested by the lice, along with infected human blood, soon became sluggish, then disappeared altogether. Or, seemed to: "Their disappearance was *only apparent*." Though they could no longer be seen, even under the ultramicroscope, the spirochetes remained, to return again after about a week to their more familiar form.[29] When they returned to their visible state, however, they were not located in any part of the louse that had direct access to the world outside its body. The spirochetes, bottled up within the louse, had only one means of escape: to be *un*bottled. In short, "the louse must be mortally wounded, so that its lacunary liquid, the only thing virulent in it . . . comes into contact with a scratch in the skin." Such an "accident," Nicolle pointed out, happened frequently enough. Individuals often scratched themselves when bitten by lice. The fragile lice were easily broken by the human fingernails that, in turn, became veritable vectors of relapsing fever, inoculating any scratch in the skin, or any contact with conjunctive tissue, with the disease.[30] In 1919, Nicolle, with collaborator Charles Lebailly, would offer what is generally accepted as conclusive evidence of this path when they found that the louse bits where spirochetes abounded were the easily broken legs and the antennae. "We thus grasped [*saisissons*] exactly how the infection was perpetuated in nature."[31]

Although it would never receive the international acclaim of his typhus studies, Nicolle's work on relapsing fever made an important contribution to the field. One might even argue that it was more innovative than his typhus work. On yet another level, it was of profound significance for the subsequent development of Nicolle's ideas about typhus, disease, and even "nature." Appreciating its significance requires a brief discussion of two additional aspects of his early relapsing fever work. First, in 1914 and with the collaboration of Georges Blanc, Nicolle showed that spirochetes in lice were virulent while still invisible.[32] Not only were they virulent while invisible; they were at the *peak* of virulence just *before* they became visible again. Once visible, the spirochetes' virulence rapidly decreased.[33] This strange combination of virulence-without-substance would play upon Nicolle's thoughts and, as we shall see, haunt him. It also encouraged him to consider more carefully whether microbes somehow *evolved* within an individual host.[34] What, precisely, was the relationship between the visible and invisible "stages" of the microbe? What, if anything, did this have to do with the symptoms a disease produced? Nicolle was not the first to think in these terms.[35] Yet, he was among those who helped press the issue to broader consideration.

In addition to its potential significance for the evolution of individual microbes, this early relapsing fever work brought the evolution of disease *species* to Nicolle's attention. What was the relationship between the tick-borne and the louse-borne forms of the disease? Was their apparent separation truly fixed, or was there something about the vector itself, tick or louse, that altered the microbe and produced the two related forms of the disease in a more temporally immediate sense?[36] If they were indeed distinct, did the louse-borne form have an animal reservoir similar to that of the tick-borne, or was it, like typhus, a disease exclusive to humans in nature? If exclusive to humans, where did it go between epidemic outbreaks?[37] This was not, in fact, the first disease Nicolle investigated to raise such questions: his work on kala-azar, for example, focused on a Tunisian variation on the standard disease. Relapsing fever enticed him to examine the evolution of disease species more explicitly, guiding the questions he posed for further research and the places he looked for answers. Perhaps the presence of Ludovic Blaizot, enthusiastic student of zoology, reminded Nicolle of his earlier passion for natural history and encouraged him to look beyond the intentionally fixed limits of bacteriological causality for a broader understanding of the evolution of disease species. For the remainder of his active research years, Nicolle would be drawn back again and again to relapsing fever. Gradually, he would come to see the histories of this group of diseases less as absurd exceptions within an otherwise rational and orderly world and more as a window into the real workings of an unpredictable and opportunistic "Nature." He would help bring *biology* to the understanding of infectious disease.[38]

Like his childhood interest in natural history, Nicolle's love of literature had never been wholly eclipsed. As Blaizot and relapsing fever had helped remind him of his passion for the former, Marthe Conor would encourage him to engage with the latter. Indeed, after Nicolle moved to Tunis, Marthe, whose youthful interest in literature he had helped cultivate, became a central source of his French cultural news. She was nineteen when Nicolle left Rouen; the next year, she married his student Alfred Conor, then approximately thirty-three. Despite their distance in geography and age, Marthe and Nicolle kept in close touch, writing to each other about books and ideas; she sent him reviews of the exhibits she had attended and copies of journals he did not otherwise receive. Their animated correspondence skipped playfully between subjects, evincing their mutual delight in witty turns of phrase and general irreverence. Nicolle even sent her copies of his sonnets. He attached to one the following aside, lamenting the cultural isolation he felt in his new home: "one of my admirers (!) simply wrote this: that Tunisia's greatest scientist was at the same time its greatest poet. And I repeat this without blushing (or maybe just a little), because there are neither poets nor scientists in the Regency."[39] Through their shared interests, Nicolle came to expose to Marthe—with evident glee—his darker humor. In so doing, he demonstrated his awareness of, and general disregard for, the religious structures that permeated French culture and even the very form of his own Pasteur Institute.

Nicolle was well aware of Catholicism's influence on Pasteur's Institute. Drawing ironically on clerical categories, Nicolle often referred to himself in letters to Marthe as the "Reverend Pasteur Elias Murphy." In March 1909, after he had persuaded the Conors to move to Tunis, Nicolle addressed a heretically playful description of his institute to Marthe, whom he called "dear sister." He referred to his staff as the "reformed troop that elected me its pastor" and the institute as "our evangelical temple." He promised her that she would find "at the I.P. a small but select evangelic society," headed by himself, the "Pasteur Elias Murphy."[40] Nicolle invoked this pseudonym many times, and Marthe occasionally employed it when writing to him. Thus, he found in his charming correspondent a partner in a self-conscious semiheresy; they drew on their literary skills to extract the cultural categories informing the social structure of the Pasteur Institute.

The Conors arrived in Tunis in the spring of 1909. It is not a coincidence that Nicolle began writing his first novel shortly thereafter. His hearing had declined to the point that listening was painful, and he had been lashing out with biting sarcasm at others' words (when, in fact, he had misunderstood them).[41] Whereas conversation took sustained effort, in literature, Nicolle found pleasure and communion. And in Marthe Conor, he found his link both to a hidden inner world and to a distant outer world. In the course of their exchanges, Marthe became intrigued by the adversity Nicolle had faced in Rouen. At her encouragement, life, art, and need merged into Nicolle's first novel. Years later, she told Nicolle's son of the stories his father had told of Rouen. Upon hearing them, "I . . . asked your father to tell me stories like that of *Heurtebise*. From this exchange was born the *Pâtissier de Bellone*, which is why your father dedicated the book to me."[42]

The step from writing the book to publishing it was not an easy one. Huet notes that, in 1912, Calmann-Lévy initially rejected Nicolle's manuscript as interesting, but not so widely interesting as to be a promising prospect for future sales. Huet credits the publisher's subsequent reversal of this decision to two factors: the intervention of no lesser a luminary than Anatole France; and Nicolle's agreement to pay the publication fees personally.[43] Final fees, he points out, came to what would have been just over two months' salary for Nicolle in his role as director of the IPT.[44] Huet rightly notes that Nicolle's willingness to take on this financial burden underscores the significance this literary publication held for him. He does not, however, speculate about how Nicolle, with a wife, two children, and no family fortune, sustained this burden. Chronology suggests a possible source of supplemental funding. The book was published in the spring of 1913.[45] Later that summer, Nicolle and his collaborators, casting aside Pastorian tradition, embraced a plan to *profit* from their medical research.

Seated with brioches, chocolate, Blaizot, and Alfred Conor at the Café de la Régence in 1913, Nicolle announced an important decision: he would sell to the Paris-based pharmaceutical company Poulenc *frères* the right to distribute their "stabilized atoxic vaccines"—the aforementioned *vaccins fluorurés*.[46] By September, the three men had negotiated a contract with François Billon—in correspondence, they referred to him as "the Cardinal"—at Poulenc, promising them personal and institutional remuneration for each dose of vaccine Poulenc sold.[47] Blaizot would stay in Paris to help establish a new lab for vaccine production; Marthe Conor, Beatrice-like on many levels, would attend to marketing strategies and contract negotiations; and Nicolle would serve as Poulenc's "bacteriological super-advisor."[48] Poulenc would in turn supply materials for production, attend to the costs of advertising, and distribute the vaccines. In all, the contract promised a profitable alliance, as was reflected in Blaizot's praise of Nicolle's entrepreneurial savvy: "Thanks to you, I will soon be cured of [my poverty]."[49]

By March 1914, Billon placed a newly furnished laboratory, located in an industrial area just outside Paris, at Nicolle's disposal. Blaizot immediately set to work manufacturing serum while Billon applied to the Académie de Médecine's Serum Commission for approval of vaccine sales. At this point, however, an apparently simple story of contractual exchange takes a provocative turn: Emile Roux was on the Serum Commission; and Blaizot, Billon, and Nicolle were going to great lengths to conceal all evidence of their alliance with Poulenc from him. In late February, just before Billon intended to petition the Serum Commission, Blaizot wrote to Nicolle:

As for the best approach to take with Roux at this time, Billon believes that complete abstinence should be the rule . . . . Now that we have published our method of vaccine production, Poulenc's request for authorization to use it might be regarded as independent from us. You have taken care to strike the Institute's name from the boxes of Dmégon [it has sent to Poulenc] so that all evidence of our contract is destroyed. Nothing overtly divulges our ties to the *maison* Poulenc. Roux . . . can only speculate.[50]

Poulenc managed to obtain the Commission's approval by late spring, but Roux soon learned of Nicolle's actions.[51] The financial policies of the two Pastorian directors clashed, bringing Roux and Nicolle into direct confrontation. Nicolle's growing autonomy at the IPT sheltered him from the direct consequences of Roux's wrath, and the Tunis-based Pastorians went forward with their profitable alliance.

To appreciate the novelty of Nicolle's actions, one must examine them in the context of pharmaceutical policies then current in France. I have noted the importance of nineteenth-century nonprofit ideals for Pasteur's policies at his new institute. Human pharmaceuticals were never to be sold at a profit. The underlying ideology might have faced a serious challenge had a lesser man than Emile Roux helped develop the potentially profitable diphtheria antitoxin. The Academy of Medicine soon responded to medicine's growing therapeutic potential by establishing a Serum Commission, on which Roux himself played a guiding role. By 1906, the Serum Commission had expanded its mission: it was in charge of approving all sera *and vaccines* (the two different kinds of products that had been brought together by the Pastorians, to the greater glory of Louis Pasteur[52]) that were to be used in France. Roux's presence helped ensure that the traditional nonprofit ideology continued to be applied to twentieth-century pharmaceutical developments. It was a policy that tended to stifle the growth of French pharmaceutical companies much beyond family businesses. It also stifled medical research (outside the Pasteur Institute).[53] If research labs were uncommon in French industry in general, they were almost unheard of among French pharmaceutical companies.[54] The Pasteur Institute remained alone in its combination of (cost-recuperative) pharmaceutical sales and research until 1903, when Poulenc established its own research laboratory.[55] Roux's IPP and the nascent Poulenc had cordial but informal relations, with the IPP avoiding all formal association that even hinted at commercial taint.[56] It expected a similar commitment from its internationally scattered outposts, including the Tunisian government funded IPT.

The events of World War I would challenge the continued viability of the French government's industrial research policies.[57] Alternative models existed not only in foreign countries but also, to some extent, in the French colonies, which were often used as laboratories for new social policies.[58] In the case of Pastorian vaccine policies in Tunisia, the colonies—or, more specifically, Nicolle and his collaborators—went far beyond the presumed pattern of passive colonial technology transfer, in which ideas of the center were exported to the periphery, where they were tested, refined, and sent back to France. Instead, the IPT group was returning to the metropole with an approach to vaccine production and distribution that they had developed in Tunisia. It was an approach that challenged France's nonprofit approach toward the distribution of human pharmaceuticals.[59] At the time, Nicolle was not so much looking to persuade the IPP of the benefits of this laissez-faire model as he was seeking to establish a more immediately beneficial working relationship with the ideologically sympathetic Poulenc *frères*. He sought financial gain—for his institute, his collaborators, and himself. Only later would he begin to think seriously about transforming the IPP.

How did Nicolle come to break so soundly with Pastorian tradition, risking, as he did, alienation from Roux and the IPP in the process? The circumstances surrounding the writing and publication of his novel, whether or not the driving force behind his heretical vaccine-related actions, suggest an interrelated series of explanations. Marthe Conor had inspired Nicolle to write fiction by reminding him, on a number of levels, of his time in Rouen. These were, for him, the early days of his faith in the Pastorian mission and his first real exposure to the importance of institutional autonomy. There was in Nicolle, Marthe would later tell Pierre, "always a bit of [Don] Quixote": the man who took on social injustice and backwards administrations.[60] Nearing his fiftieth birthday, Nicolle was reminded of the idealism of his youth by a woman nearly seventeen years his junior. Indeed, at this time and throughout the rest of his life, Nicolle would surround himself with close friends and collaborators a generation younger than himself.[61] It is clear that Marthe Conor and Ludovic Blaizot, in addition to reminding him of passions past, also encouraged him to rethink his attachment to certain traditions he had held out of sheer respect for tradition. Achieving desired ends might necessitate the abandonment of socially sanctioned means: means such as an unquestioning devotion to nonprofit ideals. Nicolle's novel required funding. So too did his institute, if he wished to ensure that he would have full autonomy over its direction, even in the context of the Tunisian government's technical control.

Another factor at once motivating his novel production and illuminating his unconventional stance on medical profit is more abstract. Throughout his life, Nicolle felt removed from the social world around him. "*L'isolé*"—the isolated one—is perhaps his most common autobiographical trope. As a child in Rouen, he had felt isolated from the bourgeois world surrounding him; as a young man, he had confronted a more external (if still internal) force of social isolation in the form of his growing deafness. It is clear that writing, and being read, were central to his feelings of connection to the world around him. Nicolle's sense of isolation was heightened by his cultural and geographic distance from Paris. This colonial isolation, however, had positive consequences to counterbalance the negative ones.[62] His distance from Paris may have obscured his accomplishments from the view of his esteemed colleagues, but it also blunted the force of their disapproval. Meanwhile, his successes, if perhaps not earning him the credit they would have done had he been in Paris, did heighten his self confidence and elevate the status of his institute. And so, sitting at a café in Sidi Bou Saïd, overlooking the sea and surrounded by collegial colleagues, Nicolle was emboldened to challenge a few traditions—not just professionally, but personally.

Until around 1910, Nicolle had endured life with wife Alice with resignation. Thereafter, he began to complain to his mother with more insistence about his domestic circumstances. His mother eventually confided to son Marcel that "Charles has repeatedly complained that life with such a person [*une mentalité*] is impossible."[63] Nicolle filed for a separation by September 1911, although he hoped to forego the financial and emotional expense of a legal procedure if Alice would simply agree to leave Tunis permanently and preserve his rights concerning their children. Nicolle's mother, who was attending to the legal paperwork from Rouen, strongly encouraged her son to resolve his problems outside the courts.[64] Alice resisted both the separation and the request that she leave Tunisia.[65] Yet, three years later—just *before* the Great War began—Alice and the children moved back to Rouen.

Nicolle's breaks with Pastorian and familial values thus followed in rapid succession. Just as his profit-oriented administrative style increased his estrangement from Roux, his personal choices alienated his family. Despite earlier tensions between Mme. Nicolle *mère* and her daughter-in-law, the two initially lived together with the children in Rouen. Later, Alice took a Paris apartment. As the Nicolle family drew closer to Alice and the children, they grew more critical of her estranged husband. Tensions were evident even before Alice left Tunis. Mme. Nicolle despaired that Charles might be blind "at the bottom of his heart to how detrimental his conduct is to his family."[66] References to Charles, which had filled Mme. Nicolle's correspondence with Marcel for years, grew rare; gradually, they were replaced by passages about Alice and the children. Maurice was so infuriated by brother Charles's behavior that Mme.

Nicolle withheld information to keep peace between them.[67] Nevertheless, Charles and Maurice suffered an irreparable break in relations. After Maurice's wife, Valentine, died in 1915, Alice helped the widower care for his young son, Jacques. At the same time, Maurice grew closer to his gifted niece Marcelle. Indeed, the generally arch-conservative Maurice championed Marcelle's scientific aspirations. At a time when both her father and her grandmother were plotting strategies to make her "fulfill seriously and with joy her 'feminine mission' (wife, mother, mistress of the house),"[68] her uncle Maurice was offering her space in his Parisian lab.[69] Alice's place in the Nicolle family was further solidified in 1921, when Maurice suffered the series of strokes that essentially ended his scientific career. She tended to her ailing brother in law, even playing the piano "to distract him from his solitude."[70] Thus, Charles Nicolle, stepping outside his family's values, became "*l'isolé*" in his own family.[71]

Nicolle's novel and its related motivations and implications may well have precipitated his decision to challenge Pastorian dictates, but a more concrete event certainly induced him to take drastic familial measures in the early summer of 1914. On April 4, Alfred Conor, who had fallen mysteriously ill some months earlier, died. Although many attributed his condition to an unspecified laboratory infection, Nicolle apparently had his doubts about this vague diagnosis.[72] Whatever its cause, Conor's death left Nicolle short a valued collaborator and Marthe without a husband.

Marthe Conor left Tunisia shortly after her husband died, but she returned again late that year. By this time, it was clear that the world's war would not come to any rapid resolution. Nicolle was desperately short of collaborators in Tunis, and Marthe, who in addition to her literary and negotiating skills was adept at laboratory work, assisted at the IPT. Nicolle and Marthe not only collaborated on research but also cowrote scientific papers.[73] If an outside reader of the early Marthe-Charles correspondence had not already suspected that the two loved each other deeply, her suspicions would have been raised by the timing of the events of 1914. They would have been strengthened as well by the number of letters, sent by a wide array of friends and colleagues to Nicolle in Tunis, that subsequently included "best wishes to Mme. Conor" in their conclusions. If any doubts remained as to Marthe's status as Nicolle's mistress—indeed, as his great romantic love—they would have been dispelled in reading her later letters, still vibrant but deeply melancholic, to Pierre Nicolle.[74]

The other opening created by Alfred Conor's untimely death was among Nicolle's formal staff at the IPT. Georges Blanc arrived in Tunis to fill this position that May and was named a *chef de laboratoire* on 1 July.[75] Though Conor's formal position as assistant director of the IPT was to remain unfilled until late 1920, it is clear that Nicolle quickly came to think of Blanc as his heir apparent.[76] He would later write that Blanc was "another me."[77] It is interesting that his newest colleague achieved this status despite the fact that one of his first acts at the IPT was to challenge the "bite" element of Nicolle's famed typhus transmission theory.

By mid-July, Nicolle was so evidently delighted with his life's direction that colleagues even commented on his positive mood.[78] A new world of possibilities, defined on his own terms and outside ill-fitting traditions, seemed open to him. Blaizot had helped remind him of his natural-historical inclinations, with their promise of illuminating the intriguing complexity that lay just beyond the narrow constraints of bacteriological specificity. Blanc and Marthe Conor both reminded him of an idealized version of his past self: creative, dynamic, passionate. Blanc's presence would soon inspire Nicolle to dream of a kind of Hellenic immortality for himself and his institute; Marthe Conor's had already encouraged him to express publicly desires long hidden. Poulenc promised a more autonomous and secure future for them all. Indeed, Nicolle had gotten his houses in order that summer. Then "war came and disrupted everything."[79]

Know Thy Enemy

> History proves that epidemics of the two typhuses have almost always accompanied great wars. In spite of the progress of civilization, and although France appears to have long remained unscathed by these two diseases, the ordinary conditions of their development can appear in the current war. These conditions are: louse infestation and the existence of typhus reservoirs. . . . If care is not taken, reservoirs of the virus will be imported sooner or later by the indigenous contingents, especially those from North Africa . . . and by prisoners coming from manifestly contaminated regions: Silesia, Galicia, and the Slavic provinces.
>
> —Nicolle and Conseil, 1915

Just days before Georges Blanc was officially appointed *chef de laboratoire* at the IPT, Austrian Archduke Franz Ferdinand was assassinated in Sarajevo. By late July, Austria had declared war against Serbia; by August, most of Europe had joined the fray. National alliances, colonial relations, and technological "improvements" helped ensure that this war would become a "Great" War—a World War. Initially, optimism abounded, with both sides predicting a rapid victory that would culminate in a glorious homecoming by Christmas. Doctors were similarly optimistic, secure in the knowledge that bacteriological and surgical advances would give them new power over disease and death. The IPT, like other medical institutions, offered its staff to the cause: Blanc and Blaizot left Tunis almost immediately; Conseil soon followed. Subsequently, Nicolle, like directors of other medical institutions, was faced with constant staff shortages and struggled to keep his institute functioning profitably and his distant staff well shepherded and supplied.[80] Despite the multitalented Marthe Conor's return to Tunis late in 1914, Nicolle would constantly feel that his resources were stretched to the breaking point.

Sustaining resources in wartime became a common difficulty from late autumn, when fast-moving armies on the Western Front stopped moving and dug themselves into trenches. This great line in the dirt (and mud), which zigzagged from near Ostend in the north to near the Swiss border in the south, remained essentially fixed for the next few years: despite all the artillery shells, machine gun fire, and chemical weapons called upon to dislodge it. The entrenched line would take a steady stream of men and supplies to sustain it; but life in the trenches itself, even between battles, was hazardous. Soldiers were exhausted, cold, hungry, and crowded together, troglodyte style. Lice abounded. The Great War, according to Paul Fussell, is where the English word *lousy* got its present meaning.[81] The persistent and ubiquitous pests even inspired their own wartime ode, "The Immortals."[82] Nicolle, who took the lessons of history seriously, knew that conditions were ripe for a typhus epidemic. Here, then, was something he could contribute directly to the war effort, even from his colonial distance: his expertise.

In the winter of 1914–15, Nicolle and Conseil coauthored a number of papers urging military doctors to take seriously the threat posed by lice.[83] By taking the louse as their focal point, they were able to make a few important moves. First, they made an epidemiological grouping of two diseases that were, etiologically, quite distinct: typhus fever and relapsing fever. This then allowed them to claim broad credit for the recent discoveries made by "French research, confirmed in other countries," in a manner that (at least in the shorter articles) did not give priority to any particular French researcher.[84] Third, they could introduce a wide international audience to "the results obtained in Tunis by the application of rational measures" that had been derived from this new knowledge, and—finally—they could outline "the means that must be employed to fight against the introduction and the possible diffusion of these two diseases among our armies."[85] This "battle against the parasites" was, in part, a battle against the reservoirs of disease. Specifically, the "exchange of troops" from places like Morocco "with the *métropole* must be closely supervised." Moreover, as "prisoners of war constitute another possible path for the introduction of the virus into France," it would be "prudent" to "treat all prisoners as suspects."[86] The French were thus being endangered not only by the Germans crossing their borders, but also by their own overseas troops. They would defeat the enemy from within by controlling the louse; and they would control the louse by extending that favored tool of Western civilization: by "redoubling . . . the measures of cleanliness of the whole body of troops [*tout le corps de troupe*]."[87]

Despite its abundant lice, the Western Front remained relatively free from typhus. The story was quite different in the East: severe epidemics followed, almost sequentially, in Serbia, Poland, and Russia. Typhus struck Serbia first. Serbia had been in a state of war almost constantly since 1912.[88] Typhus took hold early in 1915; it raged for six months, killing at least 150,000 people. An already beleaguered medical staff was cut down by more than a third.[89] As the United States had not yet entered the war, its Red Cross responded with humanitarian aid. The American Red Cross Sanitary Commission to Serbia was funded by the Rockefeller Foundation, which had just funded a successful study of hookworm in the southern United States and was looking for similar projects to support.[90] Harvard's Richard Pearson Strong was the commission's director; Hans Zinsser, then at Columbia, was appointed bacteriologist. In fact, an international medical contingent descended upon Serbia that spring, including representatives of Great Britain, Russia, Belgium, Holland, and France itself.[91] Georges Blanc saw a circular for the French mission while stationed in Campiègne that February and asked Nicolle for his help in obtaining a transfer to the unit.[92] By April, Blanc was heading up a laboratory in Nich. Conseil, too, went to Serbia, where he directed a lab in Valjevo.[93] There, they soon discovered that Nicolle and Conseil's articles on typhus had been quite necessary but only marginally effective. Much skepticism remained as to whether Nicolle had truly demonstrated the louse to be the sole (or even principal) vector of typhus: "Certain experts," Conseil complained, were "always ready to declare that one has not yet demonstrated that 2 + 2 does not equal 4 + a fraction."[94] Indeed, as late as 1915, some continued to argue for the miasmatic origins of typhus: Colonel Jaubert, head of the French mission in Serbia, had assured Conseil that "putrefying cadavers, etc., had created typhus, as I would see. I tried to protest. 'Wait,' he told me; 'you will see.' "[95]

Nicolle went to Paris that spring, to give a series of lectures on typhus to the French segment of the Serbian mission.[96] For a time, it looked as if his role in wartime typhus control would be more than simply instructive. Strong wished to appoint him as an official consultant to the American Red Cross Sanitary Mission.

Blaizot, temporarily back in Tunis and overseeing the institute while Nicolle was in Paris, asked the Director of Agriculture to grant Nicolle permission to accept the prestigious offer.[97] While awaiting a response, Nicolle rather optimistically signed and returned his contract, and began to negotiate his terms, including the appointment of Mme. Marthe Conor as his assistant. He was sent his official appointment letter on April 12.[98] As late as April 28, official Red Cross publicity still had Nicolle, "the French expert on typhus," listed as a consultant.[99] By May, it was clear that Nicolle would not be going to Serbia. The Director of Agriculture in Tunisia had decided that he was needed at home. Conseil consoled Nicolle, telling him it was best he didn't come: after the excitement of the journey had worn off, he would have found there was little equipment and little to do. Conseil himself had "nothing to do but cross my arms."[100]

In Tunis, there was plenty to keep Nicolle occupied. A faithful correspondent and an attentive *patron*, he sent letters and guinea pigs to both Blanc and Conseil and even wrote regularly to their mothers; when necessary, he attended to their finances as well.[101] After the Serbian mission ended that autumn, Nicolle became relentless in his efforts to retrieve his distant colleagues to assist him at the IPT. His letters indicate that there was more behind these efforts than simply his desire to keep his institute functioning. He was lonely. His family had departed; his assistants were scattered; the war made the Mediterranean feel vast indeed. Particularly at those times when Marthe Conor was not in Tunis, Nicolle lamented his status as "*l'isolé*," faced constantly with his own "solitude." It was a feeling that escalated over the years. More immediately, a handful of replacements from the IPP or drawn from the pool of colonial doctors in Tunisia were temporarily appointed to assist him at the IPT.[102] In annual reports, Nicolle was effusive in his praise for their assistance. But private letters make it clear that, with perhaps one exception, these "replacements" could begin not replace Blanc and Conseil, either personally or professionally.

Despite staff shortages, the IPT continued to function—profitably—during the war. It even took on several new functions. When Parisian supplies of antidiphtheria and antitetanus sera threatened to run short, Nicolle began to produce them in Tunis. His institute also supplemented the production of smallpox vaccine when Algeria's Centre Vaccinogène de l'Hôpital Militaire du Dey, which had until then supplied the army, couldn't meet wartime demands.[103] Moreover, Nicolle continued to supply his *vaccins fluorurés* gratis to military personnel and civilians in Tunisia, as Blaizot was working to supply them, through Poulenc, to France. Early in 1916, Nicolle was officially appointed "technical counselor of the African army."[104] The military bacteriology laboratory, which he and his colleagues had been running informally, was officially incorporated at the institute.

Indeed, this incorporation even facilitated temporary returns by Blaizot and Blanc. Additionally, the IPT "loaned its scientific and technical assistance and supplied useful materials to the laboratories" of the naval hospital at Sidi-Abdallah, and other hospitals.[105] With Blaizot and Général Alix, Nicolle urged the military to establish a laboratory in southern Tunisia, near its border with Libya, because of its triple vulnerability to military attacks, sanitary breakdown, and bacteriological isolation from Tunis. The Parisian Pastorian Edouard Chatton was sent to direct the lab, which was established in Gabès.[106] This frenzy of military-medical activity appears to have been given a strong push by the impending arrival of soldiers from the Serbian Third Army. Evacuated from Albania in January 1916, these Serbian soldiers soon began arriving in the Tunisian port of Sidi-Abdallah. There, many were treated for cholera and, eventually, for typhus fever.[107]

Form and Substance

After 1913, Nicolle continually emphasized that the only cases of typhus in Tunisia were those originating from endemic reservoirs *outside* Tunisia.[108] To continue his laboratory studies of the disease between such importations, he needed to maintain an uninterrupted chain of contaminated animals. Although wartime saw the growing acceptance of the extremely tiny microbe described by Henry Ricketts as the causal agent of typhus,[109] it was still impossible to cultivate the disease outside very specific, living bodies. Publicly, Nicolle did not much engage in discussions about the microbial cause of typhus. He was, however, a Pastorian and, as such, was deeply interested in retaining the virus in order to perfect a curative serum or a preventive vaccine. This was not as simple as his earlier published accounts might suggest: from the time of his first successful transmission of typhus to laboratory animals, Nicolle had been tormented by the threat that his cherished virus would disappear.[110] There was a double threat. On the one hand, continued animal passage appeared to weaken the disease for subsequent infections. On the other, the inoculated animals would randomly fail to exhibit signs of subsequent infection. At first, he attributed the latter problem to the natural resistance of individual animals (by this time, he was using guinea pigs) and suggested that two or three be inoculated at once. But the problem persisted. And then, typhus again came to Tunisian shores along with the Serbian soldiers.

Initially, the hospital staff at Sidi-Abdallah were unaware that their new patients had typhus. Expressing neither the characteristic rash nor the fever pattern, "they initially passed wholly unnoticed ['*entièrement inaperçu*']." Then, the French staff who came into contact with them began to fall ill with classic typhus.[111] The pattern was familiar to anyone who had read Conseil's earlier papers on typhus reservoirs in Tunisia. Conseil, too, had described the benign expressions of typhus that tended to come out of the nomadic foyers. He, too, had noted that cases often passed "unnoticed." Nicolle had in turn described these as "silent" infections.[112] Now, the Serbians had arrived, expressing an even milder form of typhus: a typhus without *apparent* typhus symptoms. Moreover, this clinically silent infection was found to have normal virulence when inoculated into a more susceptible host, such as a French medical attendant. Viewed from the outside, it is striking that, just after completing studies with Blanc suggesting that the most virulent stage of relapsing fever in the louse came when the spirochetes lacked apparent substance, he was again visited by cases of typhus, evidently virulent, but lacking the substance of observable symptoms.

The Serbian typhus importation gave Nicolle the opportunity to test some of his latest laboratory developments. He had, in fact, been working on the efficacy of the blood serum of convalescents (animals and, later, humans) to prevent or cure active typhus from the time he had found viable experimental animals.[113] By 1916, he had developed a convalescent serum preparation that he hoped would stave off infection in healthy but exposed individuals. The hospital staff working with typhus patients at Sidi-Abdallah offered him the perfect opportunity for a small trial of his preparation's efficacy.[114] Moreover, the Serbian typhus samples in themselves allowed Nicolle to engage in a growing debate over whether there was one typhus throughout the world or many partially related varieties. At the time, and in contrast with his thoughts on relapsing fever, Nicolle came down firmly on the side of unity: "typhus fever is . . . a unique disease, identical over the whole surface of the globe."[115] Clinically, the Serbian typhus importation gave Nicolle further evidence in support of his laboratory-directed program of rational hygiene. By April, he, his IPT collaborators, and their colonial/military colleagues had successfully contained the outbreak.[116] Now, Nicolle could boast that they had not only extinguished the typhus foyers endemic to Tunisia, but also contained each imported epidemic—even in wartime.

His 1916 typhus investigations required nearly constant movement between clinic and lab. In the lab, they relied fundamentally on the continued passage of typhus between guinea pigs. By this time, however, Nicolle's earlier concerns about the nonexpression of typhus in inoculated guinea pigs was escalating. Nearly 16 percent of these experimental animals appeared to be resistant.[117] Might the virus be lost because of a few too many "resistant" guinea pigs?

Nicolle began to look beyond individual resistance as an explanation for the unsettling phenomenon. Could it be an effect of the seasons? The number of passages? Faulty technique?[118] In May 1917, Charles Lebailly was sent to Tunis to augment Nicolle's beleaguered institute staff. In less than two years, the team of Nicolle and Lebailly had made great progress. Not only had they published what many consider to be the conclusive demonstration of Nicolle's "absurd" relapsing fever transmission hypothesis; they had also provided similarly persuasive evidence that the causal agent of the devastating 1918–19 influenza epidemic was a filterable virus.[119] Moreover, they had devised an interpretation of the nonexpression of typhus in apparently susceptible experimental animals.[120] The interpretation rested on a conceptual shift concerning the relation of disease symptoms and microbial virulence: they called it "inapparent infection." The conceptual shift itself was part of a broader series of interrelated challenges and changes Nicolle was experiencing at the time. He began to work out their various meanings not just in the laboratory, but in his own works of fiction.

The Persistence of Memory

Nicolle's long-standing interest in history was particularly focused on two periods: "antiquity," which extended to include Carthage in the third century C.E.; and the eighteenth century. One of his dearest friends in Tunisia was the archeologist Alfred-Louis Delattre, a *Père Blanc* who specialized in Punic, Roman, and Christian Carthage.[121] Delattre was excavating the area and Nicolle was an ever-eager student, frequently visiting not only Carthage but also the ruins of Dougga with his expert friend. Nicolle was thus principally interested in "enlightened" historic eras that were considered to have advanced the cause of "rational," Western civilization. He would often hold up the Middle Ages as a true dark night of the soul for civilization, a return to which was to be avoided at all costs. He also situated much of his own fiction in antiquity, and in the eighteenth century.

Enlightenment ideals had a number of tangible expressions in France. Following their famous political expression in 1789, they met up with religion in the nineteenth century to help shape the new French Church of Reason, otherwise known as "positivism." Central to positivism was an unwavering belief in the march of progress, fuelled by the power of scientific reason. Elie Metchnikoff, Nicolle's more romantic mentor, was a fierce believer in the redemptive power of science: "If there can be formed an ideal able to unite men in a kind of religion of the future," Metchnikoff wrote in 1903, "this ideal must be founded on scientific principals. And if it be true . . . that man can live by faith alone, the faith must be in the power of science."[122] This statement was the culmination of a religio-positivistic sociology, in which humanity had raised itself up slowly over the ages, holding first to magic, then to religion, and finally to science. Science, believed Metchnikoff, was the pinnacle of progress: it would fulfill the potential of civilization and ensure that people acted reasonably. Once a truly scientific world view had been adopted, there would be no more war or injustice. Though aware that the West had not yet wholly embraced this scientific approach, he believed that it had made tangible strides in its direction and would, naturally, continue along its path to perfection. Emile Roux shared this faith in science, even if his version of its form was (as we shall see in more detail later) far more monastic than Metchnikoff's. In short, Nicolle came honestly by his faith in scientific medicine, as defined by the laboratory and enacted by rational hygiene.

War challenged such simple beliefs. An eloquent testimony to this fall from faith came from Metchnikoff's widow, Olga. Metchnikoff died in 1916, well before the war ended but well enough into it to appreciate its devastating consequences—and its significance for his belief in the power of science to perfect humanity:

> Metchnikoff felt as if he had suddenly been dropped into the abyss of centuries, into the times of human savagery. . . . And as, one by one, the news came of the death in action of several of the young men who had left the [Pasteur] Institute, Metchnikoff's grief knew no limits. He could not bear the idea, now a terrible reality, that these brilliant young lives should be sacrificed, victims of those who should have directed the peoples towards peace and a rational life, and who, instead of that, threw the most precious part of humanity into the abyss of death.[123]

A generation of young men was lost; an older generation, brutally detached from its comfortable moorings, had been set adrift.

Nicolle's faith in science was not as fervent as that often witnessed among his mentors' generation, yet it was not as pragmatic as was common among his juniors—those of Blanc's generation and those younger still, who were now fighting the war.[124] We have seen evidence of Nicolle's faith in scientific medicine and in the Pastorian mission it informed. The control of typhus in Tunisia, which focused, rationally, on the destruction of the louse, was his favored illustrative justification for this faith. As the war went on, however, Nicolle found that their successes in Tunis did not simply translate into success in Serbia or

Poland or Russia. His collaborators in the field kept him apprised of the difficulties of typhus control outside Tunisia, and visitors from ravaged areas came to Tunis to understand more clearly how Nicolle had achieved his results.[125] Through these witnesses, Nicolle began to suspect that knowledge conferred only limited power to control nature: particularly where *human* nature was involved. With time, Nicolle would develop his frustrating realization into a broader, pessimistic philosophy about progress, "nature," and civilization. His wartime experience encouraged him to pose the questions that would eventually point him in this darker direction. More generally, the war acted upon Nicolle as it did on so many others, casting a shadow over the bright light of past certainties. For Nicolle, this occurred at a time when he was already trying to reconcile a number of conflicting duties, desires, and convictions.

Sometime in 1915, Nicolle wrote a short story, entitled "Comme un Souvenir Qui ne Vieillit Point" ("Like a Memory That Does Not Age").[126] It is one of his better known literary works, largely because Georges Duhamel himself later interpreted it as an effort to work out the concept of inapparent infection.[127] Alternatively, it has been read as Nicolle's attempt to think through ideas about immunity.[128] Both interpretations are viable. Given its timing and themes, however, I believe it served a larger and more complex purpose. It was a part of Nicolle's efforts to come to terms with a number of unsettling or contradictory elements in his life. Thus, it gives us a window into his thoughts (and actions) at a pivotal time in their development. Far from historical fiction, "Souvenir" is closer to a dark romance—not in the modern "Harlequin" sense of the word but, rather, in its early-nineteenth-century, "reaction-against-Enlightenment-Romantic" sense. Nicolle set the story in an undefined year, though it is roughly "present-day." The action unfolds between April 12 and an unspecified date in mid-July, with a brief postscript from several years in the future. It is presented in the first person, as the journal entries of "an unknown" ("*un inconnu*") and is dedicated, presumably by Nicolle rather than by the "unknown," to a "woman who is absent" ("*à une absente*").[129] The journal itself is devoted to the unknown author's attempts to understand a "phenomenon" he first witnessed on April 12.

Our narrator opens, not with a description of the mysterious phenomenon he had seen that day, but with an urgent declaration of his need to determine exactly what he saw and with a plan of action as to how he would make that determination. He can tell no one what he saw, because anyone else would either dismiss it as a hallucination or try to explain it away. Instead, he turns to a kind of scientific account. In so doing, he reveals important information about himself. First, he seeks to give an exact time and date to his experience. However, he is not in the habit of wearing watches: they merely underscore the fleeting quality of life. Nor does he immediately know the exact date: "The calendar . . . is not much better than the watch. In their pursuit of time, the one is like a soldier; the other, like an army corps." He personally prefers to "hold to the present."[130] Later in the journal, he notes, in passing, that his fiancée, Lucie, had found several "white" hairs on his head. He would prefer to have the graying process stop at a dozen: "It does not amuse me to grow old."[131] Having established his distaste for the passage of time, he finds that "today" is April 12 and that his encounter took place at approximately (he meticulously chronicles all the mundane events that transpired between his encounter and the official time of sunset, to make the most accurate determination possible) 4:05 P.M. He then makes note of the weather: seasonal, without a cloud in the sky: "This is an important point."[132] Finally, he describes the phenomenon.

He was walking alone in the woods when he saw "what I will call *the object*." This object "seemed to be a kind of elongated body, flat, without density, at once black and transparent." It moved silently—"glided"—but its motion seemed "incoherent." As it moved, it "changed its shape . . . elongating itself to double or triple its length; shortening itself a moment later, reducing itself to something almost round." Eventually, it merged itself in his own shadow: "My first thought was that it was a shadow, the shadow of something overhead, a bird or a cloud. I looked at the sky; it was clear and empty. . . . this was not a shadow [*ombre*]."[133] Nevertheless, over the next few days, he refers to the manifestation as a shadow—but also as an "object" and a "phenomenon" ("*phénomène*"). After sleeping on his speculations, he continues to investigate possible explanations. Several weeks pass without discovery of an explanation or reappearance of the object, and he is just about to give up his quest and go to the oculist. Then, on May 9, it reveals itself to him again. The shadow—he finally settles on the term—begins to present itself to him more frequently, materializing within his own shadow, adapting itself more closely to his form, and generally growing more comfortable with him. As he continues to add descriptive entries to his journal, he reflects, with some bemusement and a touch of concern, that "if a reader were to glance over this journal, he would think me a madman [*fou*], hopelessly insane, irrevocably mad."[134]

Meanwhile, life with fiancée Lucie has become strained. Lucie's "uncle" had been visiting, and she appeared inappropriately attached to him. Our narrator confronts her with his suspicions, but she dismisses them. Her uncle then leaves for Aix. A few days later, on May 25, Lucie leaves for six weeks in Bretagne: "Six weeks is a long time!" he laments. Before departing, she makes her nervous fiancé promise to write her regularly.[135] Five days after Lucie's departure, "a miracle! the *shadow* speaks!"[136]

Once beyond the initial shock of this new development, the narrator asks the shadow many questions. It tells him, in its "shadow of a voice," that, if he prepares his house with soft light, it will visit him that night. It promises to tell him all.[137] He does as instructed and the shadow comes. It is "a unique night; a marvelous night."[138] He does not have to ask questions: the shadow reveals everything he wants to know. It recounts a kind of origin-myth. When humans are born, it tells him, they are given a shadow. The human protects its shadow by day; the shadow—an obedient and willing servant—protects its human by night. Normally, human and shadow die together. However, in certain cases—such as suicides—the body departs, but the shadow is fated to linger on, with nothing to protect it from the harsh and destructive light of day. By day, then, it floats about in dark spaces, in woods or in caves, to protect itself until nightfall. These shadows are perpetually tied to the form and mental state their departed human exhibited when he or she chose to leave the world: "We remain faithful to your final image."[139] In this sense, shadows live in a "perpetual present."[140] Yet, their existence is not eternal. They do not age, but are gradually worn away with time: "Slowly, our substance is erased . . . we become increasingly indistinct. This is our old age. Any light hastens this fatal process [*composition fatale*]."[141] There is even a society of shadows, which governs itself similarly to human society: "the old shadows lay down laws to constrain the passions and endeavor to strangle the fertile genius of their juniors."[142]

The shadow continues to visit him at night; when it departs before dawn, it leaves behind only the faint scent of verbena. Gradually, it becomes clear that this is the shadow of a woman, and that she is fiercely jealous of her host's continued correspondence with his absent fiancée. At the same time, he is increasingly suspicious of his fiancée's actions. On June 5, a letter reveals that Lucie is not in Bretagne, as she had told him, but in Aix, where her "uncle" had gone. The shadow insists that he break off all contact with Lucie. He refuses: "Lucie perhaps has her weaknesses, but who doesn't? she is charming [*délicieuse*] and I love her."[143] Lucie continues in her deceptions; the shadow persists in her insistence on absolute fidelity. Finally, on June 14, he writes Lucie with an ultimatum. Choose: your "uncle" or me. He then decants verbena throughout his house.[144] June 15 is the last dated entry in our narrator's journal. The shadow comes to him again and tells him that she was once attached to a young woman who "killed herself out of despair over love." The woman committed suicide by drowning at sea, abandoning her shadow to its solitary fate: "Pale, almost immaterial, I am the ineffaceable memory [*souvenir ineffaçable*]."[145] She then asks if he would like to see her. He turns off the lights and she reveals herself to him: "floating before me was a form, supple, young, and ravishing. . . . I saw in her as much the beauty of a dream as the perfection of a statue and the mortal grace of the living. She danced. . . . Imperceptibly, she captured my soul."[146] She is now more confident of his fidelity, telling him that she has "faith in your fear of decrepitude. . . . I am eternal youth."[147]

In a subsequent, undated entry, he describes his life in the "perpetual present" created with his shadow-love.[148] He had closed himself off in the house, sleeping by day and spending nights with her. "My neighbors think me mad."[149] Finally, "I fulfilled her desire. My shutters, closed from now on, will make the evenings and days into one solitary night."[150] The two pass an undetermined amount of time together in this indeterminate existence—indicated by a number of blank pages in the journal—when suddenly, the windows were "opened wide. Rays of light pierced and flashed; not a corner did they spare." Lucie had returned; the "poor wounded shadow" had "fled" forever. His reaction is perhaps unexpected: "How beautiful the light is!"[151]

Apparently, Lucie had used her long vacation as a test of her fiancé's commitment. The uncle was a ruse. Pleased by her lover's jealousy, she was even more pleased to learn, through spying neighbors, that he had been so despondent over her absence that he had shut himself away from the world: "a true proof of love." Without hesitation, he embraces her return: "Lucie, woman, flesh, my desire, my. . . ." A flicker of the shadow remains in his thoughts: "Poor . . . poor little shadow," he concludes his story.[152] Some "years" later, he adds a postscript to his narrative. He and Lucie were married and had children: children who "charmed us [of] our youth to take it from us." This loss of youth no longer torments him: "Whether on them or on us, the ornament [of youth] is always beautiful, and those who remember [*souvient*] without regret do not fear the mask of later days [*le masque des vieux jours*]."[153] He then addresses the shadow directly: "what has become of you, dear shadow, brutally chased away by the light, betrayed by a disloyal lover?" Had she found a "more faithful friend"? Did she love this new friend, "dance before him" at night? Yet, even now, years later, when "shadows have sealed the night and no one is near," he wonders if she is truly gone. Sometimes, he even smells her perfume: "*comme un souvenir qui ne vieillit point.*"[154]

In "Souvenir," Nicolle arrayed the tensions in his life around the ever-popular poles of light and dark. These poles, however, do not map onto any simple moral grid of "good" versus "evil." Light is associated with the world of reason, tradition, and society. Dark represents revelation and passion outside acceptable social conventions. Dark is ravishing, isolating, and ever young. The story's oppositions could apply equally to the tensions Nicolle felt between family and mistress, between the obligations of age and the freedoms of youth (he was approximately forty-nine years old when he finished this story), between the scientist and the novelist—and, likewise, between reason and revelation. It might well extend to the constant pull of society's noisy obligations against the laboratory's silent autonomy. "Souvenir" was, on some levels, Nicolle's attempt to deal with the many ways in which he was haunted by memories—and confronted by them at the same time.

The correlation of the subject matter with the timing of the story suggests that it was "about" his recent dismissal of his family and his embrace of Marthe Conor. This reading is almost impossible to deny. In this context, the question arises: Is the "absent woman" of the dedication Marthe, or is it Alice? If Marthe, what might she have made of the fact that the tortured narrator ultimately chooses family life over the shadow?[155] Was she to have been comforted by her eternally haunting place in the writer's memory? Here, fiction presaged reality: though Lucie "wins" in a way Alice never did, Conor did indeed disappear from Nicolle's life in a flash. She clearly continued to haunt him thereafter. Still, it was Alice that Nicolle would summon back to his side in Tunis with every future cardiac crisis; it was daughter Marcelle, then herself a doctor, who cared for him, and son Pierre, then a medical researcher, who helped preserve his memory—if not for eternity, then at least for posterity. Marthe Conor has (quite unfortunately) disappeared from the historical record with little trace. Her letters to Pierre, written decades after she left Tunis, show that she, too, continued to be haunted by memories of his father. In the early 1960s, she sent Marcelle and Pierre a packet of letters their father had written to her. She admitted that there had been other letters as well: "To tell the truth—though I think you will doubt it—[the packet] is incomplete: it lacks the longest and most beautiful letters that were addressed to me. I am the only one to have read them." These letters were absent, not because she was holding them back, but because "they were too intimate . . . and I burned them all." One can easily imagine that, at the very least, Nicolle was thinking of Marthe Conor when describing the shadow's allure. The story itself gives some hint of what those charred letters may have contained. "Your Father," she told Pierre, ". . . was in no way the austere scientist that most people believed they knew."[156]

What is the reader—the historian—to make of the evident triumph of light over darkness in Nicolle's tribute to the persistence of memory?[157] There is some ambiguity in that triumph, as all the narrator's scientific efforts to understand events fail to explain them. Illumination comes only through the shadow's revelations. Yet, by the end, light has won out. The anonymous journal writer does not date Lucie's shutter-opening return from her six-week vacation. It is possible, however, that Nicolle wished to suggest that it occurred on July 14. Lucie's actions were, in fact, symbolic of the triumph of science, reason, time, and tradition, over mystery, passion, and an eternal, youthful present. It was Nicolle's reaffirmation of faith in all those values he had chosen when entering his adult life. Yet, it was also the profession of a skeptic, of a man who continued to be shadowed by growing doubts—a man who loved solitude as he despised it and who sought to reassure himself that the world—his world—was not *really* going to change, when everything was changing around him.

My struggle-oriented interpretation arises not just from the tensions evident within the story and their apparent correlation with tensions in Nicolle's own life, but also with a number of suggestive parallels that exist between "Souvenir" and another short story: Fyodor Dostoevsky's "Dream of a Ridiculous Man." Was Nicolle familiar with Dostoevsky's "Dream"? Possibly. Though first published in Russian in 1877, it was available in French by 1904.[158] We know that Nicolle was quite well read in contemporary literature, and that Tolstoy's plays were among those that influenced Nicolle and his friends during their student days in Paris.[159] In "Dream," Dostoevsky raised certain questions that Nicolle was himself struggling with in and around the years of the Great War. Whether consciously or not, I believe that Nicolle used the "Dream" as a kind of template for his own efforts to work through similar issues. At the very end of his life, he would return still more explicitly to the themes of knowledge, happiness, and innocence explored by Dostoevsky.[160]

Both "Dream" and "Souvenir" are first-person narratives, telling of mysterious events that would have branded their narrators, if their experiences had been discovered by others, as ridiculous. In both stories, these events take place in a kind of otherworldly utopia, and entry into that utopian world is, in both cases, made possible by a suicide.[161] Although this utopia is dark for Nicolle and brilliantly light for Dostoevsky, Doestoevsky's light is not the light of reason but, rather, of pure innocence, just as Nicolle's dark is not the darkness of any simple evil. Both utopias are romantic worlds of intuition, love, and peace. Both narrators, once inside their respective utopias, exist in a timeless state. In "Souvenir," time stands still within the utopia while continuing to pass normally outside it; in "Dream," it passes rapidly inside the utopian world, racing though many human generations, though the narrator is not subject to this passage of time. Here, as in "Souvenir," time continues to pass at a normal rate outside the utopian world. The narrators' utopian experiences teach them important lessons. Finally, both men are awakened to their original existences—but transformed, each with a new commitment to his old existence that is informed by the lessons he has learned in his dream-state.

Why, then, might Nicolle have been thinking about Dostoevsky's "Dream" in 1914–15? Long before the start of the Great War, and in contrast with men such as Metchnikoff, there were those who were skeptical of the power of science to effect "progress" and achieve the perfection of humanity. Dostoevsky was one such skeptic. His "Ridiculous Man" dreams of a utopian world of innocence—of Earth without the Fall from Grace, without scientific knowledge. Inhabitants of this world are healthy, joyful, and happy: "their knowledge was higher and deeper than ours; for our science seeks to explain what life is, aspires to understand it in order to teach others how to love, while they without science knew how to live."[162] Eventually, however, his very presence corrupts this Eden: "like a germ of the plague infecting whole kingdoms, so I contaminated all this earth, so happy and sinless before my coming." Bloodshed, languages, and nations emerge; happiness is lost: "They even laughed at the possibility of this happiness in the past, and called it a dream." Though this corruption does not begin with science, science is one of its products. The fallen inhabitants boast:

> We may be deceitful, wicked and unjust, we know it and we grieve over it. . . . But we have science, and by the means of it we shall find the truth and we shall arrive at it consciously. Knowledge is higher than feeling, the consciousness of life is higher than life. Science will give us wisdom, wisdom will reveal the laws, and the knowledge of the laws of happiness is higher than happiness.[163]

They go to war and make slaves of each other. Eventually, the Ridiculous Man is so tormented by the seeds of destruction that had been sown by his own insecurities and reasonings that he begs them to crucify him. They do not, and instead threaten to lock him up in an asylum. Finally, when "such grief took possession of my soul that my heart was wrung, and I felt as though I were dying . . . I awoke."[164]

Dostoevsky's "Dream" is a cautionary tale, warning of the dangers posed by too naïve a faith in reason. Nicolle was beginning to entertain doubts about the power of science and the inevitability of progress when he wrote "Souvenir." These doubts were being encouraged by his growing appreciation for the powers of imaginative intuition on the one hand and, on the other, his growing frustration with human nature and with the powers science conferred upon "humanity" to inflict unspeakable suffering on itself. As suggested by the end of "Souvenir," Nicolle would never wholly abandon the vision of the more certain world he had known to exist before the Great War. He would, however, acknowledge that it had been shattered into pieces that no longer fit together as they once had. He would spend the next twenty years trying to rearrange and reassemble them.

We have now examined how "Souvenir" can be used to illuminate Nicolle's changing thoughts on tradition, family, and science. What of its more familiar connections to the specifics of his microbiological projects: immunity, relapsing fever, disease reservoirs, lost typhus in lab animals? Here, too, the story's themes suggest connections between seemingly unrelated elements of Nicolle's life and work. The key to understanding the relations between "Souvenir" and this more immediate conceptual work lies in the *shadow*, and the nature of its relationship to human forms. First, there was immunity. Though Nicolle's brother Maurice was, technically, the family immunologist, Charles continued, in his more pragmatic way, to work on the nature of immunity throughout his life. It was central to his vaccine work and would become central to the philosophy of disease he eventually espoused. With immunity, a disease, once successfully banished from the suffering body, left a kind of shadow of itself behind that helped protect that body from future attacks of the disease. Immunity was a "memory" of the disease that—if the patient was fortunate—"did not age." Alternatively, the gradual adaptation of shadow to human form might also mirror the ways that particular hosts (or vectors) altered diseases to produce new species: such as were known to exist in relapsing fever, and would come to be known in typhus. Moreover, in his work on relapsing fever, Nicolle was struggling to understand how an invisible microbial state—"*inaperçu*"—had the *power* to produce disease. How did something without apparent substance relate to the visible and very tangible world of symptomatic patients? Perhaps the shadow knew.

The year after he wrote "Souvenir," Nicolle began treating those Serbian soldiers who were acting as "silent" reservoirs of typhus. These men were, in a sense, harboring shadows of disease capable of becoming embodied as symptoms in more susceptible individuals. And then there were all those typhus-resistant guinea pigs. In this latter case, Nicolle, aided by the able Lebailly, looked again to the shadow for an explanation. Perhaps the virus was not *lost* in these animals but, rather, was expressed silently—invisibly. If so, it might also be expressed when transferred to other, more susceptible, animals. Perhaps the apparently healthy animals were *in*apparently infected with typhus.[165]

Silent Infections

In 1919, Nicolle and Lebailly published their explanation of laboratory animal resistance to typhus in more *scientific* terms.[166] The problem that threatened the laboratory supply of typhus, they argued, was not the result of resistance in individual animals. Instead, guinea pigs that *appeared* to remain healthy after inoculation and incubation were not resistant but "inapparently infected." If one subsequently drew their blood on a day when febrile guinea pigs were virulent, then "inoculated a monkey (*Macacus sinicus*) with the blood," the monkey would indeed contract typhus. Nicolle extended his trials. Back in 1911, when he initially demonstrated that guinea pigs could act as laboratory reservoirs of typhus, he had found that the characteristic febrile curve was displayed most distinctively when one injected the animals intraperitoneally. Seven years later, and using his new understanding of disease expression, he tested a guinea pig that had remained asymptomatic after being inoculated in its thigh muscle. After an appropriate period had passed for incubation, he took a sample of its blood and injected it into the peritoneal cavity of another guinea pig. The second animal subsequently displayed a febrile curve.[167] Even rats—creatures consistently asymptomatic after typhus injections—passed typhus on to guinea pigs in this manner.[168] Thus, unlike Pasteur's attenuated vaccines, which were distinguished precisely by their *diminished* virulence, the virus striking the inapparently infected *retained* its virulence. In short, *virulence* was separable from *symptoms*. In this way, the laboratory alone could determine if an animal was truly infected.

Nicolle's first disease concept thus prioritized the laboratory over the clinic. There is a certain poetry in this: the aspiring young practitioner, taken from the clinic by his growing deafness, later comes to envision a kind of quiet disease that no clinician alone could diagnose. Yet, it seems that there was a good deal of the clinic in his movement from "individual resistance" to "inapparent infection." The key lies in "silence." In an effort to clarify the difference between his new discovery and the well-known "latent" infections, Nicolle acknowledged that both were asymptomatic: they were "*silent* infections."[169] *His* silent infections, however, went through all the normal disease stages—"a period of incubation, an infectious state (septicemia and virulence), then cure, all without a single sign to warn the observer."[170] With *latent* infections, the host merely *conserved* and passed on the virus. It did not actually go through the various stages of disease itself. The logical inference drawn from Nicolle's argument is that inapparent infection was a *true*, asymptomatic infection, while latent infection was less an acute *infection* than a chronic carrier state. True, acute, but benign infections—"*silencieuses*"; "*inaperçus*"—were precisely what Nicolle and Conseil had faced with the Tunisian nomads and, even more strikingly (because still less apparently infected), that Nicolle and naval doctor René Potel had encountered with the Serbian soldiers. It was only the transmission of the disease to a more expressive host that gave it recognizable symptoms—

a "clinical voice," if you will. Nicolle was restrained about the implications of his conceptual turn in 1919. He would delve into its applications and implications in the 1920s.

The Spoils of War

On many levels, Nicolle had a very successful wartime experience. When the war ended, he had much to boast about and, apparently, much to look forward to. His cherished collaborators, Ernest Conseil and Georges Blanc, were returned to him. Marthe Conor was still at his side. Beyond Tunis, his name was internationally attached to the louse transmission of typhus. In a postwar article published in the *Bulletin de l'Institut Pasteur*, Nicolle reviewed the progress that had been made in typhus studies. He underscored the connections between "this new knowledge" and successful "typhus prophylaxis," repeating again the striking examples (no typhus in Tunis; containment of typhus among Serbian troops in Tunis) of this success. Now, however, he could claim far broader significance for these discoveries. They "translated into the protection of many thousands, perhaps millions, of people."[171] The Pasteur Institute of Tunis was beginning to enjoy a kind of international attention that was rare for overseas outposts. Yet, in this Pastorian-oriented article, Nicolle claimed that the "experimental study of typhus was above all a Pastorian, and a French, achievement."[172] In his home journal, Nicolle was inclined to take more personal credit for his accomplishments.

Nicolle's 1918 annual report highlighted not only the institute's many scientific achievements, but also Nicolle's excellent managerial skills. Despite his limited staff, in spite of rising prices for materials, the institute balanced its budget through its frantic activity. This allowed it, "doubtlessly alone among all establishments of the Regency, both public and private . . . neither to have raised the price of sales of its products or its tests, nor to have restricted its free services."[173] Such wartime successes set up another, previously unexpected, contrast. The *Maison mère* had not fared nearly as well as the Tunis institute. Many of the IPP's young researchers were dead, profits were down, and the institute's scientific activity was reduced to one third of its prewar level.[174] Meanwhile, relations between Nicolle and Roux, though still often cordial, had become strained. Nicolle's willingness to treat human vaccines as products to be sold for profit had enraged Roux. Nicolle's further successes increased both his autonomy and his distance from Paris. In letters to collaborators, he began describing his former mentor as "dessicated" and "mummified."[175] No longer did Nicolle or his institute rely on the kind of patronage from Paris that had characterized his first decade in Tunisia.

From Nicolle's immediate postwar relations with Poulenc, it is clear that, though concerned about the status of the Paris institute, he did not yet have any real plan to use his improved position in Tunis to aid it, particularly if it was at his own expense. At that time, he was actively seeking to expand his alliance with Poulenc—to the explicit *exclusion* of the IPP. Aware that the steady demand for vaccines would subside with the end of war, Nicolle, Blaizot, and Billon began to discuss strategies for survival in the new market. They saw potential competition on all sides. In a manner uncharacteristic of the inward-looking French pharmaceutical industry, Poulenc sought adaptations that would make it competitive on the international market. Billon and Nicolle discussed in detail the possibility of creating an "*Institut sérologique,*" an idea obviously influenced by the German model of industrial cooperation with vaccine production.[176] As Poulenc increasingly lost business to foreign companies, Blaizot's brother traveled to the United States in search of approval, and a market, for their vaccines.

Meanwhile, another opportunity for expansion seemed to be opening up for Billon. It was an opportunity that threatened the IPT-Poulenc alliance and promised instead to benefit the IPP. When Metchnikoff died in 1916, his anointed successor, Albert Calmette, then in Lille, was unable to fill the position immediately because his own institute was filled with German occupiers.[177] With the war's end, Calmette was able to take up his position as assistant director to the IPP. Calmette, who was known to be more flexible than Roux, inspired hope in men like Billon that change was near at hand. Nicolle struggled to maintain his place in the *maison* Poulenc to the exclusion of the IPP, evincing a competitiveness that suggests his gaze was fixed firmly on his own institute and had not yet extended to the "salvation" of the *Maison mère*. This shift would soon follow. Meanwhile, Billion remained intent on "becoming the sole proprietor of Parisian serums"; he put off any plans to build a serological institute with Nicolle.[178]

The potential threat represented by Calmette and the Paris institute was essentially averted. Whether this was due to Nicolle's maneuverings, Roux's hesitations, or some combination of both is unclear. What is clear is that Nicolle's convictions concerning the importance of profit were crystallized during his collaboration with Poulenc. The relative buoyancy of the postwar Tunis institute compared to the struggles of the IPP served only to deepen these convictions. Despite the fact that Louis Pasteur himself had embraced a nonprofit ideology, that ideology now seemed detrimental to the future growth of microbiology. Thus, microbiology had to ally itself with industry if the Pastorian mission was to survive.

Even before the war began, Nicolle had started to question the values he had brought with him to Tunis. On the one hand, there was the Pastorian mission, as classically defined; on the other, there was his dull but socially appropriate marriage. In his first decade at the institute, he had faithfully upheld both—at least on the surface. Below that surface was Marthe Conor, a general irreverence for authority (combined with a deep need for autonomy), and a healthy dose of personal ambition. Between the two levels was a successful researcher and administrator who chose his projects carefully and marketed them strategically. By 1914, Nicolle was selling vaccines at a profit and packing his wife off to Rouen. War brought him a series of opportunities that he was quick to exploit. He expanded his institute and his own international reputation. He even began to articulate his first original disease concept, in inapparent infection. Typhus research was central to all these accomplishments. At the same time, the war shattered other beliefs that might otherwise have remained intact. Nicolle had clung, for instance, to a nineteenth-century expression of positivism that rested on faith in rational, linear progress, achievable in a world made harmonious by science. This was his teacher Elie Metchnikoff's vision. It was the vision that led Nicolle to balk at the young Georges Blanc's assertion that typhus transmission relied on anything so absurd as scratching louse droppings into the skin. After the war, absurdities seemed more plausible; disharmonies, potentially constructive. "Intuition" and "imagination" could move from the realm of literature to that of science. Nothing was quite so simple as it had once seemed.

The contrast between his own successes and the IPP's failures served to sharpen Nicolle's sense of an autonomous identity. This identity, however, emerged in a world whose certainties had been set in motion by war. In this new world, Nicolle gradually came to see Paris as having been displaced as absolute center of the Pastorian cosmos. Without a fixed center, connections between other, moving parts became at once more evident and more significant. Parts, such as his own in Tunis. One can again imagine him sitting at a café in Sidi Bou Saïd, looking out over the sea. Now, perhaps, the Mediterranean would be less a barrier between himself and Paris than a warmly engulfing opportunity, a fluid space bringing together places Pastorian and potentially Pastorian, that could work collaboratively—like a mosaic—to revive the Pastorian mission itself.

Nicolle was well on his way to becoming a heretical Pastorian.

Part Three

Antithesis
Mosaics of Pieces

4

ALLIANCES

"Emperor of the Mediterranean?" (1918–25)

> The plan to coerce the I. P. into reform without entering the place itself, to play the role of its benefactor from without, truly has a seductive elegance. I am ready to give myself wholly to it. (September 6, 1920)
>
> The goal we are after [is] to transform the necropolis that extends around your grandfather's tomb into a vital establishment worthy of his name. (February 14, 1921)
>
> Your father . . . addressed me as his "Pocket Pasteur." (September 22, 1922)
> —Nicolle to Louis Pasteur Vallery-Radot

On December 27, 1922, "the whole world" celebrated "the centenary of the birth of Pasteur." Pasteur's son-in-law, René Vallery-Radot—who had already paid tribute to his wife's famous father by naming his son Louis Pasteur— helped set the festive international tone with his hagiographic article "Why the Whole World Glorifies Pasteur."[1] Colonial extension helped ensure that the chorus of "hosannas" found voice at the earth's four corners. In Tunisia, Vallery-Radot's article was read to all schoolchildren as part of an hour-long discussion of Pasteur's many contributions to humanity. To help them remember their lesson, the children were presented with a special commemorative plate, which was a gift of the Société des Sciences Médicales—joint sponsor, along with the Tunisian government and the IPT, of the country's *grand fête*. The day itself was celebrated by a series of conferences, held—most certainly to underscore the applications of Pasteur's work far beyond medical realms—at the Agriculture School in Tunis, as well as in Sousse and Bizerte. The day also kicked off "Pastorian week" ["*la semaine pastorienne*"], which featured an exhibit on "Pasteur, his family, his disciples, and his work (photos, manuscripts etc.) organized by the Palais des Sociétés françaises." A special subscription was opened to fund a bust of Pasteur and a scholarship for study at the IPT.[2]

Although planning of the Tunisian celebration was shared by several organizations, Nicolle was clearly its prime mover. He was in constant contact with René Vallery-Radot's son, Louis Pasteur—"Pasteur," as he was more commonly known—to procure the requisite photographs and other documents for the Pasteur exhibit.[3] His own article, "The Way of Pasteur," appeared in the *Dépêche Tunisienne* on December 27.[4] This very public celebration evidently had deep personal significance for the director of the Pasteur Institute in Tunisia.

Spectacles such as Pasteur's centennial celebration may have a number of functions, but, on a general level, they present a carefully constructed image of past achievement to a public that is, in turn, expected to embrace the continuity of this glorious past with present grandeur and to extend it, through renewed faith, into a promising future.[5] Such spectacles are grand symbolic events containing a host of meanings and moments, all gathered together in a jubilant present. For Nicolle, Pasteur's centenary offered an opportunity to help reshape the Pastorian future as it paid homage to its past. The future that Nicolle envisaged drew upon the successful present of both himself and his Institute, and was fueled by the perceived decline of the Pasteur Institute in Paris. In other words, just beneath the polished public surface of Tunisia's celebratory events lay Nicolle's far more jagged, private set of critiques of Pasteur's Institute as it was being directed in a rapidly changing postwar world. As Nicolle attempted to alter this direction—a project that would change over the years but that would greatly define the final years of his life—he began to pay closer attention to Pasteur and the shape of his original mission. Indeed, he began to participate in Pasteur's legacy more actively, drawing himself into the remnants of Pasteur's identity and, eventually, laying claim to Pasteur's plans—all the while seeking to adjust them to the contours of the world after war.

Emperor of the Mediterranean

The broad hopes for peace that had been inspired by the November 1918 Armistice appear to have extended even to long-standing personal rivalries. That very month, Charles Nicolle traveled to Algeria to meet up with his old friend and frequent rival, Edmond Sergent. During the war, the pair had engaged in their own battle over credit for demonstrating the louse's disease-transmitting capacities. Nicolle, as we have seen, was careful to attribute generic credit during wartime: advances concerning the epidemiology of typhus and relapsing fever had been made by "French" researchers.[6] Sergent was apparently far more specific in his attributions. During the war, the Algerian director pressed his claims not only for having demonstrated the louse transmission of relapsing fever, but also for having inspired Nicolle to consider the louse for typhus.[7] Sergent's assertions were picked up by Britain's George Nuttall, who reported them as fact in his thorough 1917 review of louse-related pathological conditions.[8] In November 1918, even such nit-picking divisions could be set aside for the promise of greater collaborative achievements.

Nicolle and Sergent were joined in Algeria by Pasteur Vallery-Radot. As the trio looked to their geographical left, right, and center, they saw institutional promise: Pasteur Institutes in Tangiers, Algiers, and Tunis, with more institutes on the Mediterranean horizon. As they looked northward toward the *Maison mère,* they saw decline. The war had upended earlier, simpler assumptions of linear progress into a certain future. The future now had to be taken in hand. How, they wondered, might they reshape the Institutes Pasteur so as to ensure the survival of Pasteur's memory and mission? Over the next few years, they devised two plans to achieve this goal. The first, led by Nicolle and Sergent, focused on linking the North African institutes into a powerful coalition that would at once speak to the continuing luster of Pasteur's vision and serve as a model for Paris itself. Eventually, Nicolle would expand his sights beyond North Africa, toward the whole of the Mediterranean. The second plan, led by Nicolle and Vallery-Radot, was to form a new association that would devote itself to the salvation of the Paris institute more directly.

The meeting of Nicolle and Vallery-Radot was to be as significant for the pair as were the plans they made: indeed, their growing friendship and reform concerns would be almost inseparably intertwined for years. Though Pasteur's grandson was not a Pastorian by formal appointment, he was one by birth. He was also a medical doctor. Before completing his thesis in 1918, he had studied under Fernand Widal, worked at the Institut Impérial de Bactériologie in Constantinople, and directed a number of bacteriology labs during the war.

Starting in 1922, he would publish the first volume of his famous seven-volume collection of his grandfather's complete works.[9] Already in 1918, Vallery-Radot was committed to preserving Pasteur's legacy, which included his institute. During the war, Nicolle had been kept abreast of the unfortunate developments under Roux at the IPP by his longtime friend, medical reformer Emile Leredde.[10] Now, however, he had access to someone a bit closer to the inside, someone who shared his critical assessment of the situation and had no affiliations that might compromise his reform designs. Moreover, he had in Vallery-Radot his most tangible connection to the identity of his idol, Louis Pasteur. Their relationship helped pull Nicolle out of his more narrow focus on personal successes (both scientific and institutional), and into a broader consideration of the present state and future survival of the Paris institute. For, in those early years after the war, the IPP shifted in Nicolle's mind from parent-rival to object of mission. This shift was effected not only with the persuasive aid of Vallery-Radot, but also through Nicolle's growing involvement with the "Mediterranean Pasteur Institutes." It is seen clearly in his exchanges with Pastorian insider Félix Mesnil.

Nicolle and Félix Mesnil had remained collegial over the years, despite Nicolle's tendency to find his collaborators among Brumpt's students at the Faculté.[11] In 1907, Mesnil had been appointed Chef du Service de Microbiologie Coloniale at the IPP and was consequently among the most colonially informed members of the Paris establishment.[12] During the war, a shift in relations between Mesnil and Nicolle became evident: as Nicolle's international status rose, their exchanges grew more equal and open. By the time the war ended, Mesnil was discussing institutional matters with Nicolle more directly, even asking his advice. In particular, the two discussed the staffing and structure of Mediterranean-based Pasteur affiliates. These included not just the extant North African institutes but also the Constantinople institute and the prospect of a new institute in Morocco. In their earlier meeting, Nicolle and Sergent had discussed the creation of more formal links between the Mediterranean institutes. Nicolle remained convinced that, despite national differences, shared local pathologies made the area a natural grouping. He presented their ideas to Mesnil, who particularly approved their suggestion that these institutes be referred to as the IPM: Mediterranean Pasteur Institutes.[13]

Now, however, there were plans for yet another Mediterranean institute, which was to be established in Nicolle's beloved intellectual *"patrie,"* Greece. The correspondence exchanged between Nicolle and Paris regarding the IP Athens not only charts the (relatively lengthy) path by which new Pastorian staffs were chosen, but also demonstrates the continued control Roux maintained over all

Pastorian decisions. Moreover, it illuminates the emerging conception of a "Mediterranean" grouping of Pasteur Institutes. In so doing, it indicates the extent—and the limits—of Nicolle's influence in Paris. Ultimately, those limits would cost him an important piece of his own future plans for the IPT.

Shortly after wartime hostilities had ended, the senior Pastorians engaged in the flattering but consuming task of establishing a new Pasteur Institute. The creation of the "Pasteur Institute of Athens" had been proposed by the director of the Greek Army's Health Services: a French doctor who had procured private funding for the institute's establishment.[14] Might the Paris institute please send a director to set up the new institution? Emile Roux was initially inclined to send Constant Mathis as director, but by February he had changed his mind. The field of candidates was thus open.[15] Through the late winter and early spring of 1919, Nicolle and Mesnil corresponded about the staffing problem. Nicolle had suggested Mesnil's former student Edouard Chatton (who had been sent to Tunisia to assist during the war) for the position. Mesnil thought Chatton an excellent choice but warned Nicolle that Roux preferred the future director to have an MD: a qualification Chatton lacked. Roux was now leaning toward Etienne Burnet or Georges Abt. Nicolle emphasized to Mesnil that the new director, whoever he might be, "must know Mediterranean pathology."[16] Again, Mesnil agreed, but told Nicolle that Roux was not persuaded, preferring instead "someone with administrative and diplomatic qualities, as the director will have no time to conduct research."[17]

Springtime brought Albert Calmette, newly installed at the IPP, into the Athens discussions. "Installed" is an overstatement. It was March, and Roux had still had not even found his new assistant director any laboratory space.[18] Calmette, like Nicolle, was skeptical about the increasingly probable choice of Abt as director and encouraged Nicolle to present his case for Chatton directly to Roux. Still, he was not optimistic about their ultimate influence. Roux, Calmette complained, "preferred to continue to reign *alone* and as *absolute master*." By May, Calmette was deeply concerned. Roux, he lamented to a sympathetic Nicolle, "fears innovators" and despised anyone who intruded upon his tranquil universe. The Pastorians were in part to blame: "we think of him as an icon that one invokes with fear and respect."[19] Their recent exchanges over Athens had brought Calmette and Mesnil to a position that began to approximate Nicolle's own views about Roux and the status of his institute. Finally, as they all had feared, Roux disregarded the opinions of his subordinates and appointed Abt director. The position of assistant director remained unfilled. Here, Roux was more open to suggestion. The suggestion he took came not from Nicolle but from Calmette: that Georges Blanc be moved from Tunis to Athens.

Georges Blanc's arrival in Tunis in 1914 had crystallized Nicolle's vision of the IPT's future. It was a classical vision of immortality: creating something enduring that could be passed down to your children—or, in the case of Nicolle and Blanc, your intellectual children. It was Nicolle's most fervent wish for the IPT that Blanc would eventually succeed him as director. Blanc's absence in wartime seemed only to strengthen Nicolle's resolve. Perhaps it was the appreciation of the transience of life that is so commonly felt during war; perhaps it was the temporal proximity of the 1920s, when he would turn sixty. Whatever the cause, by the time war ended, Nicolle was intent upon completing his institute so as to prepare it for Blanc's impending guidance. "It is thus to you," he confided to Blanc, just days after the end of the war, "that the highest place here falls, on that not so distant day (in seven or eight years) when I retire. Would this place please you?"[20]

Blanc, however, did not rush to embrace Nicolle's vision of the future. He had returned to Tunis after the war ended, but the Athens prospect was more immediately autonomous and clearly appealing. His interest in the position could only have been strengthened by Calmette's suspicion that Abt would not last long as director and, therefore, that the assistant director would soon become director.[21] In December, obviously with Roux's blessings, Calmette asked Nicolle for the "sacrifice" of Georges Blanc "for the greater good of the Mother House."[22] (Calmette would include in many a future letter to Nicolle his sincere apologies for taking Blanc from him.) Blanc—acting perhaps more like Nicolle than even Nicolle would have wished—accepted the appointment and was officially appointed assistant director of the Pasteur Institute of Athens in February 1920. The following year, when—as Calmette had predicted—Abt asked to leave Athens, Blanc succeeded him as director.[23]

Not one to accept the dealings of fate (or the decisions of others) passively, Nicolle bade Blanc farewell, then proceeded to beg him—literally until his dying day—to return to Tunis. Blanc did not have to tax himself by reading between the lines of Nicolle's letters. Any and all topics, from research discussions and institutional updates to emotional encouragement (Blanc, like Nicolle, complained of isolation and depression), could be turned into an appeal for Blanc to come back to him. At times these pleas took the form of warm tributes, proclamations of Nicolle's affection and esteem for his distant colleague; at times they were sharpened with mock anger or paternal guilt. When Blanc was named director of the Hellenic Institute, Nicolle wrote, "Of course I am proud to have given the Athenian institute its director, but I would have preferred to have kept him near me."[24] Occasionally, he heightened his pleas with the rhetoric of Greek tragedy: "Alas! and again, alas! why have you, the best researcher I have known, left me?

You were our future. What a beautiful establishment I would have left you."[25] If Blanc was flattered by Nicolle's adoration, he rarely acknowledged the request that underlay his mentor's relentless entreaties.

As devastated as Nicolle was by the loss of Blanc, he soon found—as so often seems to have happened in his life—that the opening allowed him to make an influential addition to his institute. Calmette himself presented the opportunity: in his letter warning Nicolle that Blanc's appointment to Athens was probable, he also mentioned that the Pastorian Etienne Burnet, suffering from hemoptysis, intended to spend the coming winter in Tunisia. (Calmette's diplomatic skills were justifiably acclaimed.)[26] Burnet had been a student of philosopher Henri Bergson at the École Normale Supérieure. Leaving philosophy for medical research, he had been working at the IPP for more than fifteen years. Calmette suggested that the well-rounded Burnet join Nicolle at his Institute while wintering in Tunisia. And so it was that Blanc's final months overlapped with Burnet's first months at the IPT. By early January 1920, as Blanc was preparing to depart, Nicolle sought "to attach [Burnet] to us" on a more permanent basis. There was, of course, Blanc's position as *chef de laboratoire*, but it was, in itself, not quite senior enough for Burnet. Yet, there was also a new position that had recently been approved and would draw on Burnet's interest in public health and hygiene.

As it was with Tunisian power structures in 1903, so it remained in 1919: the *Résident Général* was the key to any real political change. After his wartime successes, Nicolle was enjoying "the trust" of *Résident Général* Flandin (and Flandin's wife), which gave him "an authority over what happens here" in a way he had never before known. With this authority, he had "decided to create a Direction Générale de l'Hygiène."[27] Conseil remained as director of hygiene for Tunis, but the new position would extend to the whole of Tunisia. Calmette, having just finished restructuring hygiene in Lille before taking up his post at the IPP, wistfully expressed his appreciation for his colleague's accomplishment: "You have an excellent opportunity to realize the goals to which France aspires but cannot attain because of petty bureaucratic interests."[28] Nicolle only had to think back to his years in Rouen to understand Calmette's envy. The "colonial laboratory" still offered far less (effective) resistance to social change than did France. Tunisia's new hygiene position would be controlled by the IPT and would thus also serve to increase the Institute's power.

With plans drawn up and approved, Nicolle faced the problem of filling the new position. An early and strong choice was his talented wartime collaborator Charles Lebailly. Lebailly's position in Tunis had ended January 1, 1919, at which time he took up a position at a bacteriology laboratory in Caen. Two months later, when Nicolle tried to tempt him back to Tunis with a position as one of his Institute's *chefs de laboratoire*, Lebailly declined.[29] In December, Nicolle offered him the position of Tunisia's new Director of Hygiene. This time, Lebailly told Nicolle that the sole attraction Tunisia held for him was working with Nicolle himself—and, enticing as that collaboration might be, he would not leave his position for Tunis.[30] Subsequently, Nicolle offered the position to Burnet. Burnet's response at once annoyed and amused Nicolle: "This damned man, who is otherwise an excellent sort, has remained indecisive. Some days, I think he will accept; others, he appears to have changed his mind."[31] Burnet was finally named to the position in March.[32] He was also named *chef de laboratoire* at the IPT.

By the following winter, Nicolle had further strengthened his institute—in part, again, through hygiene:

> On 15 December 1920, a decree officially attached the Pasteur Institute of Tunis directly to the General Secretary of the Tunisian government. In a second decree, dated 31 December, the Director of the Pasteur Institute was named Technical Counselor to the Tunisian government for all questions concerning hygiene and public health: a position he delegated to his Assistant Director.

In short, "the Pasteur Institute of Tunis was no longer under the Director of Agriculture"[33] but, instead, was under the Director of the Interior—and was given a new function. The new structure, however, posed an apparent difficulty. Nicolle had delegated the new coordinating hygiene position to his assistant director: yet he had had no formal assistant director since Alfred Conor's death in 1914. Now, the long-vacant position was given to Etienne Burnet. Gobert was named to Burnet's former position as Director of Hygiene for Tunisia: and Burnet, Gobert, and Conseil were all claimed under the Pastorian umbrella.[34] It is no wonder that Nicolle privately noted with pride that changes had effectively gathered into a single department "Hygiene, Welfare, Labor, and Pasteur Institute."[35] He now controlled half of a government department, thereby striking the balance between autonomy and profitable alliance he had worked so long to achieve.[36]

To Nicolle, however, hygiene remained "mere" hygiene when not properly guided by the laboratory. Indeed, expressing contempt for those shortsighted Pastorians who focused exclusively on public health, he hissed that they were "leading the Institute into the cemetery of hygiene."[37] The IPT needed to be the leader of laboratories as well as of hygiene and statistics. Throughout the 1920s, Nicolle expanded his influence to include the creation and regulation of laboratories. In 1922, the Regional Laboratory of Sousse opened, "placed under the patronage of the Pasteur Institute of Tunis" and subsidized by the Direction Générale de l'Intérieur and the communes of central Tunisia. Headed by pharmacist Hector Diacono, the Sousse lab diagnosed syphilis and conducted medical tests for the hospitals of Sousse, Kairouan, and Thala.[38] A similar laboratory opened in Sfax in 1925.[39] Two years later, the laboratory of the Hôpital Civil Français was placed under the Pasteur Institute's control; Nicolle appointed Mme Vuillier, who had been trained at his institute, to head that lab.[40] He published the annual reports of these laboratories in the *Archives;* he counted their directors, with Conseil and Gobert, as *membres associés* of the Pasteur Institute. Meanwhile, his own institute was producing ever more vaccines and carrying out ever more analyses. Nicolle was pleased to reap the profits, both in currency and in accolades.

At the same time, another piece of Nicolle's IPM project fell—temporarily—into place. Shortly after his meeting with Sergent and Vallery-Radot in Algeria, Nicolle published in the *AIPT* an article Sergent had written on the IP of Algeria. The Tunis director announced that the article "inaugurated the collaboration of the North African Pasteur Institutes on a common publication."[41] In 1921, the *AIPT* was subsumed into a new journal: the *Archives des Instituts Pasteur de l'Afrique du Nord* [*AIPAN*]. Editing alternated between Tunis and Algiers.[42] Burnet, too, became involved in the cross-country meetings with Sergent, traveling to Algeria when Nicolle was otherwise engaged. He clearly had gotten into the spirit of the project, proclaiming that Nicolle would soon be "Emperor of the Mediterranean."[43] Over the next year, Nicolle would come to find this "empire" too limited in its scope. As his faith in Paris's ability to recover its former glory waned, his vision became more global and broadly reforming. "I am quite angry," he confessed to Mesnil, "that the resources I have here are not exploited by enough people. *Emigration to its filials would be the scientific salvation of the IP.*"[44]

Transforming the Necropolis

Soon after the war, it became evident to Nicolle that several well-placed Pastorians were not content with the direction of Roux's institute. They had come to share a *private* understanding of the Institute's problems. First and foremost, this private critique rested on the perception that Emile Roux did not believe in profit. He did not pay his researchers enough to support even a moderate lifestyle; he did not market Pastorian products with enough savvy to sustain continued research. War then came, bringing with it mounting financial problems and a reduced staff. The end of the war had not helped diminish these problems. Many of the young researchers the Institute had managed to attract, despite its policies, had died during the war. Nationally, finances were precarious, and donations were inadequate to needs. Roux was doing nothing to improve matters. Clearly, many highly placed Pastorians were concerned with the apparent decline of the *Maison mère*. Even the normally reserved Mesnil conceded to Nicolle, "it is apparent that the autocracy (however it is softened!) must disappear with the *Patron*." However, he felt compelled to conclude with conspiratorial fear: "keep this *strictly* to yourself; we would all be demolished if it were discovered."[45] With his usual flair, Nicolle stated things more bluntly. In a letter to Vallery-Radot, he asserted: "the goal we are after [is] to transform the necropolis that extends around your grandfather's tomb into a vital establishment worthy of his name."[46]

It had been just over a year since Nicolle and the younger Vallery-Radot had met when the two began to write to each other frankly, and regularly, about the state of the IPP. In January 1920, Nicolle complained that all his recent news of Paris—"even from Calmette"—was discouraging: "the ruin grows." So dire was the state of the IPP that it needed nothing short of "a complete revolution" to rejuvenate it. Unfortunately, he knew of "no one who could bring it about."[47] Later that month, Nicolle suggested that Vallery-Radot might himself be able to help effect that revolution. In February, Vallery-Radot responded in kind: "oh! how I wish you would devote yourself to the *maison mère!*"[48] By summer, the two had begun to collaborate on a plan. They would assemble a society of influentials—Pastorians and non-Pastorians alike—that would work to *coerce* Roux to change his policies and reform the Institute. Nicolle was in France in July and August. He took advantage of his proximity to Vallery-Radot to clarify precisely what was needed to save Pasteur's house. The new association would work principally to raise public awareness and public funds. Where would those funds best be used? "We always return to the same two principal needs: *recruitment; payment*."[49]

The planned association would attend to the problem of raising funds so that typically underpaid research positions would be more enticing to young men and women. Nicolle's personal function would then be to inspire the youth to consider such positions, with visions grander than money. He would undertake "missions to Paris to fan the flames of enthusiasm in the young by showing them how discoveries are made, by making them love experimental medicine and discovery."[50] This succinct formulation is more revealing than its brevity might suggest. It was informed by a crystallization of Nicolle's own self-image, articulated alongside his more considered conception of the identity of the Pasteur Institute itself. The clinically trained laboratory researcher who had so relied on his more clinically oriented colleagues in his earlier years was coming to see himself principally in terms of the *laboratory* and of "discovery." He began to complain that he'd lost poor Conseil to the clinic.[51] When Blaizot wished to take on private patients, Nicolle was furious. Blaizot was being paid a good salary so he could devote his time to *research,* not dilute it with patient care. (The two suffered a break in relations shortly thereafter, and Blaizot left Tunisia in 1921.)[52] Nicolle drew justification for his position from Pasteur himself: Pasteur's grandeur had come from his research. The spectacular achievements of hygiene, of vaccination, of serotherapy—all were made possible by research. It was research that differentiated teaching-oriented, state-funded university laboratories from the private Pasteur Institute: "those who teach are scholars; different is the mentality of the researcher."[53] The more he identified Pasteur with pure research, the more he prioritized "discovery" and "the laboratory" over daily patient care and the clinic. Eventually, he would tell romantic tales of discovery—of his *own* discoveries—to audiences of young medical students, and even to the general populace. All this would work within a concept of "mission" that was redirecting the object of its focus, from periphery to metropole.

The plan to save the Pasteur Institute had two other broad components. The first expanded upon Nicolle's plan to form a coalition of Mediterranean Pasteur Institutes. The larger network of institutes radiating out from Paris had to become more than beacons of Pasteur's radiant glory. They needed to be more active, better coordinated, more research-oriented. This kind of cooperative, international identity would in turn help sustain the Paris institute by training more researchers and contributing more discoveries. The second component addressed the need for funds and, by implication, Roux's tendency to approach his administrative position as if he were the IPP's king—or pope—instead of its director. Nicolle himself had profited from an alliance with industry. Leaders of industry were far more adept at generating profits than were heads of private medical institutions. His personal experience clearly guided his longer term plan for Roux's coercion: "the Pasteur Institute can only be truly saved through industrial reform. . . . we must bring together a group of industrialists and businessmen who will approach the Institute's Director and brutally propose that they manage his commercial affairs, leaving him with power of direction and inspection, and promising him in return increased profits. This conception captivates me."[54] The Pastorian mission could only be saved by adapting the nineteenth-century methods of the IPP to the realities of a postwar society. Specifically, they had to exploit their connections and their resources, both actual and potential, if the mission was to survive.

As Nicolle and Vallery-Radot drew upon their own resources to assemble a group fit to inspire large public contributions to the Pasteur Institutes, Nicolle made *his* first public appeal that autumn. It came in the form of an article in the Paris newspaper *Le Temps* (now *Le Monde*). Entitled "The Peril of Microbiological Studies in France," it appeared in October. Although the title did not mention the Pasteur Institute by name, it loudly implied it, for the Pasteur Institute essentially *was* (research-based) "microbiological studies" in France.[55] The article opened with a statement of the glory the Pastorians had brought to France, then proceeded to defend the Pasteur Institute as the sole institution capable of providing France with true bacteriological research. The problem, Nicolle argued, lay not with the institution but with its terrible financial standing and its inability to recruit promising young people. This was no more than had already been made public. Yet, he pressed his case further.

The fine line between public and private is more often felt than articulated. When making a private critique public, it is understood that there are simply those parts of the story that are not to be told. Dirty laundry, then as now, was to be neatly tucked beneath a well-appointed frock. Although Nicolle did not actually reveal those private unmentionables, he did provide enough hints that any reader with imagination could clearly envision them. He had described the shameful financial destitution of the institute's researchers and the deprivations faced in laboratory experiment. He had then blamed the public for expecting glorious discoveries without having to pay for them. Finally, he hinted at the existence of a culprit other than war or public apathy:

> Scientists, my colleagues, you do not merit your fallen position, but you are in part responsible for it. Scientific disinterest is indeed a virtue: it gives authority to scientists' thoughts and actions. But the deprivations that you tolerate, do you think that it is fair to impose them on others? Are the material interests of your family and your colleagues not as important as the ascetic standards of an anonymous [pressure] group?[56]

Here, clearly, he was attacking the nonprofit policies of Emile Roux and those scientists who failed to challenge him—or, worse, who perpetuated his values and extended them to future researchers. Nicolle had made the private quite public.

So flagrant was Nicolle's transgression that Roux himself responded. Roux argued that his policies protected researchers from a hedonistic excess that would hinder their productivity: "had I started to work in Pasteur's laboratory with a salary of 30,000 fr. instead of 1,800 (an amount that did not change for twelve years), I might have been tempted to rush out to see what lay beneath dancers' tutus instead of devoting myself tirelessly to my laboratory work."[57] Roux's sarcasm highlights his monastic mentality: "The past shows that the best work has come out of laboratories where researchers were not covered in gold."[58] It had been nearly five years since Nicolle had tried to sneak his profitable vaccine production methods past the Paris director. Now, he was suggesting to readers of *Le Temps* that Roux's monastic mentality toward profit was compromising the very future of the IPP. For the remainder of the decade, relations between the two directors were publicly respectful and even supportive.[59] Yet, despite appeals by a number of well-placed Pastorians, Roux never offered Nicolle a permanent position in Paris.

Despite Nicolle's October miscalculation, the Association pour l'Extension des Études Pastoriennes [AEEP] was officially founded on November 15, 1920. Vallery-Radot orchestrated the enterprise in Paris; Nicolle supported him by writing to sympathetic Pastorians of their plans. The two stirred Pastorian interest. Calmette gladly helped establish the Association, as did Mesnil.[60] The Association was an independent organization chaired by the Countess Albert de Mun, but staffed with a select group of Pastorians—in particular, Nicolle and, by familial extension, Vallery-Radot—on its advisory panel. Its stated mission was to supplement the dearth of young bacteriological researchers by providing stipends that would encourage entry into the Pasteur Institutes of Paris and its *filials* alike. To that end, its assistance (a promise of 12,000-franc research scholarships) was accepted with gratitude by the Pasteur Institute as "intelligent and effective aid . . . in a difficult time."[61] It raised this money through subscription and membership dues. If the AEEP included members who sought to use it for more covertly revolutionary ends, its public face exemplified the persuasive *official* formulation of the Institute's peril.

The inaugural publication of the AEEP abounded with the rhetoric of patriotism and humanitarian responsibility. It reminded readers that Louis Pasteur himself, who had brought great glory to France, had proclaimed that laboratories were "the temples of the future." In the recent war, these temples had saved many lives. Yet, the war had in turn taken the lives of many Pastorians. Having established the public's debt to the Pasteur Institute, the Association made its plea:

> How will we restaff these many empty spaces in our laboratories with young scientists educated in the pastorian tradition, when a spirit of insecurity,

hardly conducive to the nurturing of scientific vocations, reigns in their hearts? This is a difficult task, because worry about the future, about what will be lacking as the result of current economic conditions and the effect this will have on caring for a family, makes disinterested scientific work particularly arduous.[62]

This was again the public face of the Pastorian critique, acknowledging that society had changed after war. It made its claim for generous funding from the debt of past responsibility and the promise of future service. Without such assistance, the *cultural* glory of France itself was at risk. Pastorian discoveries had "bathed France in a light of incomparable brightness." The institute's current crises of researchers and finances threatened the very existence of French science: "the country of Lavoisier, of Claude Bernard, of Pasteur, risks seeing extinguished—perhaps one day soon—the scientific beacon it has shone on the world."[63] The AEEP, with funds raised for its just cause, would ensure the hearty survival of the Pasteur Institute and, with it, the glory of France.

Yet, just months after the Association was founded, it began to stray from Nicolle's vision of it. In a February 1921 letter, Vallery-Radot informed Nicolle that the Comte de Polignac, the Association's enthusiastic treasurer, seeking a larger and more prestigious technical council, asked Roux himself "to play a part." With simple optimism, he concluded, "this isn't a bad thing."[64] Nicolle, however, thought the move catastrophic. The AEEP was now thoroughly pasteurized: "whenever Roux is present, the pastorian members will follow him in the Society just as they do at the *I. P.* . . . . We will therefore be in a constant minority."[65] In giving a place to the Pastorian hierarchy, the AEEP had given up any real chance to change the Pasteur Institute. Though sympathetic to Nicolle's fears, Vallery-Radot supported Polignac's position. Polignac had taken steps toward a more Pastorian board after he was rejected for support by potential contributors who argued that he didn't have enough important scientists in the AEEP.[66] They were trapped. If they were to raise money, they needed a prestigious (defined as this was in Parisian terms) board, but the acquisition of this prestige would cost the AEEP its potential influence. The need for this move could only have reinforced Nicolle's feeling of alienation from the Parisian core. The AEEP compromised; Nicolle despaired. Further deepening his despair was the threat of Rockefeller intervention in the Association's dealings.[67]

The Rockefeller Foundation, which had earlier looked to Paris as an institutional model, was now debating whether to offer the ailing institute funds to help resuscitate itself. The Foundation's executive committee was aware of both the public face *and* the private critique of the Pasteur Institute, citing war and "bureaucratic mediocrity" as causes of the institute's decline. Relying on Calmette's evaluation, the Rockefeller committee decided that the combination of its funds and Calmette's rise to power would save the Pasteur Institute. It therefore agreed to provide a three-year grant to be used primarily for fellowships for young researchers.[68] The question was, who would receive these funds: the fledgling Association or the established institute? While Polignac argued the Association's case, Calmette threw his considerable weight behind the Pasteur Institute. The Rockefeller Foundation sided with Calmette.

Nicolle was furious. He condemned Calmette and the institute for accepting foreign charity: "we French—we Pastorians," he protested to Mesnil, "must not become an American colony like the Philippines."[69] Moreover, the Foundation's grant was assigned the function that Nicolle's Association had defined for itself. To Calmette, the important point was that young researchers received money, regardless of its source; but to Nicolle, Calmette's maneuvers belied a fundamental resistance to any real change. That which Nicolle had initially envisioned as an external force capable of coercing Roux to modify his policies was increasingly internalized under Calmette at the very institute it was meant to reform. Such movement helped ensure that Roux's model would remain intact, protected by a Pastorian insularity that guaranteed that private critiques would not be acted upon. Still, although Nicolle's plans for the AEEP may not have been realized, the newly established grants did provide him with a number of grant recipients, two of whom would become long-term collaborators: Charles Anderson and Paul Giroud.

The AEEP, which had failed in its larger, covert goal to transform the Pasteur Institute even before it gave its first grants, soon faltered. A decade later, after Roux's death, it was formally dissolved and its remaining funds were given over to the *"fondation Roux,"* which took over the process of granting scholarships. Nicolle, who had held firmly to his missionary aspirations and the categories of reform he had set out in the 1920s, could not have failed to notice the irony.

Identities

This, then, was the backdrop to Nicolle's frantic planning of the Pasteur centennial celebration in Tunisia. His writings on the event are put in sharp relief when set against it. By late 1922, when he contributed "The Way of Pasteur" to the *Dépêche Tunisienne,* and mid-1923, when he spoke at the ceremony inaugurating Pasteur's bust at the IPT, Nicolle was thinking about ways to alter the course of the IPP. In so doing, he was increasingly identifying with Pasteur and his goals for microbiological research. Both aspects of his thinking are evident in these scripts.[70] In the more broadly read *Dépêche* article, he again appealed to potential researchers and encouraged society to ensure that these young men and women were paid sufficiently.[71] He also held up the example of Pasteur's genius as a way to appeal to prospective students of microbiology.

It is hardly a coincidence that Pasteur's brilliant methods, as presented by Nicolle, were not all that different from those Nicolle himself espoused. He used history to set the stage. At the time Pasteur was born, Nicolle told his readers, medicine was in a state of confusion. Doctors were "ensnared by absurd doctrines." It was not that they continued to believe, "as did their *moliéresque* ancestors, that all their science could be found in Aristotle; however it was in vain that Bacon instructed them on observation." Nineteenth-century French doctors remained the "ever faithful disciples of Descartes," confident that "they would find the key to all phenomena in reason. They moved away from the facts to discuss it and, on arguments of pure reason, they built up unreasonable conclusions."[72] Then, "Pasteur came." A "stranger to all doctrines," the chemist was not under the spell of medicine's "received ideas and learned speculations." Instead, "he brought a fresh mind, a mind of a luminous perspicacity. He examined, he saw, and at once he understood what none who had previously looked could understand."[73] Baconian induction, which Nicolle had long believed was the supreme determiner of scientific truth, now had an indispensable companion: intuitive genius, embodied by Louis Pasteur.[74]

When addressing the doctors and government officials who had assembled for the inauguration of Pasteur's bust in the IPT garden in June 1923, Nicolle paid special tribute to his clinical colleagues. The "perfect understanding" that existed between the "Tunisian medical corps and the Pasteur Institute" had produced not only valued friendships but also scientific successes. Moreover, this collaboration took place between doctors from different countries: "Pasteurian science does not distinguish between races. How could it do so it without contravening its mission? Are not the disease and misery that we fight a plague common to all men?"[75] Having completed his inclusive praise, Nicolle went on to establish his identity *apart from* the Tunisian medical corps. He was a Pastorian. As proof of his pedigree, he told, at some length, the story of his sole exchange with the great Pasteur. This was the aforementioned single encounter, in which Pasteur chanced upon the young student Nicolle and asked him if he was working. Nicolle replied that he was. Pasteur blessed him with his reply: "It is good to work." Nicolle explained that he had long kept this encounter to himself: "So many people had such beautiful stories about Pasteur" that he feared his paled in comparison. One day, however, he decided to relate his anecdote to individuals who had been close to the "great man": "To my surprise, it was quite well received." He had been unaware that this was Pasteur's signature conclusion to his professional discussions. Nicolle had thus been ordained a Pastorian by the Master's words.[76]

The centenary may have encouraged Nicolle to think again about Pasteur and his plans; at the time of the bust inauguration ceremony, however, he had a more immediately pressing concern: his two-year alliance with Edmond Sergent had fallen apart. It was perhaps a bad sign that Sergent, in the very first volume of their jointly edited *Archives de l'Institut Pasteur de l'Afrique du Nord*, insisted on including an article on earlier typhus experiments he had conducted with Foley and Vialatte—experiments that Nicolle regarded as poorly conceived and considered. Originally conducted before the war, these experiments rested on a misdiagnosed case of typhus: an indigenous man was diagnosed as having pure relapsing fever when, in fact, he had *both* typhus and relapsing fever.[77] Because the latter was mild and curable, Sergent and his colleagues did not hesitate to conduct experiments on the disease's possible transmission by louse eggs. They collected up the nits, crushed them, and inoculated them (through scarification) into healthy individuals. Eventually, they found that they had inadvertently transmitted typhus. (Fortunately, the recipients of the disease did not die.) They concluded that they had demonstrated the possibility of louse transmission by the nit and, consequently, the hereditary transmission of typhus in lice.

Nicolle was incensed. His colleagues in Algeria had, in the first place, based their conclusions on a "grave diagnostic error, which is nothing to boast about."[78] Second, when inoculating their subjects, they did not first remove traces of louse droppings from the surface of the nits; and, as was well known, typhus was frequently transmitted through louse droppings.[79] He warned Sergent that, if he insisted on publishing the article, Nicolle would himself be forced to respond in print. Sergent insisted; Nicolle responded.[80] Then, in 1922, Britain's *Lancet* published a positive review of Sergent's discoveries.[81] Somehow, the North African collaborative journal managed to continue over the next year; however, Nicolle's contributions to its pages (and those of his collaborators at the IPT) dropped considerably. By June 1923, the *AIPAN* was officially dissolved. The *AIPT* picked up publication from the number of its last volume, and the Algerian institute started its own journal. Not wishing to abandon his Mediterranean vision wholly, however, Nicolle continued to name Georges Blanc, in Athens, as an "associated member" in the IPT in annual reports.

Vallery-Radot was perplexed by this seemingly sudden rupture. Nicolle responded to his friend's queries frankly and at length: "That which you perceive to be an abrupt action is in reality the much-delayed conclusion to an old and oft-repeated conflict." He then recounted the details of his ongoing louse-related disputes with Sergent. He took personal credit for their brief rapprochement ("the entente that led to the creation of the *Arch. des I.P. de l'A. du N.*"), then blamed Sergent for publishing his erroneous article. Throughout the letter, Nicolle insisted that Sergent's proprietary stance towards the louse was of no real concern to him: "I have not responded. I will not respond, unless he further insists. I could only respond by accusing him of poor collegiality, of childish vanity, which I find distasteful; or by demonstrating the inanity of his experiments on relapsing fever, which would be serious, but easy to do." He appears to have kept his word. As far as I have been able to determine, he never went public with the details of these disputes over priority and interpretation. (Nicolle and Sergent reestablished relations in 1925 but suffered another rupture around 1930.) In a final defense of his dissolution of the *AIPAN* to Vallery-Radot, he appealed to the example of Pasteur himself: "Your grandfather would have protected his independence, and if it had been compromised, he would quickly have reclaimed it."[82]

In her later correspondence with Pierre Nicolle, Marthe Conor tended to couple Sergent with Calmette. Both men, she told him, were jealous of his father's successes and were in constant competition with him over who would become Roux's successor. Would the next director of the IPP be Calmette—or Nicolle? Conor's letters make it clear that she believed Sergent to have been Calmette's ally in the ongoing (if largely unacknowledged) power struggle.[83] Later events, combined with the ongoing louse disputes, suggest that schisms among Pasteur's followers ran deep—and along fixed personal and institutional lines that continue even into the present.[84]

By the time Nicolle and Sergent experienced their journal-related falling out, Marthe Conor was not there to witness the events. She had left Nicolle and returned to France back in 1919. Even decades later, however, she could not quite articulate the reasons for her departure. The closest she could come to an explanation was an anecdote. Some time before she left, she had needed surgery.[85] Before she underwent the operation, Nicolle had asked her if she wished him to summon a priest—presumably to hear her sins. Perhaps she realized at that moment that Nicolle felt uneasy about their involvement, or that he would never divorce his wife. All she could tell Pierre in 1963 was that, after she had recovered from the operation, she knew she had to leave.[86] A final, undated letter from Marthe to Nicolle suggests that she was still very much in love with him when she left, and that he had become bitter toward her.[87] Her letters to Pierre make it clear that even a subsequent remarriage did not prevent memories of Charles from haunting her until the end.

Nicolle had, by the early postwar years, found two great modes of self-expression outside the laboratory: novel-writing and institution-building. Marthe Conor had acted as his conduit to culture and literary expression. Etienne Burnet, who arrived in Tunis the same year Marthe left, would have helped fill at least part of the cultural void her departure left in Nicolle's life. Burnet also helped fill the institutional void left when Blanc accepted the Athens position. Yet, it is clear from his correspondence that Nicolle, despite his many activities, was feeling increasingly isolated in Tunis. He was far from France, he continued to be alienated from much of his family, and, despite his regular visits to Sidi Bou Saïd and his tours with Père Delattre, he was isolated from (French) cultural life in Tunisia. Strangely, an old Rouen connection and the war itself would present him with a solution that would not only fill much of that emptiness, but would even transform his vision of the world and himself. Early in 1923, he met the French novelist and critic Georges Duhamel.

Georges Duhamel was born in Paris on June 30, 1884. Having completed his studies at the Sorbonne, he became *docteur en médecine* in 1909, after studying at the Faculté de Médecine.[88] Like Nicolle, he was torn between science and literature; while studying medicine, he also was writing poems and plays. With a select group of talented friends, he founded the Abbaye de Créteil, a "lay monastic community"[89] that drew upon the teachings of Whitman and Tolstoy to create a community of thinkers and artists who aspired to "escape from the traditional framework of bourgeois attitudes and the inevitable individualism of man, back to the earthiness of the simple life."[90] The group founded its own press so that its members would not be alienated from the manual aspects of book production and so that its untested authors would have a chance to reach a broader public.[91] Soon, however, the group disintegrated as a result of internal tensions. Saddened that the Abbaye's reflective souls had been unable to live in harmony, Duhamel became more of an individualist. His humanism, though, preserved in him a strong nostalgia for the simplicity of a less technological world.

During World War I, Duhamel served as a surgeon in the French army.[92] He found the war to be the pinnacle of technological tyranny. Turning his despair into literature, he wrote a series of short stories, all of which focused on caring for the wounded soldier, but each told from a different perspective: stretcher bearer, surgeon, colleague, mother. This chorus of voices harmonized around a central theme: that war has no glory except in the humanity that remains in spite of it. Even the hospital was no unambiguous symbol of the progress of civilization. On the one hand, it "was civilization's reply to itself, the correction it was giving to its own destructive eruptions; it took all this complexity to efface a little of the immense harm engendered by the age of machines."[93] On the other, it was a central participant in the war process, patching up soldiers only to send them back into war. It was the provider of the flesh the war needed to keep running. Collected together under the title *Civilisation, 1914–17*, Duhamel's war stories won the Prix Goncourt.[94] After the war, Duhamel abandoned medicine and devoted himself to leveling critiques of "civilization" in books, speeches, and essays.[95] Several of these essays appeared in the *Mercure de France*, which he edited.[96] He also wrote novels that were each pieces of larger stories that unfolded over a series of books.[97] These were quite popular in the interwar period and Duhamel became a well-known and respected intellectual.[98] He was elected to the Académie Française in 1935.[99]

The war not only established Duhamel's place in French literature, it also—if indirectly—brought him to Charles Nicolle.[100] One of Duhamel's surgical colleagues during the war was Albert Martin. Martin was convinced that Duhamel would find his former Rouen colleague (and fellow student during hospital internship), Charles Nicolle, a congenial acquaintance. In 1922, Nicolle sent Duhamel a copy of his latest novel. That winter, Duhamel announced that he and his friend René Arcos had been invited to come to Tunis and speak (on the effects of the war on French literature!) to the local cultural group, l'Essor.[101] The invitation had been extended by Alexandre Fichet—a "man of conscience and great merit"—who had founded the group some twenty years earlier.[102] Duhamel would be in Tunis for two weeks.[103] Nicolle invited Duhamel to stay with him at the institute, and Fichet invited Nicolle to preside over the lectures. All appears to have gone brilliantly. Nicolle was delighted to learn later that year that Duhamel and wife Blanche planned to return to Tunisia that winter. Nicolle eagerly attended to the details of their accommodation and welcomed the visitors gladly.[104]

Duhamel's return to Tunis was motivated by more than his simple desire to revisit a new friend. As he appears to have done on many other occasions, he was there to combine business and pleasure, completing research for a forthcoming novel based on his experiences in Tunisia. The novel itself, *Le Prince Jaffar*, was published in 1924. He dedicated the book to Nicolle, who appeared as the character Arnauld:

> Of all the world's charms, Arnauld's smile was one of the most exquisite.
>
> Whenever Arnauld was unhappy or upset, his smile vanished. On those days, we would suffer a feeling of despair and abandonment. Our courage would leave us.[105]

Conseil appeared as "Loti." Habib, too, informed a character: "Habib."

Evidently, it was Habib who stole the novel, making the real Habib into a bit of a local celebrity. Duhamel was particularly taken with the language Habib had created in his efforts to communicate with his French employers, and with his distinctive manner of storytelling. He was also amused by the details of Habib's biography: "Were it not for his extreme curiosity about European beverages," Duhamel wrote of the character, "Habib would pass for the model servant."[106] Although Nicolle's deep affection for his *chaouch* was apparent even before Duhamel made him famous, it is clear that Nicolle became more expressive of that fondness after Habib had so enchanted Duhamel.[107] When Habib died in 1926, Nicolle wrote to Duhamel with a grief he knew would be shared: "My friend, our Habib is no more."[108] Five years after Habib's death, Nicolle completed a biographical essay in tribute to his friend.[109] He had hoped that a literary magazine would be eager to publish the firsthand account of the life of a man whom literature had made famous. When no magazine editor expressed such an interest, Nicolle persisted—with Duhamel's repeated assistance.[110]

After their initial meeting, Nicolle and Duhamel corresponded regularly. Nicolle's grown children, Pierre and Marcelle, became frequent dinner guests at the Duhamels' home, and Nicolle himself stayed with them for a few days when he visited France. During the first few years of their friendship, the two also arranged occasions for longer and more intimate visits. Until the end of Nicolle's life, Duhamel would remain one of his dearest friends. He also became Nicolle's new conduit to French cultural developments, his connection to French publishers, and his greatest promoter to the "well-informed" French audience that consumed Duhamel's abundant writings.

Moreover, Duhamel's visits encouraged Nicolle to participate far more actively in Tunisian cultural circles. In particular, he became friends with the Fichets. Fichet and his equally active wife, Eva Noelle, extended their energies beyond literary realms: they were also members of Tunis-Socialist, which "campaigned . . . for the equality of all human races."[111] Nicolle, who avoided overt political affiliations, nevertheless participated in some of the pair's gatherings and frequently dined with them at his institute.[112] In 1926, the friends joined another cultural group: l'Abbaye de l'Ane d'Or. In a manner that must have seemed quite natural to Nicolle, the Abbaye drew upon Catholic structures to promote secular culture. Formed by two professors at the Lycée Carnot, the Abbaye sponsored literary and philosophical discussions and welcomed visiting writers to Tunis. Nicolle was named "*Abbé*," Mme. Fichet "*Abbesse*," and M. Fichet "*Frère Portier*." Its members, referred to as "brothers and sisters," were "among the principal personalities of the Tunisian intellectual elite, both French and Muslim."[113] Nicolle reported to the group on his work; when in Tunis, Duhamel also gave presentations.

Nicolle's participation in some of these societies was brief, but his interest was constant, and led him to the Société des Ecrivains de l'Afrique du Nord (SEAN), which had been founded by Arthur Pellegrin in 1920 for " 'the study and protection of the moral and economic interests of its members, and the propagation of the French language and North African literature.' "[114] SEAN strove for a cultural harmony throughout North Africa that would, of course, express itself in French.[115] In 1918, Pellegrin had sent out queries about interest in such a project; the response he received encouraged him to compile a series of articles in 1919: *La Littérature Nord-Africaine*. SEAN solicited support from the Tunisian, Algerian, and Moroccan governments.[116] Establishing links with l'Essor and the Institut de Carthage, it sponsored lectures by both local and visiting luminaries.[117] Moreover, it quickly acquired enough prestige to offer, starting in 1921, the Prix de Carthage. Decided by a jury of government and community leaders along with at least one of its own delegates, the Prix was given annually to honor works by North African residents on North Africa. The award alternated between literature and science. In 1922, the first Prix de Carthage in science was given to Nicolle.[118] SEAN also published selected literary works by writers residing in North Africa. From its small initial bulletin, *Les Nord-Africains*, SEAN grew to publish a true literary journal: *La Kahena*.[119] Nicolle was among its regular contributors of short stories and even served a term as the society's president. Shortly after Nicolle's death, *La Kahena* dedicated a volume to his memory.

Silent Nights

Late in the summer of 1924, Nicolle and Duhamel traveled together to Greece. Technically, Nicolle was undertaking a formal scientific mission to the Pasteur Institute of Athens. Of course, Georges Blanc—who was now married to Blaizot's sister—was director of the Athens institute. Given the place both Blanc and classical Greek history held in Nicolle's personal conceptual hierarchy, it is unsurprising that he wished Duhamel to accompany him.[120] In Greece, the pair not only visited the Blancs but also made pilgrimages to assorted places of myth and history. Nicolle, ever the diligent and thoughtful correspondent, reported on their discoveries to Duhamel's wife, Blanche.[121] For both Duhamel and Nicolle, the trip became a symbol of shared intellectual communion. After spending their days exploring their intellectual *patrie,* they spent their nights discussing civilization, reason, nature, and science. Duhamel later recalled: "It was at the end of the summer; the nights were sweltering, radiant, and not at all conducive to sleep. We spent long hours at the front of the ship, in perfect solitude, and Nicolle would tell me of his dreams and his work."[122] One can well imagine the heavy, heated night air, muffling their animated conversations.

As we have seen, from his childhood onward, Nicolle often felt disconnected from the world around him. To survive, he created. As he grew older, he found that certain friendships also helped him bridge the gap between his inner world and the outer one. Although he craved solitude, he found that solitude could too easily turn into isolation, which in turn bred depression. He described his frequent bouts of depression as "asphyxiating clouds"—clouds that, happily, often "dissipated" when confronted with the enthusiasm that came with new discoveries.[123] In this same spirit, Nicolle had moved to Tunisia hoping to create something enduring. In Tunis, however, he found that the very things he created also served to keep him far from family and friends, and made access to necessary information (and recognition) difficult. Moreover, during the early 1920s, he complained more frequently about his growing deafness.[124] Communication was increasingly difficult. And so, on those quiet summer nights of conversational communion with Duhamel, he spoke at length about his cherished conceptual creation: inapparent—*silent*—infections.

Nicolle had essentially set his new disease concept aside since 1919.[125] Five years later, just before embarking on his Hellenic voyage, he had returned to it.[126] That August, he presented a note on his work to the Académie des Sciences. Though he expanded upon the potential applications of inapparent infections to the production of new vaccines and the explanation of disease reservoirs, he was still restrained in his assertions about the concept's significance.[127] Then, he and Duhamel went to Greece. Shortly after the pair returned to their respective countries, Duhamel made a passionate appeal to Nicolle about inapparent infections:

> The more I think about it, the more I am convinced that such a discovery has the capacity to overturn not only pathology, but also, and I would say principally, psychology. If I dare to express myself to you here, it is to beseech you not to waste so beautiful a discovery on [scientific] notes or communications. It seems to me that you must make a full and complete memoir of it, exposing all the facts, but also announcing all the consequences. You are perhaps the only living scientist capable of giving so grand an idea its full

development and to break with the absurd practice of dividing things into pieces [*compte-goutte*]—which is to say of the small communications of loquacious societies.[128]

Nicolle appreciated the advice, and the faith in his concept that underpinned it. Yet, the empiricist in Nicolle was not quite prepared to spin out its consequences just yet.[129] He would continue to work on the details of inapparent infection, which would bring him back to "ultramicrobes," relapsing fever, and experimental biology in general, before discussing it more broadly in his first book of "popular" medical science, *Naissance, Vie et Mort des Maladies Infectieuses* (1930). It would be further developed with yet another return to typhus research and was fully articulated in his classic 1933 text, *Destin des Maladies Infectieuse*.[130] Years later, Duhamel recalled the time when he had encouraged Nicolle to develop and share his thinking about inapparent infections: "If I have done anything to serve that great man's ideas, it was not through the articles on him that I have written and published, nor through the lectures I have delivered in his honor, but through my efforts on that night in Greece when I persuaded him to reach out with his ideas to kindred intellectual spirits."[131]

Georges Duhamel not only served as public champion of Nicolle the Grand Man of Science, but also as private confessor of Nicolle the Isolated Soul. In rhetoric (and probably also in fact), the two roles often overlapped. Shortly after the pair returned from Greece, Nicolle wrote to him:

> My friend, to know solitude for better or for worse, one must experience it. It is an animal who is always pregnant and who gives birth—according to your humor, the humor of the heavens, and of other events—to different kinds of monsters. . . . I believe that solitude and Arnauld are like an old couple who have little more to learn from each other. *They too fade into inapparent exchanges.*[132]

Solitude, in Nicolle's description, was inherently productive—although the fruit it produced was not always sweet. It was a creative, imaginative force that had motivated him to be active and ordered, yet had given birth to both his greatest discoveries and his darkest depressions. After almost sixty years, he had come to know and accept its power and its cost. His language, however, belies the long struggle with solitude that had preceded this fragile truce: the mother of invention is cast as a disease. Nicolle's use of "inapparent exchanges" implies that solitude first came upon him like a disease, made him suffer its unique symptoms, and that only after years of mutual struggle did they come, through adaptation, to a more peaceful coexistence. Nicolle had thus applied his poetic disease concept to his own inner struggles.

Duhamel acted as a bridge leading Nicolle beyond his solitary world. Witness the intimate thoughts he shared with his new friend shortly after Duhamel left Tunis in 1923:

> The tenderness of your pen prolongs the beneficial effect your presence has on my solitude. Whenever those dearest to me—my children—leave, I experience a painful emotion. This same emotion, to a degree hardly less sharp, I felt the other day when leaving you. To attenuate it, I ask of you what I ask of them: write to me.[133]

Nicolle's images—"the beneficial effect," "to attenuate it"—reveal his guiding assumption: if solitude is the disease, Duhamel is the cure. To overcome the symptoms of solitude at a distance, Nicolle asked Duhamel to use his pen. The pen, to Nicolle, was both tool and symbol. It was the agent of imaginative expression; it had the power to create an alternative "center of gravity" and thus to effect "action at a distance";[134] it was the means by which a moment or a thought was preserved for posterity;[135] and it was a soothing balm for "ennui."

To Nicolle, the pen was an instrument of expression that externalized an inner, silent world. He used the pen both to transform the external world and to bring that world back to him. This need was illustrated by his almost obsessive concern with publication. Writing in itself did not suffice. Once he began publishing his literary efforts, Nicolle found deep satisfaction in this expressive process. Duhamel assisted Nicolle by introducing him and his work to his friend Jean Richard Bloch, who worked at the publishing house Reider. Although Reider did publish some of Nicolle's novels, the negotiations behind those publications brought their own trials. Once Nicolle began sending his materials to Reider, he faced a constant string of delays; these in turn became the subject of long and frequent discussion in his correspondence with Duhamel.[136] Nicolle's geographic isolation from Paris forced him to rely on Duhamel's interventions to prod Bloch into action on editorial decisions and printing. Not entirely comfortable asking his famous friend to assist him with hesitant publishers, Nicolle was nevertheless driven by frustration on several occasions to address Duhamel as sympathetic confessor and plead his case in a manner that clearly revealed his needs:

> You know why I write, and why I seek the natural end of writing: publication. It is a treatment for my infirmity. The laboratory sometimes exasperates me;

I am courteous to it. I cannot have any social distractions; I cannot simply read all the time. I write to occupy myself, and if I am not published, it is probable that this distraction will finally leave me all together. I fear this possibility. That is all.[137]

Couched within this rhetoric of finalism is Nicolle's need to know that his writing was reaching a world outside his own. His was not "art for art's sake," but a kind of creative therapy for his isolation. Hidden in this rhetoric, however, is the importance of *control* in this expressive process. Nicolle was an ambitious man who often felt he had to deny the existence of that ambition; its object was the fulfillment of his need for self-expression. How better to overcome isolation than to transform the world according to your own image of it? Moreover, such a process would, if successful, guarantee one's cultural immortality, much as Pasteur had guaranteed his. Yet, one could hardly admit this aloud—even to one's confessor.

After Greece, their time together tended to be limited to those few days at the Duhamels' home when Nicolle visited Paris. The choice appears to have been Duhamel's. It reflects the mentality of a writer who enjoyed traveling to new places, learning and writing about them, then moving on.[138] Nicolle struggled against this tacit decision in a way that further reveals Duhamel's place in his life. In addition to frequent entreaties that Duhamel visit him in Tunis or travel with him to Morocco or Athens or Egypt, Nicolle all but begged Duhamel to accompany him on his forthcoming mission to Buenos Aires in 1925. In mid-June of that year, Nicolle wrote to Duhamel with the details of his intended mission and asked him if he would be interested in accompanying him. Duhamel politely declined, mentioning the cost of such a trip and a previous commitment to lecture in October.[139] Through July and August Nicolle pressed on, making inquiries about official positions in spite of Duhamel's resistance. Finally, in late August, Duhamel was forced to repeat, with finality, that he would *not* be going with Nicolle: "I think it would be wisest to turn down this magnificent folly."[140]

New World Missions

In mid-September 1925, Nicolle departed for Buenos Aires on the *Lutecia*—with Charles Anderson, not Georges Duhamel. The duo traveled "deluxe and first class," arriving at their destination (with a small menagerie of infected animals) on October 7. During their two-month stay in South America, they visited not only Argentina but also Brazil and Uruguay, and they were kept busy with research, talks, and the general business of extending the Pastorian mission. Indeed, while preparing for the trip earlier that summer, Nicolle had confided to Vallery-Radot that he was "fulfilling one of our goals by becoming an *outward* Pastorian agent. Last year Athens; this year, Buenos Aires."[141] The trip itself was the product of Nicolle's personal *and* Pastorian status. During the war, Carlos Chagas, newly appointed director of the Oswaldo Cruz Institute in Rio de Janeiro, wrote Nicolle to establish professional relations with him and his institute. The connections were typically Pastorian: Chagas's "glorious master," Oswaldo Cruz, had trained at the IPP.[142] They were thus filially related. Nicolle apparently followed through on the invitation, as 1925 saw him making arrangements to pay an official visit to his distant colleagues in Brazil. He was also invited to visit Argentina.

Once in South America, Nicolle rapidly blazed a Pastorian trail—with a personal flair. First, he brought with him the agents of typhus and canine kala-azar.[143] Transported in guinea pigs and dogs, respectively, these diseases were emblematic of Nicolle's success as a researcher, embodying (literally, as well as figuratively) his interests and ensuring that his work would be carried on around the world. He visited the city's laboratories and hygienic establishments, praising his colleagues and the "durable links" that had been formed between South American bacteriological research and the Pasteur Institutes. Such international connections, he later noted in his official report on the trip, were essential to the future of medical science: "an indispensable element in the enrichment of knowledge."[144] With a small team of assistants, Nicolle went into the countryside to conduct experiments on local diseases—not only for the sake of knowledge, he explained, but "to demonstrate my work methods to my Argentine colleagues and to sketch for them a plan for their own investigations."[145] In true Pastorian fashion, he was ensuring that Pasteur's techniques—and his own—were disseminated around the globe. Moreover, to facilitate a properly *French*-led international scientific exchange, he helped found the Sociedad Argentina de Patología Medical del Norte. Functionally similar to the Paris-based Société de Pathologie Exotique, the Sociedad met annually to present laboratory and other medical investigations that had taken place in the past year. This in turn led to the establishment of a new research institute in Jujuy.[146]

In addition to microbiological samples and French medical models, Nicolle brought with him evidence of his own microbiological contributions. Moreover, he tied it all together within his revised approach to the Pastorian mission. In his many talks during his two-month visit, he spoke of subjects dear to his heart: typhus, relapsing fever, and inapparent infections. It was at the Centre des Etudiants en Médecine of Argentina, however, that he most clearly revealed his new vision of microbiology's future. The Argentine medical students listened to Nicolle's sales pitch for the joys of "experimental" medicine.

He began by establishing his *clinical* credentials: "I am not only a man of the laboratory, but I am, above all, a doctor. . . . My father was a doctor; I have a brother who is a doctor; my children are studying medicine."[147] Nicolle and his audience were therefore a kind of family. And, as one would do with family, he had come to them to appeal for their aid: "The old world," he told them, "is going through a terrible crisis. The atrocities of the war have spent its force, its energy, its conscience." Given "the immediate necessities of a precarious life, fatigue" and "a general slackness," young people were no longer devoting themselves to medical research: "We are the last of our species."

From this point, his message diverged from one he might have given a Parisian audience. Within his (sometimes paternalistic) words, one sees the emerging product of his continued reflections on the true power of civilization and the proper nature of international interdependence. He was rearranging the pieces of his old beliefs. "Humanity," he informed his young potential converts, "has come to rely on European nations" for making "progress" in science."What would happen if, as he feared, his generation was the last of a kind? if European civilization was in decline? There would be a "return to barbarism" that could only be prevented if young people, from "young nations," picked up the standard: "In our concern, we, your elders in the old countries, turn to you. You are the youth of a new people. War and its consequences have not touched you. . . . Your reservoirs [*foyers*], your forces, remain intact. You are rich. It falls to you to put yourself to the task and take the place of the old workers, who are tired and dispirited."The epidemiological and neurological metaphors are striking. More striking still, however, was the fact that Nicolle had finally come to believe that France was unlikely to recover its past glory.

Also taking a far more explicitly defined place in Nicolle's recruitment of foreign youth was his growing reverence for genius—and his growing conviction that the West had special (if not quite exclusive) access to the talent. He assured his audience that they wouldn't have to work terribly hard to bring experimental medicine to South America. The models had already been created: "Young nations have only to put into practice that which they have learned from older peoples."[148] Naturally, they would eventually have to find their own geniuses to carry the project forward: "A nation is made great by the beneficent geniuses it produces."The history of Tunisia itself testified to his claim that material wealth and military power paled next to the accomplishments of genius. No country could find lasting acclaim without creating works of genius. Indeed, when Argentines visited France, they were "astonished" that the French knew so little of their country. The visitors attributed this to ignorance—and, certainly, it was in part that. But it was something more as well: "if Argentina had produced a genius in letters, or in the arts, or a great scientist, the whole world would know the place where that man[149] was born . . . the town where he led his useful life."[150] Perhaps, if they were to come to Europe's aid, Argentines, too, would be known as citizens of a country in which genius thrived. Informing Nicolle's plea was a clearer vision of the assumptions he had made in forming the AEEP and the AIPAN. The Pastorian mission—indeed, the civilizing mission itself—needed to be saved; but, that salvation might well come from *outside* the "old" establishment. Further, civilization would be preserved through the efforts of its *geniuses*.[151]

In early December, Nicolle departed from Buenos Aires. He left his kala-azar and typhus strains at the Bacteriological Institute of the Department of Hygiene for its researchers to study and returned home with a sample of the local variety of leishmaniosis.[152] He also returned with a "tranquil soul, knowing that I have fulfilled my mission well."[153] When he returned to Buenos Aires in 1930, Nicolle participated in the ceremony inaugurating a new bust of Pasteur.[154]

Journées Médicales Tunisienne

Despite his increasingly international focus (and reputation), Nicolle was not neglecting his Tunisian commitments. Indeed, the IPT's prestige and his staff's achievements, combined with the country's improving salubrity, were centrally important to his plan to revise the structure of microbiological research worldwide. They were both model for, and means to, the ultimate triumph of his missions. As early as 1922, he began making plans for renovations to his institute.[155] With an original government subvention of 300,000 francs and a goal of reconstructing the institute's labs, Nicolle oversaw what was to become a long and expensive venture. Pushing his long-standing desire to annex veterinary services to his institute, he decided to add animal buildings to his reconstruction plans. This doubled the 1925 estimate to 1,000,000 francs.[156] The 1926 collapse of the franc further delayed construction, but the project—gradually—went forward.[157]

In the midst of these expansions, the IPT structure as first opened in 1904 celebrated its twentieth anniversary.[158] Nicolle published a special report on the institute, similar in structure to the 1906 "Notice." Besides the intriguing addition of dates in the Muslim calendar, the new publication initially showed little change from the first edition. Then, it shifted. Adrien Loir's founding role in the institute was still undermined, but now he was dismissed in a sentence that did not even mention his name.[159] The dismissal was possible because Nicolle could replace the vague promises of future glory he had made in 1906 with examples of actual accomplishments that had subsequently taken place at the IPT. These accomplishments tended to be listed principally as *his* accomplishments. Extending over almost nine pages, the list of the institute's scientific work was divided, by disease or treatment, into sixteen sections. In only one of those sections was Nicolle not listed as a specific contributor, and, in that section, no one person was named.[160] Whether Nicolle was indeed the principal investigator in all of the institute's research, as the list suggests, is certainly a valid question. Nevertheless, Nicolle's point was clear: the IPT was the institution *he* had made. Earlier emphases on local and national collaborations faded in the bright light of his own accomplishments. This tendency may have annoyed his collaborators, but it did not dissuade increasingly eminent visitors from traveling to Tunis, to work in the laboratory Nicolle had built.[161]

All, with the exception of construction delays, appeared to be going exactly as Nicolle planned. He had perfected his institute, strengthened the medical cosmos rotating around it, even attracted international attention to its achievements. He was eager to invite the world to examine his accomplishments firsthand.

In April 1926, Nicolle hosted a gala event to showcase the medical accomplishments of France in Tunisia. "Journées Médicales" had already been held in Morocco and Brussels. Nicolle headed up Tunisia's efforts, assisted—again—by his colleagues at the Société des Sciences Médicales.[162] The event brought together international doctors and medical researchers to discuss topics of interest and to examine the scientific and cultural benefits of their host country. Delegates and official invitees arrived from eight countries; some six hundred doctors participated. One evening, Nicolle's friends in l'Essor provided the French contribution to an evening of international drama, which also spotlighted Tunisia's Italian opera company and its Troupe du Théâtre Arabe. After the formal meetings ended, attendees were offered a choice of day trips to the ruins of Carthage (where they could admire the archeological expertise of Nicolle's friend Père Delattre) or of Dougga, during which they could enjoy the architectural splendor and traditional charm of France's acquisition. In short, from program to speeches to recreation, Tunisia's Journées focused on the literary and scientific benefits that France's "civilizing mission" had brought to, or had brought out in, its protectorate.

At the conference, Nicolle, as was his tendency at such public, Société-cosponsored events, offered a spirited tribute to Tunisia's colonial doctors: "the premiere laborers in the work of extending civilization."[163] He held up for particular attention the efforts of one colonial physician who had "exhausted his 'life-force'" through selfless devotion to typhus control and hospital-building. To this martyr of modern medicine, who died at the theologically significant age of thirty-three, Nicolle added the names of other doctors who had become dangerously ill, or even died, from the diseases they were trying to banish from Tunisia. He concluded by directly comparing the work of medical missionaries with that of a more conventional missionary: "a Christian slave, M. Vincent (Saint Vincent-de-Paul)." The care the future saint had seen given to Tunisian children inspired him to "draw up his plan" for the children of France.[164] His parable's significance thus went beyond its justification of France's "mission" for its benefits to Tunisia. It demonstrated that Tunisia could provide inspiration, through the efforts of its doctor-saints, for France itself.

After Nicolle had attended to the heroics of the country's clinicians, the invited dignitaries attended to Nicolle's own glorification. Of the dozen speeches celebrating medicine in Tunisia, ten dwelled on Nicolle, his typhus work, the Pasteur Institute of Tunis, and the benefits the man and the institution had brought to Tunisia. Prof. Léon Bernard, of the Paris Faculty of Medicine, addressed Nicolle at length, praising the "school that you have created here." After listing the various diseases that Nicolle had studied, Bernard continued, "Allow me to thank you, in the name of all our colleagues, for the light you have shone upon French medicine." Others referred to Nicolle as "a great scientist of universal renown," "'the master above masters, the master of all.'"[165] Stockhlom's John Reenstierna, who had come to Tunis for the occasion, praised "the work done by your Pasteur Institute, directed with authority and brilliance by a great scientist, one of the masters of experimental medicine." More specifically, he commented on "the work on typhus fever of Nicolle and Conseil," which had "been of enormous benefit to humanity."[166] Reenstierna had also been reminding his colleagues back home of the importance of Nicolle's typhus work.

Nicolle had become his own Great Man of medical science; his institution had received international acclaim. Still, these accomplishments did not fulfill him. They were, on one level, means to a grander end. For, in the process of achieving personal success, he had used his own experience to formulate his critique of, and prescriptions for, the Pasteur Institute. The self-proclaimed *"isolé"* increasingly saw the institute's salvation in *relation*—to overseas institutes, to industry and economics, and to the wholehearted embrace of genius. Moreover, imperialism itself could only fulfill its noblest missions by integrating the world's resources. The civilizing and Pastorian missions had moved outward from Paris; they had not successfully returned from the periphery. Nicolle was *almost* prepared to go forth with his revised ideas on how France's missions might be fulfilled.

5

INVISIBLE FORCES

or, Action at a Distance (1925–28)

> To the reader who would reproach us for indulging our fragile speculations in the pages of this journal, we would reply that we have some excuse. In the great laboratories of Europe and America, no one would begrudge a "veteran" the exposition, in conversation, of tentative or impromptu explanations that were suggested to him by new observations. . . . Nothing remains of such words but the seeds that they may, by chance, disperse.
>
> Far from the common hearths [*foyers*] of our science, reduced to an elite but circumscribed audience, we have rashly written what elsewhere we might have spoken without controversy.
>
> —Nicolle, "Sur la Nature des Virus Invisibles," 1925

From the war years on, Nicolle enjoyed a steady stream of scientific visitors to his colonial institute. Members of the parasitology lab of the Faculté de Médecine de Paris—one of his favored providers of new collaborators—frequently came to Tunis to conduct research.[1] In 1923, he welcomed Dr. Salvadore Mazza, Professor of Microbiology at the Faculty of Medicine of Buenos Aires; two years later, Mazza played gracious host to Nicolle during his mission to Argentina.[2] Yet another of Nicolle's frequent visitors was John Reenstierna. A professor at the Faculty of Medicine in Stockholm, Reenstierna initially came to the IPT in late 1922 as part of a mission for the Swedish government. He returned the following summer and again in 1926: the year he paid tribute to Nicolle at the *Journées Médicales*. Apparently, Reenstierna's public praise was backed up with private activism. It can hardly be a coincidence that Nicolle first found himself in the running for a Nobel Prize in the autumn of 1923. He wrote to Vallery-Radot:

> Now, I must confess something extraordinary to you (and to you alone). I have been proposed quite seriously for the Swedish prize. Receiving it would give me greater freedom and an easier role to play, because I could return to the Parisian institute without taking anyone's place and act as a moral agent: something I find difficult from my corner of Africa.[3]

Though the 1923 run for the Nobel was to prove unsuccessful, Reenstierna's efforts on Nicolle's behalf offer a striking example of the kinds of networks that the director-*isolé* managed to create between his Tunisian institute and the rest of the medico-scientific world.[4] At the same time, as his letter to Vallery-Radot suggests, Nicolle never stopped looking to Paris—the *Maison mère*—as the ultimate source of his approval and the end of all his designs.

For the remainder of the decade, Nicolle would attend to what might best be described as invisible forces. He would draw upon his proliferating networks to increase the extension and weight of his own accomplishments, their related practical successes, and his emerging disease concepts. (The disease concepts also rested on invisible forces in their own right.) All three areas of focus would be defined in, and against, Pastorian terms. They each contained a twist that Nicolle believed at once "true" and necessary to preserving the Pastorian mission: a mission whose means he was increasingly defining in his own terms.

Invisible Virulence, I: Inapparent Infections

Although Georges Duhamel was not, technically, a "scientific" visitor, his 1923 trip to Tunis, followed by his mythic Greek journey with Nicolle, arguably did more to direct Nicolle's later thinking about disease concepts and their extensions than did any other, more conventionally scientific, visit (including the subsequent visits of Hans Zinsser). Duhamel's rapturous reception of "inapparent infection" encouraged Nicolle to think more broadly about his conceptual innovation. Though still cautious in his speculations, Nicolle was prepared to elaborate on the definition and applications of inapparent infection by 1925. Readers of his journal were informed of the full details of his latest investigations, while the more numerous (and clinically oriented) readers of the *Presse*

Médicale were introduced to a condensed version that paid particular attention to the concept's potential epidemiological applications.[5] Between them, the 1925 articles set forth a definition and a program for inapparent infection that would provide the basis for Nicolle's future work on the subject. Duhamel, though still convinced that his friend needed to press the concept's applications further, was delighted.

By the time Nicolle expanded on his concept—indeed, even by the time he had christened it—the idea that asymptomatic individuals could transmit disease was an accepted component of medical thinking. The so-called "healthy carrier" was given a public face from 1907, with the famous case of "Typhoid Mary" Mallon.[6] Previously, the possibility that healthy carriers existed had been entertained by the American bacteriologist George Miller Sternberg and by Pasteur himself; Robert Koch had examined the question closely when investigating the cholera outbreak in Hamburg in the 1890s.[7] In 1912, Frederick Novy—a founding "N" in the Nicolle-enhanced culture medium "NNN"—provided a kind of taxonomy of the concept for the journal *Science* that illustrated both how complex, and how pervasive, it had already become.[8] Within this expanding carrier concept, however, there was no apparent place for Nicolle's inapparently infected animal—a creature that displayed no symptoms but nonetheless "suffered" through a disease in its standard course. Nicolle insisted on the point in every public presentation of the subject: the inapparently infected animal was *not* a healthy carrier of disease. This was no "latent" infection. It was an acute but clinically invisible infection, and as such was characterized by "two essential points: *absence of any fever, and virulence of the blood in the period of virtual fever.*"[9]

The intriguing term "virtual fever" helps illuminate the concept for the historical visitor to the subject. Inapparent infection *was* infection—infection without symptoms. Although an animal's inapparent infection was certainly "hidden," it was not hidden in the commonly accepted sense of the term. Unlike a hidden carrier, an inapparently infected animal transmitted disease at precisely the time that any other, more conventionally symptomatic, animal would transmit it. Both the inapparently and the apparently infected animal could pass disease to others *only* when it was *virulent*. Experiments had demonstrated that both sets of animals were virulent at the same time. Thus, when a symptomatic animal was displaying fever, an asymptomatic animal was "displaying" a "virtual" fever. Blood drawn at this time would infect other animals, an observation that Nicolle presented as proof of its virulence. Moreover, the blood of both animals ceased to be infectious at about the same time. And so, while Pasteur and his disciples had made their name by inducing a *diminished* virulence in assorted disease species—they *attenuated* disease—Nicolle produced a similarly asymptomatic state by keeping virulence intact: "Adaptation [of disease sample to experimental animal species] having been achieved, virulence seems no longer to play any great part [in determining whether a disease will be apparent or inapparent]. It remains constant."[10]

In short, virulence remained virulence, even when it produced no symptoms. Though but one step removed from symptoms—proof of continued virulence came from the ability to produce symptoms in the subsequent inoculation of another animal—Nicolle's "virulence" was, in an important sense, *detached* from symptoms. This detachment would prove to be enormously important for his future ideas about disease, power, and civilization. In 1925, however, Nicolle—still empirically cautious—was content to outline more limited significance for his conceptual shift. He drew attention to three subjects that his new knowledge illuminated. First, it challenged the strict application of one of Koch's postulates. Second, it held great promise for vaccine development. Finally, it helped explain the endemic conservation and epidemic spread of typhus—and promised to do a similar service for other diseases.

Despite the obvious historical convergence of Nicolle's clinical and experimental work on typhus that had led him to formulate the inapparent infection concept, by 1925, he chose to emphasize the laboratory-oriented dimensions of his discovery process.[11] From this perspective, he presented his early work on the transmission of typhus to the guinea pig as an illustration of how "attenuated" symptoms in lab animals demanded the qualification of part of the "law, said to be of Koch." It was Koch's "Postulates," as we have seen, that permitted microbiologists to lay claim to having demonstrated that a particular microbe caused a particular disease. Nicolle argued that his investigations challenged Koch's third postulate: that "the inoculation of a pure culture of a microbe will reproduce, in susceptible species, a typical infection."[12] The existence of inapparent infections naturally threw such a strict formulation of evidence into question. It was quite plausible that an inoculated animal exhibiting no evident symptoms was still infected. Yet, Nicolle's concern extended beyond asymptomatic infections to include reduced symptoms or even an uncharacteristic display of symptoms. Two things, he explained, had enabled him to use the guinea pig as a laboratory reservoir for typhus: a specially crafted thermometer (a design later improved, according to his specifications, by "Poulenc *frères*, through the kindness of M. Francis Billon"!) and the realization that a febrile curve alone was enough to demonstrate the existence of typhus in the animals. Other researchers had assumed laboratory animals to be uninfected when they did not display the main symptoms that characterized a disease in humans. Using inapparent infection as an extreme example, Nicolle encouraged his fellow microbiologists to take a more nuanced approach to interpreting Koch's third postulate.[13]

Starting again in the laboratory, Nicolle had explored the potential links between inapparent infection and vaccination. Here, the contrasts with Pastorian vaccination methods, though not yet explicitly explored, are evident. The Pastorians had been able to inoculate individuals with live vaccines by first *attenuating* the vaccine's virulence. Nicolle's inapparent infection, as I have noted, produced a state similar to the Pastorian attenuated vaccine state. This raised a number of questions. Did an inapparent infection confer an immunity to disease similar to that produced by a live, attenuated virus? Would its certain production be safer than using a live, attenuated virus? Finally, if the first two questions could be answered in the affirmative, might he be able to devise a method that would result in its certain production?

Using an array of experimental animals, Nicolle concluded that inapparent infection did confer immunity to subsequent infection, but a *weak* immunity. This result did not discourage him from continuing to explore vaccinating possibilities. Vaccines might be given in small, repeated doses.[14] In particular, they could be given during epidemic outbreaks of typhus, to protect healthy individuals in the short run—"for several weeks"—while lice were destroyed.[15] Though lacking decisive proof of the viability of vaccines based on inapparent infections, he believed he had enough positive evidence to consider *how* such infections might be provoked, and provoked consistently, in the laboratory. As the sample's virulence remained constant, it was, he argued, "the *quantity of germs inoculated* that plays a role, if not unique, than certainly primary."[16] His experience had shown that the blood of an inapparently infected guinea pig regularly conferred symptomatic typhus to the next guinea pig inoculated with it. This, he speculated, was "a step in the restitution of the activity of the virus." The first animal had received too few germs to provoke a fever; however, "these germs multiplied in it during the course of the disease and their number became high enough to cause classic febrile typhus with its next passage."[17] Inapparent infection differed from symptomatic infection in *degree* rather than *kind*.[18] Accordingly, inapparent infection might be reproduced experimentally either by ensuring that a reduced quantity of the virus was transmitted, or by inoculating it into parts of the body in which the virus did not easily multiply. Nicolle had experienced some success with these methods by 1925, but not with the kind of consistency that allowed him to claim positive proof that the procedures were truly applicable—particularly in humans.[19]

Having explored the etiological and immunological significance of his disease concept, Nicolle turned to its epidemiological implications. He had, of course, a long-standing interest in determining the natural reservoirs that conserved diseases between epidemics, and the factors that encouraged diseases to leave their endemic foyers and take on epidemic form. The larger understanding of several of the diseases he had researched, including typhus and relapsing fever, was closely tied to the more particular understanding of their interepidemic reservoirs. His interests in evolution further encouraged him to think about disease reservoirs. In the years after the war, epidemiology as a discipline had begun to follow much of the rest of biology in earnest, with its practitioners looking beyond observation and toward the laboratory, for clarification of epidemic patterns.[20] Nicolle, never one for statistical study, took his laboratory-based concept into the field (in theory, at least) to provide his own explanations for the rise and fall of infectious disease.

We have seen that it was particularly difficult to explain how typhus was preserved between epidemic outbreaks. Nicolle felt confident that louse transmission explained the historic coupling of misery and the rise of such epidemic outbreaks. Yet, if the louse, as Nicolle had demonstrated, did not pass the infection on to its offspring, and if, as thus far seemed to be the case, humans alone harbored the disease in nature, how could science explain what happened to typhus *between* epidemics? (Similar questions existed for relapsing fever, though Nicolle was increasingly convinced that the disease was hereditary in the louse.) Conventional wisdom assumed that typhus was preserved through the infected louse's continued discovery of receptive hosts. Moreover, it was assumed that, *occasionally*, a previously infected person lost the otherwise durable immunity the disease tended to confer upon its recipients, and contaminated others. Nicolle offered his own opinion. Without dismissing conventional wisdom, he expressed strong doubts as to whether such explanations could possibly account for the actual facts of typhus preservation. Inapparent infection, he argued, expanded the explanation. Perhaps, alongside visible infections, there also existed individuals with clinically invisible infections. As these individuals would enjoy only a brief immunity after recovery, it was possible that, between epidemics, "inapparent infection, an unsuspected form of recurrence [*récidive*], takes the lead. It permits the conservation of the virus, *creating a chain* between one epidemic and the next."[21] There might be a kind of sub-pathology [*sous-pathologie*] existing alongside known pathological conditions.[22] (Or, to employ a more figurative expression, one might well argue that Nicolle believed inapparent infections *shadowed* normal infections.) In the end, Nicolle argued that "*inapparent infections* seem to constitute a new chapter in general pathology."[23] Demonstrating the plausibility of his hypothesis would take a number of years—and a number of investigators.

Inapparent Infection, in Practice

Nicolle's quest for the perfect typhus vaccine, which began in earnest when he found a viable experimental animal back in 1909, would continue until he grew too sick to conduct any further research. Thereafter, it was carried on by his collaborators, past his death and into World War II.[24] It was his interest in vaccine development that made the interepidemic preservation of typhus in laboratory guinea pigs so important to him, and that led him to conduct the experiments demonstrating inapparent infection. Back in 1916, during the Serbian importation of typhus into Tunisia, Nicolle had been particularly pleased to have the opportunity to test his "convalescent serum" on hospital workers who were caring for the infected patients. The serum had seemed to be effective: the hospital staff remained healthy.[25] The problem with the procedure, however, was that it depended on a plentiful supply of convalescent serum. As this serum was taken from human patients, it was difficult to procure in sufficient supply for general use. (Tiny guinea pigs were hardly a solution.) In 1925, Nicolle returned to the problem with Ernest Conseil and inapparent infections. The pair now hoped to produce "typhus in a large animal normally considered refractory to the disease" by approaching its refractory status *as* an inapparent infection. If an animal underwent an inapparent infection, it should be left with some (weak) immunity that could be passed on, in inoculations, as convalescent serum. Might some donkeys, like some guinea pigs and most rats, undergo an inapparent infection when inoculated with typhus? They found this indeed to be the case. However, they were stopped short in their hopes for serum production because the inapparently infected donkeys did not produce antibodies sufficient to prevent typhus in inoculated humans.[26]

It was a Polish researcher who then intervened in the Tunisian vaccine experiments. Hélène Sparrow, who was collaborating with typhus (and louse) expert Rudolf Weigl at the University of Lwow, was sent to follow the famous Pastorian *Cours* in Paris in 1924.[27] There, she heard Nicolle lecture on typhus. The two came to discuss Sparrow's research; by 1926, Nicolle was asking Calmette to procure her for Tunis.[28] Sparrow soon became an annual visitor at the IPT, even accompanying Nicolle on his 1931 mission to Mexico. She was finally appointed *chef de laboratoire* at the institute in 1933.[29] During her early trips to Tunis, Sparrow brought with her instructions on Weigl's technique for experimentally inoculating lice with typhus. She also shed a new light on the IPT's typhus vaccine efforts with her finding that the intraperitoneal inoculation of infected guinea pig *brain*, as opposed to serum, brought about a consistently mild infection with fixed virulence.[30] This permitted the inoculation of humans with small, but increasing, doses of the material, which conferred an immunity durable enough to last through an epidemic. Though far from a viable general solution to the typhus problem, the vaccine was promising. Sparrow and Nicolle continued their collaborative efforts to convert this experimental success into a working, preventive vaccine. More immediately, however, the qualified triumph increased Nicolle's optimism about the applicability of inapparent infection to vaccine development.[31]

Research supporting Nicolle's epidemiological reading of inapparent infection came from assorted international corners. First to come to his support was Georges Blanc himself: "one of our own," as Nicolle proudly reminded his readers.[32] Dengue was epidemic in Athens in 1927 and 1928, and Blanc and his collaborators had been attempting to inoculate guinea pigs—and, sometimes, other humans—with the serum of patients suffering from the disease. Initially, they concluded that their guinea pig inoculations (and, again, some of the human trials) had been negative. Thinking about Nicolle's cautions and his demonstrations of typhus in asymptomatic guinea pigs, however, they returned to their experiments. Drawing blood from their apparently uninfected subjects, they inoculated a second group of animals and found that guinea pigs did, indeed, suffer from inapparent dengue. Moreover, certain humans, *after* an initial, symptomatic attack, could suffer from inapparent dengue. Nicolle asserted that his protégé's findings were "doubtless of importance for the conservation of the virus outside epidemics."[33]

Further evidence in support of Nicolle's predictions came the following year, from S. Ramsine of the Central Institute of Hygiene in Belgrade.[34] Ramsine had been investigating "the immunobiological properties of the endemic and epidemic virus of typhus and . . . the inapparent forms of this disease, in the sense defined by the Ch. Nicolle school," within a kind of socionaturally created laboratory.[35] This human laboratory consisted of a group of nearly one hundred workers living in barracks outside Belgrade. Already isolated from the general population, they were strictly quarantined when two cases of typhus appeared among them. The workers were immediately deloused and disinfected (two procedures, Ramsine noted, that were greatly needed in the population). Despite these precautions, the epidemic lasted forty-five days, with eleven new cases appearing. How could the epidemic become so pervasive when they seemed to have detected it so early? "An investigation and serological and biological research permitted me to establish the conditions of the epidemic's development." Each worker was asked his place of origin, the date he arrived in Belgrade, and whether he had suffered from typhus previously. Each worker's temperature was taken twice daily. Finally, the Weil-Felix test was administered on samples of their blood.[36]

The Weil-Felix test is a serological test for typhus that had been developed in 1916 by Edmund Weil and Arthur Felix.[37] It was later estimated to be about 90 percent accurate,[38] though it did for a time serve to confuse the search for the agent of typhus: it tested for antigens to the "Proteus" organism rather than for rickettsia.[39] Ramsine found that 12 percent of his *healthy* subjects gave positive Weil-Felix reactions.[40] The results were far outside any normal range of false results. "So strong a percentage," he observed,

> . . . made us think that, among these subjects, we would find inapparent forms of this disease. The hypothesis of the existence of inapparent cases was also supported by the existence of so great a propagation of the virus among workers, even though delousing had been undertaken immediately after the discovery of the first two cases. It seemed probable to us that the first cases of typhus appeared in atypical form, essentially inapparent, and that these forms had spread the virus by the intermediary of the louse among members of the colony.

Ramsine inoculated guinea pigs in accordance with Nicolle's instructions and found that the blood of his normal patients was virulent for guinea pigs. "I was able to prove experimentally that my hypothesis was valid."[41] He concluded that "inapparent typhus *truly exists in humans*. It develops and evolves without a single symptom, subjective or objective."[42] It explained a naturally occurring typhus epidemic and thus was a plausible candidate for interepidemic reservoir of the disease.

Nicolle, who published Ramsine's article, was elated. Taking advantage of editorial privilege, he added his own commentary on the findings from Belgrade. He reminded readers that, ever since he and Lebailly had first noted the existence of inapparent infection, they had "very firmly stated the opinion that it played an important role, perhaps the most important role, in the natural conservation of the virus." Indeed, "each time we took up the subject, we asked epidemiologists to give us experimental proof of a fact of such importance for prophylaxis." They could not undertake such research themselves, because they would have had to take "prolonged trips to typhus foyers" (the evident subtext containing a reminder that typhus was no longer endemic in Tunis), which simply wasn't possible, given the constraints of their other work. Finally, "S. Ramsine has brought us what is in effect unquestionable proof" that their assertions were correct.[43] The combined evidence of serological test and guinea pig inoculation gave the results particular credibility. In light of this evidence, doctors, epidemiologists, and microbiologists would now have to "consider all individuals met in an active foyer as dangerous, able to secretly carry or to contract without evidence the germ of the disease." Prophylaxis would have to be made more vigilant still.[44]

Nicolle encouraged further investigations into the natural occurrence of inapparent infection in typhus and other diseases. Such evidence was to follow in 1930 from W. Barykine, director of the Institute of Microbiology of the Commission of Public Health in Moscow.[45] Barykine, who had found that inapparent infection was particularly common at the beginning and the end of epidemics, concluded that inapparent infections were "just as important from an epidemiological perspective" as were symptomatic infections.[46] Other evidence of inapparent infection would follow, mostly from Germany, Russia, and eastern Europe.[47] It appeared that the mystery of the interepidemic reservoir of typhus had been solved. The disease moved silently between humans, in the benign cases of children and in the inapparent infections of the population in general. Nicolle's ideas were also being discussed in the United States and Mexico, where typhus research had been expanding since 1928.[48]

Invisible Virulence, II: Inframicrobes

At the same time that he was working out his concept of invisible infections, Nicolle was working through what he knew—and what was more generally known—of invisible infective *agents*. Eventually, the temporal juxtaposition of these subjects would seem more than a coincidence, as his understanding of both inapparent infection and filterable viruses (he called the latter "inframicrobes") came to play central parts in his theory of the "birth, life, and death" of infectious disease. Moreover, his changing ideas about the filterable viruses provide us with insight into how a successful medical researcher attempted to make sense of the enormously complex terrain that was experimental biology in the interwar years, and of how a successful *colonial* medical researcher drew upon extended networks to assist him in these efforts to impose order on a disordered world.

Nicolle first became interested in filterable viruses while working on louse-borne relapsing fever before the war.[49] Though technically neither invisible nor filterable, the disease's causal agent did appear to go through an invisible stage while in the louse-host.[50] Nicolle and Blanc had further determined that these microbes were at their most virulent while invisible. In the decade following their relapsing fever work, a few more diseases had been added to the list of ultraviruses: Nicolle's own demonstration (with Lebailly) that the causal agent of influenza was not, as previously thought, the bacillus discovered by Pfeiffer, but, instead, a filterable virus, was one of these additions.[51] Indeed, a growing number of diseases appeared to have both a visible and an invisible "microbe" associated with them. This intrigued Nicolle. So too did the discovery by Félix d'Herelle, just two years after he had worked at Nicolle's institute, of an invisible microbe that appeared to be pathogenic for other microbes.[52] In 1925, Nicolle gathered up the assorted studies of diseases whose microbes were at least sometimes invisible and the latest interpretations of d'Herelle's "bacteriophage," and, setting these in an evolutionary framework, offered his own—provisional—interpretation of invisible viruses.

At the time that Nicolle began writing on the subject, the filterable viruses were known also as "ultramicrobes." Wendell Stanley's isolation of tobacco mosaic virus[53] was ten years in the future and the settling of virus studies into anything resembling a disciplinary field was more distant still.[54] Most researchers—Nicolle included—still regarded the invisible agents of diseases like rabies and smallpox simply as very tiny microbes. Within this framework, Nicolle was displeased with the accepted terminology and sought to alter convention. "Ultramicrobes," he noted, had been given the name because it was only with the aid of an ultramicroscope that some of them could be made at all visible. Unfortunately, "the word *ultra* (beyond) has come to mean *above* [*supra*] in our language. . . . As we are speaking of entities that are smaller than microbes, of under-microbes [*sous-microbes*], it seems to us better to create the word *inframicrobes*."[55] In this linguistic campaign, Nicolle was rather spectacularly unsuccessful.

It had been over two decades since Emile Roux had published his review of filterable viruses.[56] In the interval, basic knowledge of their structure and function had not much changed. Nicolle, like his former teacher, stressed the provisional nature of the category of "filterable virus" in itself: it rested on the limits of technology—microscopes and filters—rather than on any known quality of the entities themselves (beyond their pathogenicity). Even for those few inframicrobes that the ultramicroscope had successfully made visible, nothing beyond a scattering of dust could be seen.[57] Nicolle continued to think of inframicrobes fundamentally as tiny microbes because "we have discovered nothing thus far that would support separating them from microbes that one can see under a microscope."[58] He was not, however, wed to this conclusion. As with the remainder of the ideas he put forth in this article, Nicolle qualified his interpretations as highly speculative. He was, however, reasonably confident that the broad framework in which he was interpreting inframicrobes was strongly suggested by the existing evidence: "It is true that an evolutionary character has not previously been considered applicable to bacteria; the facts that follow will shake this classic opinion."[59]

Nicolle was particularly fascinated by instances of diseases whose causal microbes had been discovered to have both a visible and an invisible stage. This "recent chapter" in disease knowledge had been "opened by Fontès's findings on the tuberculosis bacillus." While listing a number of such cases, Nicolle focused on an example that had recently come to his attention: typhus. In 1924, Friedrich Breinl, a professor at the University of Prague's Institute of Hygiene, paid a research visit to the IPT.[60] Earlier, Breinl and Weil, of the Weil-Felix test for typhus, had collaborated on a study of the strange fact that Proteus X-19 was so closely connected with the causal rickettsia of typhus that it could be used to test for its presence. They argued that "the specificity of the [Weil-Felix] reaction was due to the specificity of the pathogenic agent." They believed that Proteus, the larger organism that could not in itself produce typhus, and rickettsia, the nearly invisible, virulent agent of typhus, "were different states [*états*] of the same germ." Moreover, they suggested that the transformation from Proteus to rickettsia was caused by a *mutation*.[61] Though he did not extend Weil and Breinl's *mechanism* to his other examples at this time, Nicolle was clearly struck by the explanatory potential of both their general explanation and their proposed mechanism.

Nicolle found the coupling of visible and invisible microbial stages to be so persuasive that he suggested its application to the hotly contested debate over the nature of d'Herelle's bacteriophage. D'Herelle believed the invisible bacteriophage to be a microbe that killed microbes, whereas the famous immunologist Jules Bordet thought it to be a by-product of bacterial interaction.[62] Nicolle, while supporting d'Herelle's conviction that the bacteriophage was a living microbial entity, proposed another suggestion. D'Herelle had discovered the bacteriophage while working on a particular variety of dysentery bacillus. Perhaps the bacteriophage was an invisible stage of the visible bacillus? He left his hypothesis at that: "we think it prudent to advance no further on such shaky ground." He did, however, believe that his interpretation "rendered d'Herelle's hypothesis more solid."[63]

The apparent ability of a microbe to undergo different forms, or stages, during its development in a particular host was becoming an increasingly popular research topic at that time. The so-called "cyclogenic" theory of bacterial development would receive a thorough review by the University of Michigan's Philip Hadley in 1927.[64] Nicolle's ideas did not, however, fit cleanly into Hadley's interpretive frame. Hadley rejected the possibility of mutation as a causal mechanism between bacterial stages. Though Nicolle had not yet applied mutation to the relations between visible and invisible microbial states, he was already convinced that the variation was part of a larger evolutionary process. In his 1925 paper, he even sketched what might be referred to as a "great chain of microbial being." First, there were the bacteria with no known invisible states. In the second category were pathogenic bacteria that had a filterable form with apparent virulence, such as typhoid and tuberculosis. Third were the pathogenic microbes, such as the spirochetes of louse-borne relapsing fever, that not only had an invisible form but also were virulent principally while invisible. Nicolle's fourth category included typhus on the Weil/Breinl model. These diseases were still linked to their bacterial ancestors but were caused by microbes *only* during their invisible stage. Finally, there were those invisible viruses whose bacterial connections were no longer evident. In short, bacteria evolved. In their evolution, temporary "stage" became permanent state as they moved toward invisible virulence.

Nicolle offered two different mechanisms by which such bacterial evolution toward invisible virulence might occur. The first rested on viewing the living host as a kind of culture medium. In this living medium, as in artificial media, "The more favorable the conditions of an environment are to the microbes . . . the more rapidly they multiply." Living media were particularly effective because they were capable of regenerating their resources. In this welcoming environment, the "youngest individuals begin to divide: there is no effort to achieve [*effort vers*] an adult form." These younger microbes, small and active, would be well served if, in their "rapid multiplication," there was "a progressive reduction in the elements that are divided." With successive divisions and reductions, these microbes would eventually "become invisible."[65] Over time, they would be fixed in this form, wholly divorced from their microbial forebears. This was not quite the "retrograde evolution" that would come to be advocated in the 1930s, but it did draw upon similar ideas.[66] The second potential mechanism called upon the so-called "granular theory," as championed by men such as William Leishman.[67] Some saw these bacterial fragments—the "dust" made visible by the ultramicroscope, dismissed by many as mere bacterial by-products—as invisible, living entities. Nicolle speculated that, in some instances, granules might be the product of "a transformation whose goal is the most active multiplication of the germ."[68]

Before concluding his essay, Nicolle suggested—more tentatively still—that his interpretation of the evolutionary relations between visible and invisible microbes might also explain, among other things, the difference between the bubonic and pneumonic forms of plague. "It would be absurd at this time," he confessed—rhetorically—"to find proof in this reasoning. . . . However . . . [*Et pourtant* . . .]."[69] He then ended with a revealing, and again rhetorical, apology, directly addressing *AIPT* readers who might "reproach us for indulging our fragile speculations in the pages of this journal." He defended himself by reminding such readers of his (colonial) removal from the centers of scientific power. "In the great laboratories of Europe and America," scientists constantly discussed provisional interpretations with each other. Afterward, "nothing remains of such words but the seeds that they may, by chance, disperse." Yet in Tunis, "far from the common hearths [*foyers*] of our science, reduced to an elite but circumscribed audience, we have rashly written what elsewhere we might have spoken without controversy."[70] At the same time that he was developing his scientific ideas about invisible forces, Nicolle was working on ways to expand his networks and increase the weight of his personal and institutional successes, so as to increase his influence—his gravitational pull—in Tunis.

1927–29: Light and Shadow

In 1928, Nicolle boasted to Georges Blanc that

> In two years, all that can be accomplished with the help of the Tunisian budget will be. Our relations with the Administration will be again what they were before: nonexistent. I will have taken total control and will leave nothing to the administration. All of the medical corps, all of the hospital services will be ours. Every morning, the Institute is littered with the sick. . . . we will soon have our own dispensary as well.[71]

This was the realization of the plans he had made when abandoning Rouen for Tunis back in 1902. Viewed from any number of perspectives, Nicolle's life at the end of the 1920s would have seemed a success. International researchers were increasingly consulting him and visiting his institute, with his recent work on inapparent infection drawing particular interest. France had even taken note, awarding him the Osiris Prize and appointing him to the Académie des Sciences. When Stockholm nodded in his direction in 1928, Nicolle and the IPT became the focus of still broader international attention. At the time, he was sixty-two years old. Other men at that stage in their careers might well have seen these awards as welcome credit at the conclusion of a lifetime's productive work. Some part of Nicolle appears to have wished to take just this approach.[72] There was a larger part of him, however, that was not yet ready to retire. The reasons for his continued activity, as one might expect, had much to do with his continued commitment to fulfilling the missions he had brought with him to Tunis. He may have achieved the kind of institutional autonomy within Tunisia that would make his larger success possible. Yet, that autonomy in itself was more means than end.

When one examines the awards and celebrations that Nicolle enjoyed at the decade's end, one finds, beneath the glory, a very intentional dynamic. Awards did not simply fall from the scientific heavens upon an indifferent Nicolle. Though he had long been critical of the preference, so common in Paris, of rewarding excellent research with the "false money" of medals and ribbons, he actively, if often covertly, sought such rewards for himself and his collaborators. The currency of awards might be false, but it was respectfully honored in Paris.[73] Moreover, it was what he believed was necessary to finally achieve his larger, missionary goals. Yet, if intentional interventions were evident beneath all this glory, there was another force extant alongside it. This was the force of fate: conditions, developments, and decisions beyond the control of even the director of the Pasteur Institute of Tunis. They were to shadow his many successes and, in so doing, challenge his ability to attain his desired ends.

Tunis

1928 marked Nicolle's twenty-fifth anniversary as director of the IPT. Months before the chosen celebration date of April 28, plans for the Jubilee celebration were underway, overseen principally by a local committee that included Charles Anderson and Adrien Loir's Tunisian protégé Béchir Dinguizli.[74] The committee raised awareness of, and funds for, the festivities by inviting respected medical researchers from around the world to become members of an "Honorary Committee" for the Jubilee, and offering them the opportunity to purchase a commemorative copy of a special "Nicolle medallion."[75] Ernest Conseil described the ceremonies themselves, which were held at the "sumptuously decorated" Municipal Theater of Tunis, as a "majestic official manifestation" that had sprung forth naturally from the desire of great numbers of people to pay public homage to Nicolle. The array of invited delegates included Amédée Borell from the IPP and Nicolle's old friend and colleague from

Rouen, A. Halipré, along with assorted representatives of the Tunisian government and leaders of local medical and cultural institutions.[76] Even Adrien Loir turned up. Those who did not make the journey to Tunis sent congratulatory letters and telegrams, which poured in from around the world.

Despite the crowds and carefully orchestrated pomp, there was a surprisingly personal exchange within the afternoon's speeches. Ernest Conseil had fittingly been tasked with giving tribute to Nicolle's scientific accomplishments and did so by providing an inside account of their work together:

> On this day, I cannot refrain from evoking memories of this long collaboration. These are the best moments of our life—for you, I am certain, as much as for me. And then, why not recount these memories in public. One is too often presented as the scientist bending over his table, detached from contingencies; yet it was from you that I learned above all that nature reveals its secrets only to those who are able to fight, and who do not hesitate to pursue those secrets wherever they hide.[77]

To chase down such medical truths, Conseil continued, Nicolle knew he had to integrate himself into the extant medical community: "You were too much of a doctor to think that experimentation could do without the clinic; you deemed it necessary that there be a close collaboration among all the country's medical resources." (This was, of course, the positive spin on Nicolle's Tunisian medical cosmos.) At the heart of it all, however, was the institute, which Nicolle rapidly ensured was "the center of attraction for all those interested in scientific research." To achieve this status for the IPT, "you recruited your collaborators. I had the honor to be among those chosen."[78]

Nicolle in turn chose this particular occasion—a public ceremony in his own honor—to honor his longtime collaborator and friend: "Conseil, this moment is dear to me. . . . without you, without your intelligence, your ever alert activity, your devotion . . . the work of the IPT, and my own work, would be significantly diminished. . . . Your name is indissolubly linked to mine."[79]

Besides his personal address to Conseil, Nicolle parceled out the kinds of thanks one would expect. There were a few twists. He chided Loir for leaving him "quite a mediocre institute"[80] and thanked "the whole Tunisian population, and above all the Muslim nation, because your confidence in us permitted our investigations."[81] Instead of reciting the contributions of his own institute, he mentioned a number of instances in which French microbiologists had improved the health of African populations more generally. Evidence of such "happy progress" could only make them "proud of the role of France" in Africa.

It should also make them proud of the contributions to France and to Humanity made by colonial medicine: "We also have the right, Africans, to turn towards [France] and say to her: Mother [*Mère*], which of your provinces has done as much for the health of humanity as your adoptive daughter, Africa."[82] Although Nicolle had started referring to himself as "Tunisian" many years earlier, his identification with his "adoptive" homeland deepened over the next few years, and especially in the months immediately preceding his death.[83]

Nicolle also paid brief tribute to a number of his collaborators, past and present. There was the "enthusiastic" Blaizot, the "calm" Lebailly, and "Georges Blanc, who among all of them is doubtlessly most like me."[84] Conspicuously absent from Nicolle's list, and even from his *fête*, was his assistant director, Etienne Burnet. Relations between the two had been crumbling since 1926. Nicolle complained of Burnet's indecisiveness, but there appears to have been more to the growing rift than hesitancy of character. Burnet, who had studied under philosopher Henri Bergson, quickly moved into the Tunisian cultural and literary circles that Nicolle had begun to dominate. When Burnet wrote a novel in 1926, Nicolle shared his biting critique of the effort with Duhamel. Duhamel's reply, a lengthy defense of Burnet's work, could only have annoyed Nicolle further.[85] Apparently, Burnet's novels were generally seen as being far superior to Nicolle's ongoing efforts. The following year, Nicolle abruptly ended his participation in l'Essor when the group met in his absence to "inaugurate" the Burnets' new villa.[86] By 1928, relations were dire. The two men suffered a bitter break, and Burnet departed for a new position in Geneva that same year.[87] Only near the end of Nicolle's life did he reach out again to his former second.

Nicolle may have been relieved by Burnet's absence, but the departure left him without an assistant director in an increasingly busy institution. The man who had created a Tunisian medical cosmos with himself at its center complained to Duhamel that he was bending under the weight of his institute: "I could well compare myself to Atlas. I cannot continue to carry this entire institute on my back."[88] Yet, Burnet's departure also gave him a certain emotional leverage in his continuing efforts to lure Blanc back from Athens. He announced his intentions to Duhamel's wife, Blanche, that autumn: "I am going to call upon Blanc. Were Blanc to come, I would taste a pleasure sweeter than that of the Swedish prize. Peace, and the future, would be assured."[89] Throughout November, Nicolle cajoled Blanc. He sent salary estimates, promised Blanc that he would press for his appointment as *directeur adjoint*, and offered him power and independence. As a final incentive, Nicolle reminded Blanc of his duty to his former teacher: "My tireless efforts to augment this institute, its budget, its research, its personnel, were all done with you in mind."[90]

Carefully preparing his response, Blanc finally replied to nearly a decade of entreaties: "The profound affection I feel for you is the sole cause of the indecision I face. . . . In all sincerity I believe that the best thing I could do would be to remain in Athens." Working conditions in Athens, he explained, were more favorable; and, further, he wished to retain his own collaborators. Moreover, the very power and grandeur of the Tunis institute (he noted diplomatically) would fill his days with administrative responsibilities that would take away from his research. He would be reduced to a functionary. Finally, he touched upon an emotional issue that Nicolle was certain to understand: "The milieu worries me; I fear that it will depress me."[91] Nicolle attempted to counter Blanc's objections with logical arguments; still, Blanc remained in Athens. After Blanc's explicit rejection of the Tunis directorship, Nicolle's pleas became less frequent, but they never ceased. When Blanc agreed to leave Athens for the newly created Pasteur Institute of Casablanca, Nicolle mourned, "The soul of Tunis has been taken by Blanc to Morocco."[92] Even on his deathbed, Nicolle did not abandon his efforts to procure Blanc for Tunis, including his long-held wish in his final testament.[93]

Meanwhile, as Nicolle had explained to Blanc, the IPT continued to expand in structure and function. Its physical renovations and additions weathered the drop of the franc, and laboratory construction began in 1927. The next year, the laboratories had moved into the newly completed building.[94] The institute's extensions into hygiene, hospitals, and labs were highly profitable. The medical analyses the institute performed for hospitals and private doctors had increased substantially over the years, rising from 1,246 in 1905 to 33,610 in 1931 (see Appendix A). A law making smallpox vaccination (and revaccination) mandatory in Tunisia was decreed in the early 1920s and put into practice by 1926. The Pasteur Institute produced and distributed the vaccine. Before the law was enacted, the institute's annual vaccine production rose with epidemics and fell with their decline; afterward, it remained steady. Further, Nicolle combined production of his own vaccines—which he had distributed free of charge until they became popular—with Calmette's newly distributed antituberculosis treatment, BCG, into a separate service. He appointed daughter Marcelle, now herself a doctor, the service's director.[95]

To run this increasingly complex institution, Nicolle required an increasingly large staff. Coupling his staff size with his budget as evidence of his institute's success, Nicolle boasted (to a journalist) in 1932 that "there were four *garçons de laboratoire* [in 1903]; I now have forty."[96] Much of this staff expansion, like the rest of the institute's growth, occurred after the war. Numbers grew particularly among supporting staff: *préparateurs, aides préparateurs*, administrative staff, and "*indigènes*" (see Appendix B).⁹⁷ They were, Nicolle frequently bragged, quite well paid: the contrast with the Paris institute was always implied, if not stated. Indeed, his successful management was evident when one looked to the growth of his institute's budget as a whole: "When I arrived in Tunis, the Pasteur Institute's budget was 30,000 fr., all total; today, it is two million."⁹⁸

From this increasingly solid center, Nicolle continued to spin connections throughout Tunisia, expanding the medical cosmos he had first begun to organize twenty-five years earlier. Here, the contrast between the Nicolle of public speeches, who praised the collaborative constellation of doctors, pharmacists, and medical researchers that guided the provision of medical services in Tunisia, and the omnipotent (and increasingly omnipresent) orchestrator of Tunisian medicine that he revealed privately to trusted correspondents, is strikingly evident. In July 1928, Nicolle was delighted to have achieved a significant increase in his power over Tunisia's laboratories. That month, on the recommendation of the *Résident Général,* the Bey decreed that all laboratories wishing to perform medical analyses needed formal approval from the Direction Générale de l'Intérieur before they could undertake the work. Petitioners were required to submit their qualifications to a special five-member Commission des Laboratoires. The commission's two highest ranking members were Pastorians: its president was the Pasteur Institute's director, and its secretary was either one of its *chefs de laboratoire* or the assistant director. The other three members could also have been de facto Pastorians: one was delegated by the Direction Générale de l'Intérieur, over whom Nicolle had great influence; one was a physician of the Tunis medical corps (and we have seen evidence of his connections with this group); and one was a member of the Pharmacy Corps. Nicolle now effectively controlled all of Tunisia's medical laboratories. No analysis could be made, no serum produced, without his permission. The system resembled France's Serum Commission, with its centralized approval, strict inspections, and dictate that actual permission to carry out analyses be granted only to the *individual* who had applied. Nicolle had manipulated the French system to his advantage when he sought a market for his vaccines and Roux sat on the commission; now, in Tunisia, he was the one on whom power rested.

Nicolle had done much to adapt *his* institute to postwar society. Yet, there was more to a weighty counterforce than a well-functioning and well-staffed institute. Nicolle was acutely aware that researchers outside Paris, particularly those "overseas," had to work far harder to garner true international acclaim of the sort that would make even Paris take note.

Acclaim

There was nothing particularly "colonial" about the efforts of medical researchers to procure prestigious positions and awards. Still, colonial distance, both geographically and culturally, made such rewards more necessary to career advancement—but at the same time far more difficult to attain. Study of Nicolle's awards-related correspondence illuminates the elaborate system of connections, posturing, and etiquette that often underlay the false fronts of merit and objective assessment in the distribution of scientific honors. At the same time, it underscores the depth of the resistance that was a common part of any bid for acclaim made from "overseas."

As director of the IPT, Nicolle was responsible for ensuring that his collaborators—and even his former collaborators—received the recognition that he thought Paris owed them. He was particularly active on behalf of Georges Blanc, even after the latter had abandoned Tunis for Athens. Nicolle counseled Blanc about admission to the Society of Biology as he wrote to friends in Paris to ensure the election of his favored collaborator. He encouraged Blanc to seek the Prix Montyon, advising him about the best documents to send to their Parisian connection for the award, Félix Mesnil. For his Académie de Médecine bid, he was to write to Calmette, with whom Nicolle had already spoken.[99] Nicolle also intervened on behalf of Burnet's and Conseil's admission to the Académie de Médecine; Calmette promised to "use all the influence that I have" to realize Nicolle's wishes.[100] Despite increasing power struggles between Tunis and Paris, the Pastorians presented a unified front when approaching French societies for the admission and recognition of their own.

For his own part, Nicolle received three great honors in three consecutive years: the Osiris Prize of the Institut de France in 1927; the Nobel Prize in Physiology or Medicine in 1928, and an appointment as a nonresident member of the Academy of Sciences in 1929.

The Institut de France combined France's five grand academies, including the Académie des Sciences.[101] Every three years, it conferred the prestigious Osiris Prize to a worthy French citizen. In 1927, when the prize was awarded to Nicolle, it carried a purse of 100,000 francs.[102] Along with its more conventional perks, the prize also won Nicolle celebratory praise from two rather unexpected sources: Emile Roux presented the official report on his scientific work, and the city of Rouen gave a reception in his honor. Roux's report was a model of how to offer public praise for an individual one holds, privately, in far less esteem. He organized the report around the themes Nicolle himself had so carefully laid out over a decade earlier. At the heart of Nicolle's work was the louse transmission of typhus, his discovery of which had allowed him to make the disease "that used to visit Tunis annually, disappear." Then, the Great War itself verified Nicolle's theory: "The delousing of soldiers . . . preserved them from typhus. Everywhere delousing was practiced, typhus was held at bay." Indeed, during the war and in subsequent years, "final proof" was offered "in the thousands, or even millions, of lives that have been saved."[103] These were basic tropes for all subsequent presentations of Nicolle's typhus-related achievements.[104]

In recognition of its native son's recent honor, the city of Rouen held a celebratory ceremony at the Hôtel de Ville in October. Nicolle, who had always taken delight in observing ironies, did not miss the opportunity to remind his hometown audience of the opposition their city had shown to his efforts to accomplish there what he had gone on to accomplish in Tunisia: "It was in vain that I persisted. . . . I left Rouen, defeated in the project that I had planned and pursued over the course of eight years of thankless labor."[105] The Institut de France appeared to be less concerned with recognizing their prize's recipient. Though Mesnil had informed him in June that he had been awarded the prize, Nicolle still had received no official word from the Institut by December. Nor had he received his prize money. Mesnil again intervened on Nicolle's behalf. Eventually, he learned that the winners tended to be notified by their sponsors rather than by the institute. The money, however, appeared to have fallen between the cracks left by absent staff members. Finally, in January, the funds were made available to Nicolle.[106]

For his 1929 election as nonresident member of the Académie des Sciences, Nicolle again relied on the intercessions of his IPP-insider champion, Félix Mesnil. Mesnil, a member of the Académie's election committee, was well placed not only to work on Nicolle's behalf but also to keep him apprised of developments in election politics. Indeed, Nicolle only received his appointment after the Pastorians were able to defeat a challenge to their hegemony. From October to December 1929, Nicolle and Mesnil were in constant communication about a vacant position at the academy. Mesnil informed Nicolle about schedules, advised him what to send to whom, and recounted the intricacies of the election process itself.[107] Debates over the candidates—with Nicolle as front-runner—began in early November, and Mesnil asked Roux himself to present Nicolle's accomplishments to the Académie. Two other men, Camille Sauvageau and Lucien Cuénot, were also candidates for the position.[108] Although they supposedly did not pose a serious threat to Nicolle's chances, they were worthy enough of entry to the Académie that some members argued that the number of nonresident positions be raised from six to eight.[109] Before the elections, those who favored Sauvageau waged "a veritable campaign against the I. Pasteur . . . and all those in the biological world who didn't like us formed a bloc." Still, Nicolle, and the Pastorians, prevailed. That December, Nicolle was elected to the Académie des Sciences. Mesnil sent him the news, along with a list of those who had voted for him—so Nicolle could send them his thanks.[110]

The Nobel Prize was, however, particularly enticing.[111] It would confer not only a substantial financial award but also sufficient recognition to allow Nicolle (he thought) to do as he wished. With it, he might move beyond distant gravitational realignments and return to Paris armed with prestige and independence, to help redirect the Pasteur Institute at close range. After failing in his earlier bid, Nicolle saw his candidacy for the Prize again raised in 1927. This time, his confidence and his interventions increased. Already officially presented by the Swedish committee, Nicolle needed to be nominated by at least one of the designated faculties of medicine,[112] but was forbidden to campaign directly. He turned again, as he had in 1923, to Vallery-Radot: "I would be grateful if you would ask the members you know to nominate me. . . . Your intervention would persuade them and would win me more votes." The passage of time had done nothing to alter Nicolle's designs on how he would spend the prestige the prize conferred: "If the projects of which we have spoken are to take shape, this title would add a great deal of weight to the authority necessary for this new role."[113] Again, Nicolle was defeated.

In 1928, once more proposed, Nicolle was forced to lobby without his Parisian champion. The Paris Faculty of Medicine had decided to back Vallery-Radot's mentor, Fernand Widal—of the typhoid test—as its candidate. Though Widal himself had told Vallery-Radot that he felt Nicolle deserved the award, Vallery-Radot was torn.[114] Nicolle gracefully released him from any obligations and praised the accomplishments of his rival. Yet he did not hide his feelings about the faculty's preferences: "An official assembly can only choose an official person. Those who are isolated must learn that they can only count on themselves and on others like themselves."[115] Nicolle's resentment of Paris's treatment of French citizens living beyond its borders—those in the provinces, but more particularly those in France's colonial possessions—fermented with age. In Stockholm, however, his recurrent IPT visitor, John Reenstierna, remained a faithful advocate. Reenstierna wrote to Nicolle, in confidence, about the most recent Nobel-related proceedings. On November 23, 1927, Nicolle had been elected to the Swedish Royal Academy of Sciences as a *membre étranger*. The election had been unanimous. This, Reenstierna informed him, was a sign that Nicolle's time as a Nobel laureate had arrived: both Willem Einthoven and

Wagner von Jauregg had been similarly honored the year before they received the Nobel Prize.[116] Moreover, "the majority" of Reenstierna's colleagues shared his opinion "that you are more worthy than those who received the 1926 and 1927 prizes. Until now, you have been the victim of bad conditions and bad politics." This year, however, they would see justice done: "the winds are turning in favor of Nicolle."[117] A month later, Reenstierna wrote to Nicolle "very confidentially." His earlier suspicions had been correct: Nicolle was greatly favored for the 1928 Nobel Prize. To guarantee success, Nicolle had again to appoint a friend in Paris to lobby for his nomination by at least one other faculty.[118] The faculty that appointed him should specify that Nicolle be considered solely for his typhus work—"not for the totality of your work."[119] Moreover, Reenstierna's colleague was writing to Jules Bordet at the Pasteur Institute, to encourage him to work for Nicolle's nomination in Paris.

The international efforts on Nicolle's behalf finally bore fruit: he was awarded the Nobel Prize in October 1928. Congratulations came to Nicolle from all corners, and Vallery-Radot mixed best wishes with other aspirations: "for the vows I have made (you know which ones) this is an excellent thing: we must carry out our project. This is essential."[120] Roux even wrote words of encouragement, alluding "(for the first time) to [my] possible return."[121] Yet no offer from Paris was forthcoming. Tellingly, the Parisian journals barely acknowledged Nicolle's achievement:

> I received a stack of journals which, often without consistency, told of my work; the Parisian journals were the most reserved. The *Presse Médicale*, to which I have contributed, devoted a blurb to me in which my first name was cut, and my last lacked one "l." *Paris Médical* didn't mention anything at all. I do not see in these omissions any hostile intent, but instead the impression that only Paris counts and that Tunis, in the end, is not France.[122]

Appalled, Vallery-Radot tried to bring Paris's attention to its distant colleague's achievements by submitting a biographical article about his friend, but Nicolle was discouraged. Once again, it seemed, his accomplishments were overshadowed by circumstances beyond his control.

When the date of the ceremony arrived, neither Nicolle nor the winner of the prize for literature—Henri Bergson himself[123]—was present. Nicolle's heart problems had returned, and he was too sick to make the journey.[124] Instead, he sent a letter to Stockholm, to be read in his absence. In it, he drew attention to the people and circumstances that had allowed him to make his discoveries, playing up his colonial identity in the process. He was but "a worker in France's civilizing endeavor in North Africa." He had been aided in his work by a "devoted, if often obscure" collection of people who facilitated his daily efforts. Above all, he belonged "to the illustrious *Maison* . . . directed by Roux, and carrying the name of Pasteur." Even Normandy received mention.[125] His formal conference talk, however, set a very different tone.

Narrative Control

Nicolle had long dealt with the isolation he experienced as a result of external circumstances—an uncongenial hometown, a distant metropole, a faulty auditory system—through writing. By the 1920s, he had begun to think of his writings as tools he might use to alter those unwieldy external circumstances. "I can write and act at a distance," he reminded Vallery-Radot, "by force of the pen."[126] We have seen that Nicolle eagerly embraced the opportunity to recruit talented youngsters into the laboratory by telling stories of his own accomplishments. Over the years, he perfected his narratives, refashioning them in accordance with the ends he wished them to achieve. As he wryly commented to readers of his work on inapparent infection, the "history of scientific progress," as "told by scholars . . . is often a purely archeological, sterile endeavor. Exposed by those who lived it, it can serve as an instructive example."[127] Indeed, in that very same article, Nicolle presented the "history" of his discovery of inapparent infection as just such an example. What followed was a discovery narrative that took rather liberal license with actual events. He pushed the concept's origins back to 1911 and stripped it of all clinical connections (at least in initial formulation). Inapparent infection was, he repeated—almost in the fashion of a Greek chorus—a discovery of the *laboratory*.[128] Subsequently, however, this story would, like the Sadiki narrative, become another example of intuitive genius—all the while preserving the importance of observation and laboratory-based inductive reasoning in *preparing* the genius to make new scientific discoveries.

The telling of any story requires the selection of certain elements and the omission of others. Within the text of his Nobel speech, Nicolle did his share of selecting and omitting. The resultant narrative was itself a kind of mosaic of his past, rather than anything approximating an accurate representation of it. Having moved through some of that history as it was recounted when it happened, we will recognize certain pieces of that mosaic. It will also be clear how the telescoping of certain elements served Nicolle's more immediate purpose: to convey his achievements as the result of careful, observation-based inductions coupled with the intuitive leaps that were possible only for men of genius. He would give order to a disordered past, and glory to Pastorian (and personal) accomplishment, by embracing the cult of genius.

Nicolle had been awarded the Nobel Prize for the whole of his typhus work. His speech—as opposed to his letter—thus focused on *his* typhus work. Gone were the *elaborations* on clinical cooperation and other debts; favorite collaborators, though named and even frequently mentioned, never diluted the message that these were *Nicolle's* achievements. All his notable discoveries were in the first person. For the discovery of the louse transmission of typhus, "there was one particular thing that occurred in this hospital, the significance of which had never been appreciated, and which struck me."[129] For inapparent infection, "[the work] brought me to the conception that I named *Inapparent Infections*" (and, further, "this new idea of inapparent infections that I introduced into pathology is, without doubt, the most important of the findings it has been given me to make").[130] Most striking in its reconstruction of facts, however, was this portrayal of the realization that louse droppings transmitted typhus: "I demonstrated that . . . the droppings become virulent at the same time as the bite. This realization dates from 1910. Clarified by the more precise research undertaken with George Blanc, it guided those who looked for the agent of typhus in the intestines of the louse."[131]

As time passed after the 1909 typhus discoveries, Nicolle came to place far more emphasis on the demonstration of louse transmission than he did on his discovery of a viable experimental animal. Louse transmission provided him with three striking narrative options that, taken together, served to reinforce the importance, and genius, of Nicolle's work. These narratives have done much to structure his historical identity. First, there was the famous "Door of the Sadiki" discovery narrative, in which his intuitive genius is clearly displayed. Second, there were both the demonstration and practical consequences of the discovery, wrapped inside the story of how knowledge of louse transmission affected World War I. Finally—and Nicolle was only beginning to formulate this particular story in the Nobel speech—there was the great "lesson for civilization" that his discovery carried with it.

The "Door" account of his realization that the louse transmitted typhus is arguably Nicolle's most famous story: it is frequently recounted in histories of typhus and biographical sketches of Nicolle.[132] Emile Roux's 1927 Osiris presentation of a version of the story indicates that Nicolle had been *telling* it before he presented it in his Nobel audience.[133] Though the account became still more detailed in subsequent retellings, it took full form in the Nobel article as a true "epiphany" narrative of scientific discovery. In it, on some oddly unspecified date,[134] Nicolle is walking into the Sadiki Hospital during a typhus outbreak. More specifically, he is walking "over typhus-ridden bodies [*corps*]" of Tunisians awaiting admittance to the hospital. In the process, he thinks about the contrast between that waiting room, where typhus is commonly transmitted, and the hospital rooms themselves, where it is not. "This observation guided me." It guides him, in fact, to his sudden intuition: "The agent of the contagion was thus something attached to the skin, to the undergarments, which the soap and water removed. It could only be the louse. It was the louse."[135]

Gone, in this narrative, is any substantive reference to the painstaking work of Ernest Conseil, who established typhus as a problem "of Tunisia" and who listed the hospital observation as one of many examples that provided insight into the nature of typhus transmission. Gone, too, is Charles Comte, who had long been involved with typhus, the Sadiki, and Nicolle and Conseil. Later, as he was increasingly effaced from the story of Nicolle's discovery, Comte would claim that it was *he* who first came up with the louse hypothesis, which he shared with Nicolle.[136] In the Sadiki story, Nicolle selected from a number of events and observations that occurred over a number of years and brought those select elements together into a mosaic of scientific discovery. It was something to inspire the youth, to entice them to turn away from the clinic and toward the laboratory. The narrative itself, however, did not contain reference to the laboratory confirmation of the louse hypothesis. That piece of the story, where Nicolle's claims to priority are far less disputable, and where one actually *finds the laboratory*, only follows. It does not merit the romantic treatment of the discovery itself. After all, if the discovery is truly a flash of brilliance, then subsequent confirmation, though perhaps necessary, is a foregone conclusion.

In addition to reflecting an idealized self-image, Nicolle's narrative mosaic had particular power because it acted as a veritable miniature of the perceived relation of France to Tunisia. Typhus had long been banished from western Europe, but it remained endemic to North Africa. In Tunis, Nicolle was not stepping over typhus-ridden bodies at the Italian or the French hospital, but the *Tunisian* hospital, the Sadiki, where, in particular, the city's *poor* would have been taken. There were indeed European typhus patients at those other hospitals, but, presumably, they were not louse infested, meaning (on Nicolle's hypothesis) they were not transmitting the disease to their neighbors and doctors. The poor Tunisian patients were transmitting typhus freely until they crossed the threshold into a Westernized, sanitized hospital—and were themselves sanitized before being treated. Once across the threshold, they acted, at least with respect to contagiousness, like Europeans. What divided North Africa from a western European typhus distribution, then, was soap and water. The Door of the Sadiki literally separated the washed from the unwashed.

World War I showed the validity and significance of Nicolle's sudden typhus intuition. As Nicolle recounted the story,

> From the start of the war, measures were taken *on my advice* for overseeing the North African military contingents. No indigenous person left African soil for Europe without first having been deloused. It was this measure, applied by all nations in similar conditions, that saved armies from typhus. The multiplication of lice could occur in the trenches, becoming a veritable plague, without, for the first time in human history, typhus having accompanied a long war. If we hadn't known the mode of transmission of typhus in 1914, if the infected lice had been imported into Europe, it would not have been by bloody victory that the hostilities would have come to an end. It would have ended in a catastrophe without example, the most terrible in history.[137]

In this way, all knowledge of typhus—with the exception of the identity of its etiological agent—and all the benefits the application of that knowledge brought to humanity, came from the genius of Charles Nicolle.[138]

All this fed beautifully into the grand conclusion Nicolle drew from his typhus work, a conclusion that "would have pleased the great heart of Alfred Nobel." Here, the more subtle morality tale contained in the Door of the Sadiki story was made explicit: "Man carries on his skin a parasite, the louse. Civilization cleans him of it. If man degrades himself, if he approximates a primitive brute, the louse will again multiply and will treat the human brute as he deserves."[139] Nicolle would come to state that lesson with more poetry later, but it would remain the grand conclusion in all future tellings of his typhus story. It is my guess that it pleased the heart of Georges Duhamel as much as it would have pleased Alfred Nobel. It also reflected, and served to reinforce, Nicolle's beliefs about the importance of Pasteur's mission within the French "civilizing mission." Unfortunately, Nicolle's heart crisis grew increasingly serious well into 1929. Between his own poor health and continued Parisian neglect of his achievements, his window into potential action to fulfill those missions closed—for the time being.

Part Four

Synthesis
Mosaics of Power

6

Reservoir Docs

Birth, Life, and Death of Infectious Disease (1926–32)

> [It has] allowed us to demonstrate something no one else has shown: variations in the agglutinating power of the same microbe when placed under the conditions of different cultures. . . . of the same microbe in diverse conditions of life.
>
> —Nicolle and Trenel, 1902

> It is thus probable that, in the course of their progressive attenuation, of their obliteration, infectious diseases have passed, pass, and will pass, through inapparent forms. . . . The first and the last stage in the life of diseases, . . . inapparent disease is the unsuspected reservoir of many evils.
>
> —Nicolle, *Naissance, Vie et Mort des Maladies Infectieuses*, 1930

Laboratory manipulation of the virulence of pathogenic microbes had been a central component of the birth and life of Pastorian microbiology. Pasteur and his disciples had fashioned their assorted vaccines by exposing microbes to a variety of changed environmental conditions—heat, cold, air, and so on. They had also found that passage through animal hosts tended, eventually, to restore such artificially diminished virulence.[1] Given this practical focus on microbial malleability (along with other cultural and certainly personal factors), it is unsurprising that Pasteur did not himself come up with a formula for a strict, "one microbe produces one disease" specificity. Pasteur and Koch roughly agreed on microbial specificity; Pasteur was simply willing to admit more flexibility *within* a species. Mazumdar has argued that it was Pasteur's disciple and successor at the institute's helm, Emile Duclaux, who attributed the "discovery" of disease specificity to Pasteur.[2] In fact, as Geison notes, although Pasteur's interest in the manipulation of microbes did not go so far as challenging the borders of their "species,"[3] he was, in *theory,* willing to push the borders of disease species still further, even suggesting that the relationships between hosts and parasites evolved over time—and that there would be *new* diseases. Emile Roux also raised the possibility of disease evolution in his *Cours;* however, neither he nor Pasteur pressed it much further.[4] Charles Nicolle did.[5]

In 1930, Nicolle published his classic treatise on disease evolution, *Naissance, Vie et Mort des Maladies Infectieuses* [*NVM*].[6] He wrote much of the book while recuperating from his long illness in 1929. In the text, the invisible forces of inapparent infection and inframicrobes found central positions—as did his father's natural-historical inclinations and his brother Maurice's immunological models. The directing roles of genius and mutation were beginning to come to the fore. Nicolle placed all these elements within an understanding of "nature," "civilization," and "disease" that was deeply influenced by the ideas of Georges Duhamel. (Duhamel, for his part, certainly encouraged Nicolle to reach out to a broader audience by writing just such a book.[7])

It was his recent return to relapsing fever research, however, that appears to have given Nicolle the remaining pieces he needed to bring his ideas together: starting in 1926, he and his collaborators at the IPT began to investigate the relations of louse-borne and tick-borne relapsing fever. As the relapsing fever work was drawing to a close in 1931, Nicolle was drawn once again into debates about typhus fever. This time, however, international attention focused on the relations between the well-known louse-borne form of the disease, and the newly recognized flea/rat, "murine" variety. In both the relapsing fever and the typhus studies, questions about reservoirs, and about the possible evolutionary influences of host upon microbe, were hotly contested and actively investigated. The typhus work, as we shall see in the next chapter, would lead Nicolle to extend, adjust, or complete many of the ideas he had worked out in *NVM*. Yet, it was relapsing fever work—work that resonated with ideas he was grappling with more generally—that brought him to his first effort to set disease in an evolutionary framework.

Return to Relapsing Fever

Nicolle began exploring the relations between louse-borne and tick-borne relapsing fever as early as 1912. Blaizot, Blanc, and dark-field microscopic study of spirochetes in lice may have brought him to consider the evolutionary development of microbes and inframicrobes, but his own long-standing natural-historical interests in disease led him to look for evidence of the relations between the two known varieties of relapsing fever.[8] He was particularly interested in the interepidemic reservoirs of the disease. If humans were the sole natural reservoirs of louse-borne relapsing fever, and if lice had only limited capacities to transmit the infection to their own offspring,[9] how did the disease survive between outbreaks? Nicolle and his colleagues began scouring Tunisia for nonhuman reservoirs of the disease; in the laboratory, they attempted to pass the tick-borne strain through a louse—presumably to determine whether such passage might explain the relations between the disease forms, and thus the interepidemic reservoir. In 1912, their efforts failed.[10] When, in 1926, Sadi de Buen published his findings on Spanish relapsing fever, Nicolle immediately returned to his relapsing fever studies: Europe, which generally housed the louse-borne variety, now had a tick-borne relapsing fever. He hoped its analysis would answer some of his unanswered questions.

Nicolle and Charles Anderson fed lice on monkeys infected with the Spanish variety of relapsing fever, then crushed the lice and inoculated them into an uninfected monkey. Ten days later, the monkey displayed a fever and had spirochetes in its blood. "This experiment," they noted with qualifications, "shows that . . . Spanish relapsing fever can be transmitted *experimentally* by lice as well as by ticks [*ornithodores*]."[11] Although such experimental transmissions did not prove that lice transmitted the disease in nature, they did suggest that the Spanish form might be "placed between the tick fever, which only ticks can transmit, and the global relapsing fever that is transmitted by the louse." Were this hypothesis to be demonstrated, Nicolle argued, it would suggest the path by which the two disease types had evolved in nature. The original form of relapsing fever was local and endemic. Borne by ticks, and closely adapted to local tick species, it tended to remain localized. Then, by chance, lice became infected by the disease's causal spirochetes. Gradually, they became infected more readily, even "conserving and transmitting" their own, unique form of the disease. The louse, unlike the tick, was "subject to the same movements as those who carry them." In short, Nicolle concluded his evolutionary hypothesis, "this change of host turned an endemic infection, attached to the conditions of central Africa, into a global, epidemic disease."[12]

Back in 1912, when Nicolle first proposed his interpretation of how the spirochetes of global relapsing fever escaped from infected lice, he believed the path to be an "absurd" exception among an otherwise fairly natural order of things. Subsequent experience, in a variety of realms, had led him to suspect that such absurdities were not as exceptional as he had thought. His return to relapsing fever, and particularly his work from 1927 to 1929, confirmed these suspicions. Certain details of the Spanish relapsing fever transmission were particularly convincing. Sadi de Buen had determined that the ticks transmitting the disease belonged to a particular species that fed on pigs. One would logically suspect that, given the disease's subsequent transmission to humans, the pigs themselves acted as its reservoir.[13] They did not. Perfectly refractory, the pigs' only role was to feed the ticks, which, quite independently, conserved and transmitted the disease. Nicolle and his colleagues, while studying the Spanish variety in the lab, had found that rodents were particularly susceptible to infection. They hypothesized that "rodents in the [pig] stables commonly acted as the reservoir of the disease."[14]

Though the Tunisian Pastorians had difficulty persuading the Spanish researchers to undertake a systematic examination of such rodents in nature, Nicolle suspected that rodent reservoirs offered a more general explanation for the historic relations between presently fixed types of relapsing fever. By 1927, he was convinced that there were indeed three distinct "groups" [*groupes*] of relapsing fever: traditional tick-borne, associated with the Duttoni spirochete; global louse-borne, with its "Recurrentis" or "Obermeiri" spirochetes (the choice of term depending merely on researcher preference); and the Spanish intermediary form, whose spirochete was increasingly referred to as "Hispanicum." Drawing upon the recent findings, Nicolle assembled a broad evolutionary description of the history of relapsing fever as a whole.[15] Originally, the disease infected small mammals and was "transmitted from one to the other . . . by an ectoparasite that may or may not have been a tick." This type of relapsing fever could, indeed, still be found in parts of Africa. Next, specific ticks intervened in the cycle, conserving the virus; eventually, the tick passed it on to the larger mammals on which it tended to feast. These mammals sometimes were, and sometimes were not, susceptible to the disease. It was only after the disease was thus established that history witnessed "the intrusion of humans." The human-tick coupling gave rise to the tick-borne variety of relapsing fever that came to be recognized in central Africa. Next, then, came the entrance of the louse into the process, much in the fashion that he had hypothesized the year before. Eventually, the louse-human variety, transported around the world in louse-infested humans, became relatively fixed in type as "global" relapsing fever. The Spanish variety gave evidence of the intermediary stage in the disease's last two evolutionary steps.[16] Nicolle spent little time speculating about evolutionary mechanisms, but he did suggest that it occurred either by "adaptation . . . over the course of years, or by mutation."[17]

In the course of this work, Nicolle came to embrace explicitly a view of nature that he had been developing over many years. We use *reason*, he noted, to understand the workings of nature. Our mistake is in thinking that *nature* employs reasonable methods.[18] Reason would suggest that the pig acted as the reservoir of Spanish relapsing fever; reason suggested that louse-scratching was an unlikely path to the perpetuation of a disease. Reason also tended to interpret the human form of a disease as, in some way, that disease's "true" end. Reason, when it came to nature, was often wrong. The "genius" of nature, Nicolle reminded his readers, lay simply in the production of numerous variations within a temporal framework large enough to permit numerous, if chance, meetings between such variations.[19] Medical researchers had to be *biologists*. "In our opinion," he urged, "one must think of infectious disease as being in a constant state of new trials. The characteristic of life is a tendency towards adaptation and dis-adaptation, in accordance with the frequency or rarity of contacts between entities that chance circumstance brings together or keeps apart."[20]

Nicolle's relapsing fever research, then, challenged his medical and philosophical presuppositions; at the same time, it both expanded and challenged cherished social assumptions. Nicolle had long believed in international scientific cooperation. We have seen that, after World War I, he had grown increasingly critical of the way Paris (or, the IPP) *directed* such cooperation between its institutes. What was needed, he believed, was a more fully cooperative exchange. Relapsing fever research presented an excellent opportunity to explore how such exchange might occur. By the late 1920s, it had become clear that there were nearly as many tick-borne varieties of relapsing fever as there were geographic locations where it was found.[21] Thorough study of the relations between these varieties brought together researchers working in France, Spain, Tunisia, Morocco, and Dakar, all exchanging samples and interpretations.[22]

At the same time, Nicolle discovered that his cooperative ideal faced challenges when put into practice. His earlier hypothesis about a rodent reservoir of Spanish relapsing fever had gone untested, despite his requests to his Spanish colleagues that they follow it out in the field. Finally, he and his colleagues found a variety of relapsing fever in Morocco that resembled the Spanish form. Nicolle felt compelled to comment. Discovery of the Moroccan strain would make it far easier to find a solution to the questions that we have posed in vain to our Spanish colleagues. Morocco is an African country, a French protectorate. There, we have colleagues of great merit who we also consider to be our friends. Not only were they interested in the goals we were pursuing; they even conducted some of this research personally.[23]

At this same time, negotiations for an IP de Casablanca were well underway. In 1932, the new institute opened, with Georges Blanc as its first director. Further close collaboration with the IPT was thus assured.

In 1927, Nicolle wrote a speculative essay that linked (ultra)microbial findings and clinical expressions of relapsing fever, then set the results in an evolutionary framework. He prefaced the article by confessing his enthusiasm for the lessons he had learned from the disease: "We do not wish to fall into the bad habits of certain historians. Prisoners of the often mediocre personality that they have elected to study, they come to see in him an excessive importance; they seek and discover certain merits and influences that he never had."[24] Still, over the years, Nicolle had come to see relapsing fever less as an absurd exception to the workings of nature, and more as a window into how diseases actually worked: "Relapsing fevers are separated from other diseases by traits that at first seem special, but in which we come to see more clearly phenomena of a general order that are less easily seen in other infectious diseases."[25]

While conducting research on the evolutionary relations between the three groups of relapsing fever, Nicolle was also continuing his vaccine research with Conseil and Hélène Sparrow. Gradually, his theoretical considerations about relapsing fever and his reflections on vaccine production and function came together, shaping his broader thinking about the nature of disease: relations of visible and invisible stages of spirochete evolution, their connections with each disease group, and their varying relations with virulence, informed Nicolle's ideas about cures, immunity, and curative vaccines. Late in 1927, Nicolle wrote a general article on dosage in curative vaccines that helped bridge the gap between his practical and his theoretical work.[26]

Nicolle continued to follow Pastorian tradition by including, within the broad framework of "vaccine," both *preventive* and *curative* substances. "Preventive" vaccines, as had been successfully produced by attenuating virulence, and as Nicolle was attempting to produce by reproducing inapparent infection, received only cursory treatment here. The main reason Nicolle seems to have included them, beyond wishing to present the full range of vaccinating possibilities, was to underscore how they *differed* from curative vaccines. Preventive vaccines were meant to provoke an *immune response* in otherwise *healthy* individuals, so those individuals would remain healthy. Curative vaccines *cured*. Immunity would follow—*if* the disease itself conferred immunity. Nicolle was convinced that curative vaccines were being made too strong by people who conflated immunity and cure.[27]

This difference established, Nicolle turned to his main subject: curative vaccines.[28] We have seen that his work on inapparent infection rested on his separation of *virulence* and *symptoms*, and that this separation, despite the claims he made in retrospective historical mosaics, appeared in publications from 1919. In 1920, Maurice Nicolle's Harben Lectures on antigens and antibodies were published.[29] In them, the eldest Nicolle divided the pathogenic power of an infective microbe into the combination of two powers: toxicity and virulence. Maurice used virulence here much as did brother Charles in his conception of inapparent infection: as an *adaptive* power. This was an uncommon, but not unheard of, distinction.[30] It was *toxicity*, rather than *virulence*, that Charles Nicolle believed to be central to the proper function of curative vaccines. Charles and Maurice may not have been speaking, but, when the younger Nicolle was in search of an immunological model that would help him synthesize his research, he did not hesitate to draw upon his brother's work. Interestingly, he did not credit Maurice for this model until he used it again in *NVM*.

Nicolle started his consideration of curative vaccination—"vaccinotherapy"—with empirical observations. Curative vaccines, resting as they did on toxic inoculations, were dangerous. Though they had often worked, no one quite understood why. One way to limit the dangers posed by curative vaccination was to understand its nature and function more clearly.[31] Answers to questions of nature and function, however, were held within that nebulous and highly contested disciplinary realm known as "immunology." *How* did the host body get well; how did it subsequently resist second attacks of some of those diseases? These were precisely the questions Pasteur was trying to answer when he brought Metchnikoff to his new institute in the late nineteenth century. In the intervening decades, schisms, particularly between the more structurally inclined Germans and the more functionally (biologically) inclined French, turned into wars that even phagocytes might have studied for tactical lessons.[32] It was generally agreed that answers to these mysteries were contained somehow in the interactions between "antigens" and "antibodies." Antigens were cellular substances that disease-causing microbes appeared to provide to the bodies they infected. They seemed to have no single physical nature, but quite a number of them, apparently specific to a number of diseases, had been discovered by 1927. These antigens *somehow* provoked the host body's formation of "antibodies," which in turn were central to the host's defenses and to any subsequent immunity.

Despite the number of unanswered questions in this formulation of antibody production, it was relatively straightforward—to this point. "Specificity" greatly complicated matters. It was evident that one type of vaccine did not cure all diseases, and that immunity to one disease did not confer immunity to all. The body's defenses, like infectious disease itself, appeared to be specific. Where was this specificity located? Nicolle, following his brother, located it in *antigens* rather than in the invading microbe as a whole. "Antigenic power" was essentially equivalent to, and perhaps even identical to, *toxicity*.[33] And it was toxicity, *not virulence*, that was at the heart of vaccinotherapy, for it was the specific antigen that was also specific to cure.[34] Though avoiding direct reference to Maurice's organizational metaphor,[35] Nicolle essentially followed his explanation of how cure was produced. Invading microbes and effective curative vaccines alike contained both the specific antigen and other similar but nonspecific substances. The nonspecific substances were in themselves "without power, or of only banal power." The specific antigen conferred upon the neutral substances "power or direction; rendered them active." The functional metaphor is striking: "The small quantity of specific antigen contained in the sick organism on account of the struggle it is engaged in against the invading microbes—this very small dose, furnished to it by its assailant—may suffice to direct the harmless antigens, contained in nonspecific bacterial products," to create specific antibodies.[36] Specific toxic power, within the invaded body, became a kind of leader of the body's own defenses, directing its troops to create the very forces—the antibodies—needed to ensure the survival of that host body. Curative vaccines acted, when properly produced and introduced, to supplement the body's own response. This was particularly important when the disease reduced, or even paralyzed, the body's ability to produce antibodies in this fashion.[37]

It was while he was in the midst of this conceptually challenging work on vaccines and relapsing fever that Nicolle was forced to deal with his own failing health. Like the persistently adaptive microbes that so fascinated him, Nicolle used this externally enforced "opportunity" to good advantage.

Disease Dynamics

> "Pasteur came, like Prometheus, bringing light to our darkness, order to chaos.... Fifty years after Pasteur's discoveries, does this foundation remain unassailable?"[38]

In 1929, the cardiac crisis that had prevented Nicolle from attending the Nobel ceremonies escalated: by March, he summoned his wife, Alice, to his bedside. Pierre, too, came to Tunis to be with his ailing father. It was during this illness that Nicolle began to write his memoirs. Although he would return to them several years later, when he again fell seriously ill, he would never take them, chronologically, beyond the early years of his medical training.[39] He also began in earnest a writing project he had long planned: a three-part philosophical study of the nature of disease, creativity, and "nature" (including human nature). The first volume of the series, *Naissance, Vie et Mort des Maladies Infectieuses*, was published early in 1930, the same year that his final novel appeared in print.[40] He dedicated the philosophical treatise to the memory of his father.

Without pressing too far into psychological realms, one can see in *NVM* an effort to reconcile the teachings of father Eugène and intellectual father Pasteur: Nicolle drew upon both to establish his own separate identity, for all the world to see. (The book was meant for a general, educated audience—and if it attracted the young to study experimental medicine, so much the better![41]) *NVM* brought natural history and medical microbiology into a proximity that may not have been wholly unique for the time, but had rarely before been examined systematically. The effect was to set infectious disease into evolutionary motion. Not only in individuals and epidemics, but also through history, diseases were "born," "lived," and "died." Pasteur and Roux may have preached the possibility that new diseases could emerge and old ones disappear; however, neither man pressed beyond the constraints of specificity—even if more loosely defined than the German variety—to consider how this might occur. Thus Nicolle, having laid out the basics of infectious disease theory, needed to attack accepted notions of specificity to make room for his own modifications. Moreover, he underscored several times that "reason and logic" alone could not determine modifications like the ones he was making: "If it is a question of a leap forward, a true discovery, it is imagination, intuition, that provides it."[42] In this way, alongside making his case for a more biological understanding of infectious disease, he was also making the case for his own genius.

Nicolle's attack on "Pastorian" specificity came only after he had sung its praises. Pasteur, "like Prometheus,"[43] had brought light to humanity—in his case, as the concept of specificity, which he had developed while studying fermentations and then "carried . . . into the world of infectious diseases." Specificity had allowed doctors "not only to find the cause of each disease, but to clearly separate one infection from another." It was the very foundation of medical microbiology.[44] Yet, it was also fifty years old. Did this foundation still "remain unassailable, does it conform to the known facts?"[45] He raised the question because he knew that it did not. Even during his years in Rouen, Nicolle knew that microbial specificity was not an absolute law. He had personally conducted research on typhoid and paratyphoid and examined how changing environmental conditions could alter the functions of microbes. In subsequent years, studies of microbial colonies demonstrated that they could be structurally varied as well.[46] Moreover, the same pathogenic agent might produce different diseases, and the same disease might be caused by different agents.[47]

Did this mean that specificity had been wholly overturned? Not quite: "We would be poorly advised to deny that specificity has its value. Our mistake is in locating it improperly." Specificity was not an attribute of the whole microbe, but only of "certain substances that compose it." It was "the antigens that, in combination, confer individuality on each microbe." As he had in his 1927 paper, Nicolle continued to think of the antigens within any particular microbe as both specific and nonspecific. Now, however, he offered a metaphor to describe their structural arrangement. It was a familial metaphor: "My older brother Maurice Nicolle defined a microbe as: a *mosaic* of antigens. With this representation," Nicolle proclaimed, "everything is explained."[48]

The "mosaic of antigens" was the structural locus of specificity. Among its component parts were the antigens that elicited a specific antibody response in the host organism. Yet, there were those many other antigens, some even associated with other microbial species, that were also present. In the end, the defining element[49] of a pathogenic microbial "species" was the very diverse array of antigens within the mosaic. An individual microbe belonging to that pathogenic "species," however, could, and would, exhibit slight variations from the idealized norm in the component parts of its own mosaic. "Species," therefore, did not *really* exist. There were only closely related *groups* of individuals, and it was these that we *called* "species."[50] (Here, again, one sees the influence of Nicolle's work on that highly individualistic set of diseases referred to as "relapsing fever.")

Nicolle pressed the evolutionary interpretation still further. The accepted classification of pathogenic microbes was itself relative, a product of the doctor's "point of view. . . . We are naturally brought to think of the agents of disease from the perspective of their pathogenic properties. We classify them in accordance with these properties."[51] Still, "a well differentiated microbe, highly pathogenic and highly toxic . . . is only the most representative type, to our eyes, of a vast botanical group." The microbes of that "botanical group" displayed a number of characteristics besides those associated with a possible "mosaic of antigens," and all of them "were modifiable . . . according to the conditions of existence of the microbes."⁵² In short, while disease specificity—the connection of microbial species (or group) with specific disease—might not be lost, it had been displaced: not only from microbe to mosaic, but from an apparent absolute, to a relative, quality. With Maurice's mosaic, microbial specificity could be salvaged, but only by placing it within a still broader evolutionary frame.

To this structural mosaic of antigens, the microbe's "pathogenic properties"—its toxicity and virulence—were attached in some as-yet-unspecified fashion. Nicolle continued to insist that toxicity was the "harmful" component in the interaction of microbe and host, and that virulence was the force that aggressively adapted microbe to host. "If a disease invades us," he observed, "it is a consequence of the ability of the microbe to profit from all circumstances. When it adapts itself to an animal species, this property becomes particularly aggressive; it merits the name *virulence*."⁵³ He appears to have assumed some close connection between toxicity and virulence but, again, did not specify the nature of that connection.⁵⁴ By the time he revised *NVM*, he would offer a fuller description of these processes and relationships. For the 1930 text, however, they were sufficiently detailed to serve his immediate purpose: to challenge "Pastorian" specificity so as to open a path for his theories of disease evolution.

This relatively lengthy prelude complete, Nicolle set to work presenting his understanding of the birth, life, and death of infectious diseases. He applied this developmental cycle to disease in its three principal manifestations: in the sick individual, in epidemic outbreaks, and in broad historical trajectory. His principal focus was, as one might expect, on the historical dimension of disease. Moreover, "history," in the epistemological sense, took its place next to "experimentation" in providing evidence for Nicolle's interpretation of each developmental phase of each manifestation. Experimental knowledge was, for Nicolle, consistently more revealing than was the evidence of history.⁵⁵ Yet, higher than both laboratory experiment and historical observation was intuitive genius. While informed by both lab and field, it was a qualitatively different way of knowing: "the revelation of a new fact, the leap forward, the conquest of that which was unknown yesterday, is an act, not of reason, but of imagination, intuition; it is an act closer to that of the artist or the poet, a dream that becomes reality, a dream that seems to create."⁵⁶ After describing individual disease, but before turning to epidemics, Nicolle detailed inapparent infection: both the concept and his discovery thereof. While preserving the experimental and observational elements of his earlier narrative, he now described the discovery itself as an epiphany: "It was then that I had the intuition of what was happening."[57] Throughout the book, he would use inapparent infection as a window into the workings of nature. Nicolle had finally found a way to integrate his literary and scientific inclinations.

The life cycle of disease in individuals is described quite briefly, reading mostly as an opportunity for Nicolle to review some of his own findings and set up subsequent sections. At the "birth" and "death" of individual disease, we find relapsing fever providing essential insights.[58] Consideration of disease birth serves, among other things, as an opportunity to emphasize the essential divide between human reason and nature's workings. How are diseases transmitted to humans? Nature does not merely follow paths we perceive to be natural; it also takes advantage of any opportunities it is presented. To illustrate this point, Nicolle held up the example of the mechanism of global relapsing fever's transmission: the tendency of louse-infested humans to scratch at the pests, breaking off their legs and antennae and, in the process, liberating the infective spirochetes that otherwise would have had no exit from the lice. It was, for the disease, a "fortuitous accident, wholly unconnected to any physiological necessity," demonstrating clearly that "there is no intelligence, no logic on the part of nature." That such chance occurrences, repeated over the centuries, sufficed to perpetuate the survival of a disease was, he thought, quite impressive.[59]

The "death" of disease in an individual had more than one meaning. At spectral ends were, of course, literal death and complete cure (ideally, the latter with immunity to further attacks).[60] Between these extremes lay chronic illnesses, relapses, and cyclical crises. Nicolle drew heavily on battle rhetoric to describe this final death match, with the human body becoming the "theater of struggle."[61] Once again, relapsing fever provided Nicolle with the substance of his discussion. Relapsing fever had been named for the disease's tendency to recur in the suffering patient. In each cycle of sickness, improvement came only after a dangerous crisis. This, he argued, was explained by the developmental cycle of spirochetes themselves: a cycle that he himself had done much to uncover.[62] He noted, as he had in his 1925 article on inframicrobes, that he and Georges Blanc had used an ultramicroscope to follow spirochetes in the course of their development in the louse. The microbes developed similarly in humans. Shortly after infection, the spirochetes disappeared from the blood—and all was quiet in the human (or louse) host. In truth, Nicolle argued, the spirochetes had fragmented into bits too small to be seen under any available magnification. Fragmentation itself was a mode of rapid multiplication: out of the fragments emerged tiny spirochetes, barely visible but highly virulent. Indeed, so virulent were these young microbes that they rendered the host body helpless. It could produce no antibodies in response: "Disarmed, it remains passive, it reacts no differently than an artificial culture medium."[63] This process translated into the host's "crisis."

The spirochetes' initial success, however, became their (temporary) undoing. In this defenseless host medium, they thrived, continuing to develop beyond their tiny young forms into the fully grown bacterial forms with which they were most commonly associated. Nicolle provided a more detailed explanation of this process than he had in 1925. In its adult form, "the spirochete returns to its ancestral state, in which it was an externally dwelling microbe, stripped of pathogenic power—a simple saprophyte."[64] Ontogeny recapitulated phylogeny in the cyclogenic development of the microbe. The saprophytic state achieved, the microbe's defenses were down and the body sprang into action, creating the antibodies to destroy its invaders. The host recovered—or, more accurately, appeared to recover. Gradually, the antibodies disappeared from the blood, and the spirochetes that had remained invisible (or otherwise hidden in the body) during the first wave now took virulent form, leading to a second attack. The process often repeated a third and fourth time before the host finally recovered.[65]

In itself, Nicolle's account is interesting for the insight it offers into his understanding of the diseased body as a kind of battlefield that had the capacity, under only certain conditions, to participate actively in the disease war. It becomes more interesting still in his attempts to generalize the process beyond the spirochetes of relapsing fever to "other diseases that terminate in a crisis"— and then, perhaps, still further: "It is possible that an analogous mechanism secretly intervenes in the cure of all infectious disease. The relapsing [fevers] are the only ones in which microbial changes and the techniques of observation can instruct us on the secret technique of certain cures."[66] Nicolle believed that invisible virulence, like invisible disease (inapparent infection), unveiled the hidden workings of nature. It was no coincidence that he laid claim to bringing both these invisible entities to light.

Nicolle's dedicated section on epidemics is still briefer than his treatment of disease in individuals. He avoided the debates of epidemiologists in the United States, Britain, and Germany on the causes of epidemics, presenting instead what he knew from personal experience.[67] Epidemic birth had two components: microbial virulence and environmental/social conditions. Epidemics were born when "the virulent properties of certain pathogenic microbes are carried to an extreme or contamination is favored by a great ease and number of contacts."[68] He elaborated on both possibilities, noting the role of potential disease reservoirs such as susceptible children and individuals who lost immunity, and of "collective suffering (wars, famine, misery)," in the transformation of a disease from endemic to epidemic.[69] Yet, amid and beyond all these quite valid explanations, "the part of inapparent infections appears to us to be great, probably predominant."[70] He reviewed the recent evidence that men such as Ramsine and Blanc had offered in support of his thesis.[71] Moreover, inapparent infection was a significant factor not only in a disease's epidemic manifestation, but also in its interepidemic conservation: "inapparent cases form a chain from one season to the next, permitting the conservation of the virus and the return of epidemics." Their clinical invisibility allowed them to pass unnoticed, making them "the most dangerous" form a disease might take.[72]

Nicolle returned to the creation of epidemics at the conclusion of his section on the birth of historical disease. More specifically, he turned to two counterbalancing examples of the intentional human creation of an epidemic. On the one hand, as Pasteur himself knew, epidemics could be used for the "destruction of harmful species."[73] On the other, they might be used as weapons of warfare.[74] Nicolle would develop his thoughts on the ability of human knowledge to be used for good and for evil particularly in the final book of his series, *Nature*.

In his considerations of both the birth and the death of historic disease species, Nicolle opened with the ever-limited evidence provided by historical documentation, then turned for more effective illumination to laboratory teachings:

> [W]e have at our disposal two methods: the first . . . is the historical method, the study and critique of documents; the second is offered by experimentation, and allows us to come to see, if not new diseases, at least the new modalities of diseases, giving us some justification to suppose that events took place at some earlier time in nature in the same way they take place today, in our hands.[75]

The study of history substantiated the idea that new diseases had appeared.[76] Laboratory investigations suggested how such new diseases might have emerged. Laboratory teachings, however, were not all equally able to disclose the actual workings of nature. Frequently, if not explicitly, Nicolle presented earlier Pastorian evidence to this end as inferior to the discoveries he and his colleagues had made.

There were several experimental investigations that suggested the paths that microbes had followed in becoming pathogenic. Indeed, the laboratory study of disease itself rested on one such path: the "extension of an infectious disease to a species that never suffered it in nature." From rats and rabbits to guinea pigs and monkeys (Nicolle naturally mentioned the example of typhus), the determination of viable experimental animals was necessary to much of the microbiological research that had been conducted.[77] Researchers had also successfully adapted, or witnessed evidence of the adaptation of, pathogenic microbes to invertebrates that did not originally transmit a given disease. (He used relapsing fever in ticks and then in lice as an extended example.)[78] Then, there were the virulence-related interventions. He and his collaborators had induced symptoms in animals that otherwise experienced only inapparent infections.[79] Similarly, naturally refractory animals had been infected by either decreasing their natural resistance—simulating "misery" and related conditions—or by augmenting the pathogenic activity of the microbe.[80] Relatedly, the Pastorians had successfully restored virulence to microbes they had experimentally attenuated by inoculating it in sensitive animals. "If we had not known the origin of the inoffensive microbe whose virulence was restored," Nicolle observed, "the creation of virulence, and thus the creation of an infectious disease, would be considered a proven fact."[81] Still, the fact remained that "no scientist has thus far been able to boast of wholly creating [*se vanter d'avoir crée de toutes pièces*] a new infectious disease."[82]

The key to understanding the birth of new diseases was to remember that all microbes were "living beings," constantly striving to "perpetuate their lives by profiting from all available circumstances." Ultimately, "infectious disease is only the adaptation, wonderfully realized, of certain specimens from an immense populace of infinitely small and inoffensive organisms to superior beings. . . . It is one of many ways to conserve life." In this process, "the adaptation of a microbe to an animal species is called virulence."[83] Here, Nicolle used "adaptation" to describe both the gradual adaptive process long described by evolutionists and the more recently discovered process of mutation. His descriptions indicate that he saw adaptation of the gradual type as the product of chance adjustments to changing environments, which were passed along to microbial offspring.[84] Over time, the relations between host and microbe became closer, and, eventually, the process we call disease "clothed" itself in its "costume" of symptoms.[85]

Nicolle had already noted that the Pastorian process of restoring virulence had never managed to turn a saprophyte into a pathogen. Now, without actually reminding readers of these limitations, he showed how his own experimental knowledge reached beyond them. The understanding of inapparent infections, he argued, might well reveal nature's methods: "While it would be impossible (and probably always will be thus) for us to demonstrate the fact, it is plausible that before revealing itself through clear symptoms, disease often cloaks itself, at least in its first expression, in an inapparent form."[86] Regardless of the actual mechanism, or mechanisms, of disease birth, conclusive proof would remain elusive. By the time we suspected the creation of new diseases, "they would already have been formed. . . . They will appear as did Minerva, springing forth fully armed from Jupiter's brow."[87]

Although it was no more likely to offer final *proof* of how new diseases emerged, there was another route microbes might take in their move toward pathogenic existence: mutation. Nicolle was clearly intrigued by this "rapid change in character": "One might wonder if the very small [*l'infiniment petit*— the microbes] also acquire virulence . . . by such rapid adaptation."[88] The man who had set aside his research on bacterial transformations nearly three decades earlier now returned to it as his career neared its end.[89] There was, Nicolle believed, strong evidence in bacteriology itself that mutations occurred in nature. The development of certain vaccines appeared to be the product of fortuitous mutations. Jenner's own smallpox vaccine—the very model of a "virus-vaccine"—was most probably the product of just such a mutation. Again, the Pastorian corrective was implied rather than stated. By the time he wrote *Destin*, Nicolle would take his evidence for mutation from the creation of the rabies vaccine itself.[90]

Finally, but without specifying an underlying mechanism, Nicolle described the possible relations between the bacterial change toward virulence—disease birth—and the methods by which bacteria reproduced themselves. To do so, he returned to his inframicrobes. In this framework, normal microbial (transverse) division was supplemented by another mode of multiplication: "transformation into granules." Spirochete studies again provided evidence. Recounting (and condensing) his earlier paper on the relations between visible, saprophytic bacterial forms and virulent invisible forms, Nicolle now offered an interpretation with broader implications. Perhaps this microbe-inframicrobe relationship "that we observed, we demonstrated for the spirochetes, might occur in other bacteria"—perhaps even "in all."[91] In support of this hypothesis, he argued for the plausibility of an evolutionary relationship between microbes and inframicrobes, underscoring the increasingly close adaptation between the two as one climbed the evolutionary ladder. With the ultramicrobe, "its adaptation [to its host] has become so perfect that it can neither revert to its [ancestral, bacterial] form nor live outside the animal organism (it cannot be cultivated on artificial media) or even infect animal species other than the one to which it is accustomed [*accoutumé*]."[92] At the very least, Nicolle concluded, one had to admit that the "acquisition of pathogenic properties by microbes is often accompanied . . . by visible changes in their structures and in their modes of multiplication."[93] Yet again, his own work acted—he believed—to illuminate the workings of nature.

As he had proceeded with the birth, he now proceeded with the death of historic disease. History gave evidence that certain diseases, such as syphilis, had diminished in severity over time. The laboratory offered far more detailed examples of diseases, diminished. Pastorian attenuation experiments for vaccine production led the list and, Nicolle asserted, showed "that a microbe can progressively lose its virulence."[94] Still, the many methods by which the Pastorians had attenuated virulence, though "excellent" for the "practical" purposes of "vaccine production, cannot explain how diseases naturally weaken and disappear."[95] Might broader human efforts to suppress individual and epidemic disease appearances throw more light on the subject? Nicolle listed the various methods that had been developed to contain disease. Thanks to medical laboratories, there was now a wide array of vaccines and antiseptic substances; hygiene emphasized the importance of cleanliness; and lab and field came together to suppress insects and disease reservoirs.[96] These human efforts, particularly in combination, had secured impressive success in the control of disease and, consequently, in the improvement of human health. Yet, for the most part, "it was hardly such means that nature, without human intervention, used to bring about the death of disease." Such efforts were the "fruit of intelligence and rested upon logical technique." Indeed, only preventive vaccination came close to following nature's path.[97]

How did disease "die" in nature? If laboratory experiments on variable virulence could shed some light on disease birth, they could do little to illuminate disease death: Nicolle argued that it was quite unlikely, even by mutation, that all microbes of a pathogenic group would suddenly lose their virulence.[98] Inapparent infection, on the other hand, offered a plausible explanation. Nicolle's "intuitive" grasp of inapparent infection during World War I had, in fact, followed his observation that typhus expressed itself in a spectrum of symptoms, from dire to benign. He (through Conseil) had further noted that populations long stricken by typhus—populations that tended to act as endemic reservoirs—generally suffered only mild symptoms of the disease. When considering nature's "path,"[99] he argued, the only imaginable possibility was that disease death occurred through "the repetition of this disease through many generations of individuals within a susceptible species, over the course of long centuries." Referring to these as "hereditary attacks," Nicolle reminded his readers that "we have demonstrated, through the example of typhus, that an increasing resistance is conferred to races that are continually stricken."[100] Eventually, those perpetually stricken peoples would lack symptoms altogether. In short, inapparent infection offered a plausible picture of how nature acted:

> It is thus probable that, in the course of their progressive attenuation, of their obliteration, infectious diseases have passed, pass, and will pass through inapparent forms. We see the capital importance of these recently discovered forms [of infection]. The first and last stage in the life of diseases . . . inapparent disease is the unsuspected reservoir of many evils.[101]

Once again, the laboratory—Nicolle's laboratory—illuminated the workings of nature itself.

In writing *NVM*, Nicolle claimed that it was his intention to demonstrate that disease was a biological phenomenon. He would then show what that meant for the evolution of disease, on a variety of levels. Within this stated project, however, Nicolle had other, less explicitly acknowledged, intentions. We have seen abundant evidence that he was attempting to establish his place as the New Pasteur: starting with the defining elements of Pastorian identity, he believed he had improved upon them, given them new direction and scope. Time and again he held up his own research on invisible disease (inapparent infection, via typhus) and invisible virulence (inframicrobes, via relapsing fever) as tools that made visible the workings of "blind" nature.[102] This personal mission intersected quite nicely with important elements of his revised conception of how the "Pastorian mission" itself might be achieved. Yet, in its beginning, its ending, and woven in between, the story of the birth, life, and death of infectious disease attached Pastorian mission to "civilizing mission" in a way that illuminates Nicolle's own evolving ideas about the future of disease and of civilization.

In Nicolle's formulation of disease, the infected body acts as the bridge, both conceptually and physically, between blind nature and human civilization. It is the point of perpetual connection, the justification—indeed, the imperative—for understanding as fully as possible how nature works. Scientific knowledge might "arm" humanity in its "battle" against disease;[103] the values of civilization, such as cleanliness, would further shore up defenses. Ultimately, however, the human body itself was the battlefield on which this perpetual war was waged. If human civilization did not call upon all its resources, scientific and hygienic—if it permitted the spread of misery, through warfare or the persistence of poor living conditions—the forces of nature would emerge victorious. Typhus fever provided an excellent example of this dynamic.[104]

Typhus was a disease that science (*his* science) had shown to be well within human control. Humans were the only natural reservoirs; lice, the only agents of transmission.[105] Western hygiene, which had controlled louse infestation, had effectively banished the disease from western Europe and parts of North America. Yet, endemic reservoirs remained in China and "certain regions of civilized countries—or countries considered to be so: Slavic countries; Mexico. From these bastions," Nicolle argued, "all humanity is menaced." The threat came less from occasional contact with individuals from outside those foyers than from certain *uncivilized* tendencies of "civilized" society itself.[106] Typhus recurred with "the extension of the collective suffering of humanity: famine, revolutions, and wars." This was the "moral lesson" of typhus from the Nobel speech, sharpened:

> Typhus presents itself to us as both a plague and a moral lesson. It tells us that man has only recently emerged from barbarity, that he still carries on his skin a disgraceful parasite such as brutes themselves carry, and that, when man conducts himself like a brute, this parasite, by multiplying and inoculating him with typhus, will prove, in effect, that he is merely a brute. The disappearance of typhus will only be possible on that day when, wars having disappeared, the work of a collective hygiene will suppress the louse. Humanity will only know this immense progress when it merits it. Will we ever merit it?[107]

With his good friend Georges Duhamel, Nicolle feared that humanity's capacity for wisdom would always be checked by its baser instincts.

Near the start of his treatise, Nicolle argued that there were "only two praiseworthy conquerors: the teacher and the doctor." All else in colonialism was "enrichment, augmentation of power, pride, sport and crime, awaiting the just returns of all offenses to natural laws: the rivalry of other nations of prey; the depopulation, and thus the ruin, of conquered regions; hatred, revolt and the extension to the vanquishers of all the diseases of the vanquished."[108] Near the end of his treatise, he warned of the dangers that threatened human health if "human civilization were to go into retreat; if peoples less civilized but more prolific" took us into "a new Middle Ages." In such hypothetical future worlds, the "human factor" in disease control would be suppressed, and "the future of infectious disease would belong solely to nature."[109] The preservation of civilization was necessary to the preservation of human health: excellent motivation for aspiring microbiological missionaries.

Nicolle's views on civilization were shaped before, during, and after World War I. He both despaired of the possibility of human progress and believed that it was our only chance at salvation. In 1930, he allowed his optimism to direct his book's conclusion: "We must trust in those who will follow us. Peaceful and better, they will increasingly know how to defend themselves, how to protect their own and the animals useful to their lives, against the Dantesque, but unintelligent and undisciplined, mob, of infectious diseases."[110]

Typhus, Recurrent

Shortly after *NVM* appeared in print, Nicolle suffered the loss of the man who had helped him lay the foundations of his typhus work: Ernest Conseil died in June 1930. In the funeral oration for his collaborator and friend, Nicolle confessed: "Our efforts have been united for twenty years; our ideas are so closely intertwined that I myself no longer know, in our work together, what belonged to whom."[111]

At that same time, typhus was returning to the international spotlight. The geographic center of the controversy was one of Nicolle's "bastions" of typhus: Mexico. Mounting evidence was strongly suggesting that typhus etiology was not as settled as it had seemed. The typhus of Mexico—commonly referred to as "tabardillo"—was producing laboratory results that conflicted with what was characteristic of the more traditional disease strain. Researchers had found, on following Mexican typhus into the field, that there also seemed to be epidemiological differences. Soon, investigations reached back in history to anomalous earlier findings and outward internationally to typhus experts in the United States, France, North Africa, Switzerland, and Poland (to take just a sampling). The question: What was the relationship between typhus of the Old World and typhus of the New World? Between 1928 and 1934, interpretations and terminology shifted frequently. Tangled inside this international research question were equally pressing questions about the nature of the relations between disease species, the mechanisms (or vectors) by which disease was altered—including the role of disease reservoirs—and the evidence one needed to make such determinations. Epidemiologists, bacteriologists, and pathologists attempted to answer these questions—and often came up with different, even conflicting, answers.

Nicolle had learned of these developments by late 1928: Harvard bacteriologist Hans Zinsser told Nicolle of the "New World" typhus discrepancies in the very letter he sent congratulating his French colleague on winning the Nobel Prize.[112] Nicolle, who was in the middle of relapsing fever research (on quite similar questions) and was about to be incapacitated by illness, did not immediately enter into the North American debates. Initially, he was suspicious of the findings that suggested that there were two distinct typhus varieties.

Given the emphasis he had placed on the louse as the sole vector of typhus (and, from this fact, on "typhus as moral lesson"), it seems a natural skepticism. By the time he joined in the investigations, however, he was inclined to believe that there were indeed two, naturally fixed groups of typhus. His research turned inclination into conviction. The remaining years of his active research Nicolle devoted to typhus. This second round of typhus work would also supply him with ideas about how to extend his earlier work on the destiny of infectious diseases.

The return to typhus that started in earnest in 1928 with questions about typhus varieties may have wrapped up active research on these questions by around 1934 (when Zinsser published pieces of his forthcoming book *Rats, Lice, and History* in the *Atlantic Monthly*); however, it quickly became connected to an active international competition to find a viable typhus vaccine. Some of this research drew on Nicolle's ideas—and on those of his colleagues. Georges Blanc, Hans Zinsser, and Rudolf Wiegl all developed competing vaccine options.[113] Nicolle, too, continued to be interested in vaccine production; however, during this return to typhus, his most significant work was on typhus varieties and their implications. The typhus vaccine work itself continued past Nicolle's death, finding particular relevance (and some resolution) during World War II.[114]

The story of typhus varieties, though escalating in the 1920s, was closely connected to certain anomalies that had been noted, but not developed, earlier. These anomalies had been discovered not in North Africa, but in North America. They would converge again in North America by 1934, with an understanding of typhus varieties that was largely in accord with Nicolle's own ideas but that, at the same time, challenged the significance of inapparent infection in maintaining endemic typhus reservoirs.[115]

In the 1910s, two U.S. medical researchers made separate, but ultimately related, observations that raised questions about the identity of typhus. Nathan Brill, the American expert diagnostician who in 1898 had employed the then-new Widal test to demonstrate that his patients were *not*, in fact, suffering from typhoid, returned to these mysterious cases in 1910. The return had particular relevance for typhus studies.[116] Then, in 1917, United States Public Health Service (USPHS) doctor M. H. Neill published the results of his laboratory study of typhus fever in Mexico.[117] The two men interpreted their findings similarly. Only in the next decade, however, would their evidence, and their conclusions, be appreciated.

In the decade after he had determined that his patients, most of whom were Russian immigrants, were not suffering from typhoid, Brill continued to compile information on similar, subsequent cases. Then, in 1910, he attempted to solve the mystery. Working at New York's Mount Sinai Hospital and armed with notes from 221 cases, Brill now suggested that the infectious disease of "unknown origin" bore a striking clinical resemblance to typhus fever.[118] Yet, because "Brill's disease," as it was dubbed, did not share the severe nervous symptoms of typhus, was rarely fatal, and showed no evidence of louse transmission, he was not convinced that his disease was, in fact, typhus fever.

Searching for further evidence, Brill took his suspicions to the laboratory (specifically, the clinician turned to colleague Reuben Ottenberg's laboratory).[119] He had monkeys inoculated with blood taken from a case of his eponymous disease, but failed to transmit the infection: all the monkeys remained healthy. Brill speculated on the possible significance of this negative trial by drawing upon earlier experiments that had been carried out in Tunisia and Mexico. On the one hand, Charles Nicolle had failed to inoculate monkeys directly with blood taken from human typhus patients: for successful animal transmission, he had first needed to inoculate chimps, then use the infected chimp blood to inoculate monkeys. On the other, John F. Anderson and Joseph Goldberger, working for the USPHS in Mexico, *had* successfully inoculated a monkey directly with human blood. The differences between the Mexican and Tunisian experiments led Brill to speculate that typhus differed in the two locations: "our experimental work in inoculating monkeys has at least so far established a fundamental difference between this group and Mexican typhus."[120] He pressed his analysis still further. If Brill's disease was, in fact, of the Old World variety, then how did so dire a disease as typhus become as "mild" as the disease he had been studying? Again, he offered a hypothesis: his patients might be suffering from "an attenuated modification of the virus of typhus." Such "attenuation in virulence" might have been "induced by environment and improved sanitation to such a degree as to change to a great extent the clinical characters of typhus fever and the biological nature of its infectious agent."[121]

Meanwhile, Anderson and Goldberger read Brill's 1910 paper and were intrigued. The pair were at that time "engaged in the study of Mexican typhus fever and, having the picture of that disease clearly in our minds, we were struck by the very marked clinical resemblance between it and the disease described by Brill."[122] They decided to conduct their own laboratory studies of Brill's disease. Using samples from Mount Sinai, Anderson and Goldberger succeeded where Brill had failed. Not only were they able to infect monkeys directly with the New York blood; they were also able to determine that monkeys inoculated with the New York strain, and monkeys inoculated with the Mexican strain, exhibited cross-immunity. They interpreted the positive results of this "cross-immunity test" as demonstrating that the two similar strains were, in fact, identical.

Anderson and Goldberger published their findings in 1912, and most medical researchers (and clinicians) considered the matter closed. The researchers in Mexico had shown that Brill's disease and Mexican typhus were identical; up in New York, it was evident that Brill's Russian patients—immigrants from an active typhus reservoir—were suffering from the European strain of the disease. Following the evidence to its logical conclusion, there was only one variety of typhus. Nicolle was among the convinced majority.[123] Brill was not. Indeed, the American cited the recent work of Pastorian Elie Metchnikoff on cross-immunity in typhoid and paratyphoid to support his doubts. "There is a great difference," Brill sagely argued, "between kinship and identity of disease."[124]

Brill finally joined the majority opinion in 1915. His student Harry Plotz had just identified what he believed to be the causal agent of typhus, and found that same organism in Brill's patients. The clinician made a dramatic farewell speech: "I stand now prepared to chant a requiem or speak a funeral oration over so-called 'Brill's Disease.' "[125] Still, he continued to wonder why one form of typhus should be "masquerading in strange garments."[126] Perhaps "some other agent than the body louse must be looked for to explain the origin and spread of the mild form of the disease."[127] Others, considering the matter closed, simply accumulated instances of "Brill's disease," which quickly became the name given to almost any mild expression of typhus that appeared in the United States.[128] There was thus severe, epidemic typhus and the milder, endemic typhus, also known as Brill's disease. It was believed that they were, in fact, expressions of the same disease.

This was the conceptual climate in 1917, when M. H. Neill observed something strange about Mexican typhus in the laboratory. It was known that when Rocky Mountain spotted fever, a disease related to typhus but transmitted by ticks, was inoculated into male guinea pigs, the animals displayed scrotal lesions. Though no such lesions had been noted in animals inoculated with typhus, Neill decided that the similarities between the two diseases merited investigation. When he tried the experiment, he found scrotal lesions on the guinea pigs inoculated with typhus. He then conducted similar tests with Brill's disease, but could find no lesions. This might be explained, he conceded, by the mildness of the disease.[129] He did not push the observation further than implication, choosing instead to focus on the similarities between Mexican typhus and Rocky Mountain spotted fever. Neill's observations might have passed wholly unnoticed by typhus researchers if Harvard pathologist S. Burt Wolbach hadn't addressed them.

Wolbach, who had led the U.S. typhus mission to Poland, further established his reputation as a leader in typhus research with his 1922 book on the disease (and the mission).[130] Wolbach, who was also working on Rocky Mountain spotted fever, dismissed Neill's findings.[131]

Questions as to the unity of typhus began to be raised again, quietly, with the work of another USPHS doctor, Kenneth F. Maxcy. In 1926, Maxcy reviewed more than two hundred cases of "mild" typhus that had been reported in Alabama and Georgia over a three-year period.[132] Weil-Felix tests made it clear that the patients were suffering from typhus. Yet, there were important clinical and epidemiological differences between the cases observed in the southeastern United States and the typhus known in the Old World and in Mexico. The former were milder and dramatically less fatal, and there was no evidence of louse transmission. Indeed, as with Brill's disease, cases tended to appear in the summer and autumn, as opposed to the springtime epidemics of more traditional typhus. For these reasons, Maxcy called the disease he had been studying "endemic typhus (Brill's disease)."[133] He did note that his cases, unlike Brill's patients, "*occurred in native-born white Americans.*"[134] Reflecting on the possible significance of his findings, Maxcy raised the question of typhus identity. While Anderson and Goldberger's conclusions on the subject seemed "to have been quite promptly and generally accepted," he now had some doubts.[135] What might one make of the differences between Brill's disease and classic (i.e., Old World and Mexican) typhus?

Of all the clinical and epidemiological differences that he had observed in his typhus cases, Maxcy was most perplexed by the strange absence of any evidence of their louse transmission. Before he could entertain the possibility of vectors beyond lice, he had, at least in a logically structured article, to account for any alternative explanations of the observed phenomena. One such explanation might be found, he noted, in Charles Nicolle's recent theory of inapparent infections: perhaps Maxcy had missed evidence of a continued cycle of human-louse-human transmission preserving the disease, because human sufferers had been suffering from inapparent infections? Maxcy found this explanation most unpersuasive. There was "little evidence to support" Nicolle's hypothesis beyond an "analogy with what occurs when certain rodents are inoculated with the virus in the laboratory." The epidemiologically inclined American commented dismissively: "The response of human beings to infection naturally acquired can hardly be compared with that of rodents artificially inoculated."[136] Further, although Maxcy believed that the louse transmitted typhus between humans during epidemics, he was unconvinced that humans—inapparently infected or otherwise—were the natural, interepidemic reservoir of the disease: "Human carriers of typhus virus have never been demonstrated, and from present knowledge it seems quite unlikely that they exist."[137] Maxcy's reasoning lay at the heart of the forthcoming debates on the nature of typhus. To what extent *could* laboratory evidence speak to how nature acted?

More immediately, Maxcy was concerned with the transmission of his mild typhus cases. He pointed out that Brill had observed a similar absence of louse transmission for his New York cases and had hypothesized that "some vector other than the louse might . . . be concerned in the transmission."[138] Maxcy followed up on this hypothesis. He eventually found evidence linking his endemic typhus to people in food-handling occupations. Then, noting the disease's epidemiological similarities with plague in the United States, as well as its classification in a disease family characterized by animal reservoir-tick vector transmission, he speculated that "a reservoir in rats or mice, with accidental transmission to man through the bite of some parasite or blood-sucking arthropod, is compatible with the epidemiological characteristics which have been revealed by this study."[139] Zinsser would later praise Maxcy's work as a "classical example of the manner in which epidemiology carefully carried out can point the direction for laboratory efforts."[140]

Two years later, a Swiss bacteriologist/pathologist working in Mexico, Herman Mooser, also returned to unresolved typhus questions.[141] Zinsser, who was soon collaborating with Mooser, commented that he had a "mind like a bell and the temperament of a Gatling gun," and was "one of the best scientific observers with whom it has ever been my good luck to cooperate."[142] As Maxcy had returned to Brill, Mooser returned to Neill, and his neglected paper of 1917. Neill's observation of scrotal lesions in guinea pigs inoculated with the Mexican typhus "so far has never been confirmed by other investigators." Mooser confirmed it.[143] Having done so, he predicted that "the finding of these lesions will probably revive in Mexico the old dispute on the nosological entity of the European typhus and tabardillo."[144]

These investigations may have remained an interesting academic aside, had Mooser not come across Maxcy's epidemiological studies of "endemic" typhus. In fact, Mooser came across Maxcy himself during a visit to the United States Hygienic Laboratory in Washington, D.C.[145] He found that the guinea pigs Maxcy had inoculated with a typhus strain from Georgia exhibited scrotal lesions. Mooser was decisive in his conclusions: "I do not hesitate, therefore, to separate Mexican typhus and the endemic typhus in the Southern States of the Union as a variety distinct from European typhus." There appeared to be two distinct varieties of typhus, after all:

> [T]he disease has been known in Mexico since the early days of the Spanish occupation and is called *tabardillo*, a name imported from Spain, but it seems now that only the name was imported and that the disease itself was already endemic upon the arrival of the conquerors, because the characteristic scrotal lesion has never been observed in guineapigs inoculated with Spanish strains or North African strains.[146]

Maxcy had classified the typhus of the American southeast as "Brill's disease" largely on the basis of its mild symptoms. Mooser disagreed with the conclusion: "Typhus has become rather a harmless disease, in Mexico too, during the past ten years, and there is no reason for changing its name because the mortality has dropped from over 25 per cent. to less than 5 per cent."[147] By the end of 1928, Mooser was certain that Brill's disease, as observed in New York, was in fact an importation of the European variety of typhus, quite separate from Maxcy's "endemic" strain. Scrotal lesions had never been observed on guinea pigs inoculated with Brill's *actual* disease.[148]

Maxcy's epidemiological investigations, coupled with Mooser's pathological studies, would indeed reopen the debate over the unity of typhus strains. Mooser's work suggested that there were two separate varieties of typhus; Maxcy had hypothesized that a rat or mouse reservoir, in combination with a vector other than the louse, fitted with epidemiological evidence for mild typhus in Alabama and Georgia. Early in 1931, R. E. Dyer, also with the USPHS, traced sporadic cases of typhus among food handlers in Baltimore to a rat reservoir.[149] Shortly thereafter, Hans Zinsser traveled to Mooser's laboratory, where the two led the search for naturally occurring rat reservoirs of Mexican typhus. With the aid of an expert rat-catcher, they soon had their evidence.[150] Moreover, the rat-flea was agreed to be the culprit in the transmission of rat typhus to humans. Maxcy's hypothesis was confirmed, and Mooser's assertion that the typhus endemic to native-born Americans in the United States was identical with tabardillo was given further credibility. However, questions about the relations between the typhus of Mexico and the southeastern United States, with its milder clinical expression and its rat-to-flea transmission cycle, and the classic, louse-borne form of the disease, remained unanswered.

Mexican Typhus Goes to Harvard—and Travels Abroad

Shortly after Mooser and Maxcy met in Washington, Maxcy left the USPHS for a faculty position at the University of Virginia. From Mexico and Virginia, the two, separately, began sending samples of their respective typhus strains to Harvard. Both samples even went to the same medical school building. Maxcy's, however, went to Wolbach's Department of Pathology, whereas Mooser's—along with his research assistant, M. Ruiz Castaneda—went to Zinsser's Department of Bacteriology and Immunology.[151] There, the samples were studied, separately, by pathologist Henry Pinkerton and by Zinsser himself. The two men weighed the available evidence (clinical and epidemiological differences, the Weil-Felix test, cross-immunity, rickettsial distribution in experimental animals) in accordance with their strongly differing assumptions about disease and the laboratory, and published their conflicting interpretations, eventually in issues of the same journal, from 1929.[152] A fair and concise statement of the differences between their positions was later given by two members of Zinsser's department:

> The point at issue has been whether the observed discrepancies represented temporary modifications of a single type, comparable to the reversible dissociation of bacteria and dependent upon passage through different animal and insect hosts, or whether each variety had become irreversibly fixed in the biological sense.[153]

Pinkerton held the temporary modification position; Zinsser, the biologically fixed varieties position.

Henry Pinkerton had come to Wolbach's attention when the latter was looking for people to take with him to study typhus in Poland. Soon thereafter, the Harvard pathologist brought him into his department. Wolbach described Pinkerton as "extremely modest, thoroughly conscientious, very persistent and resourceful in his research work."[154] It was Wolbach's guinea pig observations that Mooser had directly questioned, and Pinkerton responded to Mooser's charges. Pinkerton focused exclusively on the rickettsial agents and their distribution in guinea pig bodies to determine the relationship between typhus strains. In his initial 1929 article on the subject, he sought to demonstrate, quite in contrast with Mooser's interpretations, that the difference between rickettsia localization in the two typhus strains was one of degree and not of kind.[155] Pinkerton particularly challenged Mooser's hypothesis of a qualitative typhus strain difference by finding typhus rickettsia in the scrotal sacs of guinea pigs inoculated with Old World typhus. There was, he argued, an inverse relationship between scrotal lesions and brain lesions: a severe scrotal reaction precluded brain lesions, whereas a mild scrotal reaction allowed rickettsia to multiply in the brain. Even in a collaborative study with Maxcy,[156] Pinkerton did not look beyond the laboratory in his argument for disease identity. Cross-immunity demonstrated the essential identity of the Old and New World typhus, and the presence of rickettsia in both the scrotal sac and the brain of guinea pigs inoculated with either strain provided further confirmation: there was only one kind of typhus.

Zinsser, the future author of typhus's "biography," looked at the disease quite differently, and interpreted his laboratory evidence accordingly. He argued that such quantitative and localized etiological differences as Pinkerton discussed, if regular, might be fixed. They might thus indicate a divergence of one species into two distinct varieties: "possibly the accidental channels of transmission, determined in different regions by variations of the rodent and insect fauna in contact with man, may have influenced the development of differing disease types."[157] Zinsser's two-variety interpretation thus approximated Nicolle's understanding of the evolutionary relations between naturally distinct relapsing fever groups. Nicolle, as we have seen (and despite Maxcy's critique), looked constantly between field and lab for evidence in support of his theories. Soon, typhus labs, including Zinsser's, would be testing the viability, and the fixity, of just such host-related conversions. In the meantime, however, Zinsser was hoping to call upon the expert witness of his Nobel Prize-winning friend, Charles Nicolle, to support his two-group interpretation of typhus.

Zinsser had been in correspondence with Nicolle since 1915, when the two were slated to be in Serbia together. They finally met in 1927, when Zinsser traveled to Tunis.[158] The American would assert in his 1940 autobiography that, were he a believer in an afterlife, "the thought of death would be considerably mitigated for me by the expectation of seeing again—among others—Charles Nicolle, and renewing for a piece of eternity those summer evenings at Sidi-bu-Saïd" [sic].[159] Their friendship is evident in their regular exchange of letters that ranged over a variety of topics and returned frequently to their shared interest in the evolution of disease. Indeed, Zinsser dedicated *Rats, Lice and History*, "in affectionate friendship to Charles Nicolle, scientist, novelist, and philosopher."[160] Zinsser was particularly interested in how study of rapidly multiplying microbes could provide firsthand information about the evolutionary process. This shared evolutionary interest, along with their shared, if separate, experience of the devastation wrought by typhus epidemics, informed both men's approach to evidence about the relations between typhus strains.

Shortly after departing Tunis in 1927, Zinsser received his tabardillo samples and his new collaborator (Castaneda) from Mooser and quickly confirmed Mooser's findings. Indeed, Zinsser was so fully convinced that tabardillo represented a type distinctive from Old World typhus that he was already referring to the rickettsia of the former as "Mooser bodies."[161] Nicolle, at a distance, was unpersuaded. He had held that there was only one variety of typhus for years. Zinsser took it upon himself to engage in direct, trans-Atlantic "technology transfer." His confirmation of Mooser's work had

> depended, among other things, upon a method of preparation which was not very easily repeated. The French had failed in confirming us and Nicolle, with whom friendship played no role when it came to scientific opinion, had written a paper casting doubt on our findings. Correspondence was unsatisfactory, and the matter fundamental. So I took passage on the *Ile de France*, packed the instruments I needed for inoculation en route, and carried a hamper of a dozen guinea pigs (disguised as an ordinary handbag) into the ship. . . . Nicolle was easily convinced, and generous in saying so.[162]

Still, Nicolle did not immediately enter into the debates.

Meanwhile, the connections between lesions in laboratory animals, symptoms in suffering patients, and epidemiological disease vectors and interepidemic reservoirs, grew more complex. It seemed that mild, endemic typhus could *become* epidemic. Endemic and epidemic typhus appeared on occasion to exist simultaneously—or were they the same thing? Adding to the confusion were those who continued to refer to all mild cases of typhus as "Brill's disease." Meanwhile, there was the persistent problem of the interepidemic reservoir of "European" typhus (that is, the typhus of Europe and North Africa).[163] As Nicolle was proudly publishing accounts from eastern Europe of humans inapparently infected with typhus, North Americans continued to express skepticism as to their existence—and their ability, if they existed, to explain how typhus was conserved between epidemic outbreaks. Perhaps it was as simple as the rat reservoir. Perhaps there was but one form of typhus that existed endemically in rat reservoirs. When conditions in human society deteriorated, and people became famished, war-torn, and louse-infested, the disease was transmitted, unnaturally, between humans by those lice, becoming more virulent in the process.

Nicolle could hardly stay out of the debate, especially when, in 1931, another opportunity for travel to the New World was presented to him.[164] Early that year, Mexico's Minister of Health had invited Nicolle to come work on typhus, promising him a place at the Institute of Hygiene, a supply of all requisite laboratory materials, and even an assistant (if not a salary).[165] The French Ministry of Foreign Affairs provided Nicolle with steamer passage. Passage was subsequently extended, with some additional negotiation, to Nicolle's collaborator of choice: Hélène Sparrow.[166] By this time, Sparrow was not only Nicolle's primary collaborator on typhus, but also his mistress.

Although it is clear that Nicolle and Sparrow did not spend the whole of their time together in Mexico working on typhus, they did conduct a great deal of research in Mooser's laboratory. Soon, they confirmed his "remarkable work," writing a joint article on their findings shortly after their return to Tunis.[167] Mooser, Sparrow and Nicolle confirmed that the Old and New World strains cross-immunized. In Nicolle's words—echoing brother Maurice's— they shared a "community of antigens." Yet, the two typhus varieties did not appear to be identical. Although they were still "the same disease," they were, Nicolle believed, "dissimilar in several details."[168] Rats, in the laboratory and in nature, were central to his two-typhus convictions.

Rats were among the experimental animals that Nicolle and Sparrow were testing in Mexico. They knew that rats inoculated with typhus in Tunis suffered only inapparent infections. In Mexico, inoculated with tabardillo, they displayed a brief but clear febrile infection.[169] Moreover, typhus-infected Mexican rats had been found *in nature*. Of all the new evidence about typhus in Mexico, this discovery impressed Nicolle the most. It was "a point of the greatest importance . . . whose significance, at once general and practical, should not be underestimated."[170] The discovery raised questions about the nature and extent of the rat's role in typhus conservation, and its influence on the disease's epidemic distribution. A fuller understanding of these matters might illuminate something of the origins of typhus itself. If rats suffered symptoms from New World typhus, but exhibited only an inapparent infection with Old World typhus (a point, he stressed, that also needed confirmation in nature), it would suggest that the Old World variety was, in fact, *older*: "Inapparent forms of infectious diseases are doubtlessly forms in the process of disappearing." Mooser, they noted, argued the opposite. Because Old World typhus was so fatal for the louse, the louse must be a recent addition to the epidemiological cycle, making typhus, in its distant origins, a disease of *rats*.[171] In a follow-up article, Nicolle and Sparrow suggested that the occurrence of both forms of typhus be sought throughout the world's typhus zones, and mapped.[172] Soon, "New World" typhus was found to exist in seaports throughout the world—including Greece, Tunis, and Australia. The evidence seemed only to complicate matters further.

1931, in Tunis

Nicolle returned from his Mexican typhus trip in time to celebrate his sixty-fifth birthday. It was an active year for the aging bacteriologist. He had finished writing *Biologie de l'Invention*, his follow-up to *NVM*, in which he elaborated on his ideas about the biology of genius and the role of the genius in civilization.[173] The veterinary services he had been lobbying to create since becoming director of the IPT were finally attached that May. Lucien Balozet was appointed Director of Veterinary Services and, with Charles Anderson, assistant director of the IPT. Finally, Nicolle's institute could take over the production and sale of the veterinary vaccines and serums, previously made at the Institut Arlong.[174] The IPT's full autonomy was now assured. And, though Nicolle's wish to see Sparrow officially attached to the institute as *chef de laboratoire* was not realized until 1933, she was often present at his side, personally as well as professionally.

In other excellent institutional news, Jean Laigret was appointed as new *chef de laboratoire* that June. Laigret came to the IPT with an impeccable colonial/Pastorian résumé. He had been a student at the École Principale du Service de Santé de la Marine et des Colonies before receiving his MD (at Bordeaux) in 1919. He had then spent four years between the Institutes Pasteur in Brazzaville and Saigon before becoming a doctor in the Service d'Hygiène in Dakar, then *chef de laboratoire* in French Sudan. With Laigret on board at the IPT, in combination with Balozet heading up veterinary services, Sparrow lending typhus expertise, and Anderson's administrative skills, Nicolle was finally well pleased with the whole of his institute. Moreover, Laigret would soon offer Nicolle further substantiation—through vaccine studies—of the importance of inapparent infections. It was work that further enhanced the international reputation of the IPT.

Laigret had been in Dakar during the 1927 yellow fever epidemic. The epidemic had brought Harvard bacteriologist A. W. Sellards to Dakar as well, where he met with Constant Mathis, director of the IP of Dakar (who had also been working with Nicolle on relapsing fever), and the local French military hygiene director, Laigret.[175] Their bacteriological mission was to confirm the precise nature of the mosquito responsible for the epidemic. Using a serum sample drawn from a young Syrian man, Sellards successfully transmitted yellow fever to mosquitoes, then, subsequently, to susceptible monkeys. This sample, taken from a *Syrian* man in Dakar by an *American* bacteriologist at a French-*colonial* Pasteur Institute, was dubbed "the French Strain" and distributed to research laboratories from Paris to New York to Rio de Janeiro. Back at Harvard, Sellards passed this strain on to his colleague Max Theiler,[176] who passed it through white mice. (Laigret claimed that the idea to undertake the experiment was his.[177]) After numerous mouse passages of the strain, it could, Theiler found, infect monkeys without provoking symptoms of yellow fever. Moreover, this "symptomless infection" conferred a fairly durable immunity to the disease.[178]

Sellards traveled to France in 1931 in an effort to apply Theiler's discovery to the development of a vaccine. Unable to conduct his work in Paris, Sellards gladly accepted the invitation of Charles Nicolle—who, most certainly, just as gladly extended that invitation—to conduct his research in Tunis. There, Sellards again found Laigret, again officially a Pastorian, and the two began their work to transform the French sample into a true vaccine. In June 1934, they returned to Dakar with their new vaccine and used it to vaccinate some three thousand volunteers in two months—with apparent success.[179] The IPT was thus at the center of the creation of an efficacious virus-vaccine, based on an inapparent infection. Nicolle counted this as practical confirmation that his fully virulent yet a-toxic disease manifestation could stand next to Pasteur's own vaccines, in a new expression of power.

Reservoir Docs

Meanwhile, Nicolle continued his typhus studies. In July 1932, he devoted a section of the *AIPT* to the ongoing explorations of typhus identity. He opened with an article by Herman Mooser that raised questions about the Nicolle/Zinsser position.[180] Mooser had been influenced by Pinkerton's pathological studies of rickettsia in experimental animals and returned again to his laboratory with typhus samples. In particular, he passed Old World typhus through ongoing rat-flea transmission cycles and found that, after a large number of such passages, the Old World strain imitated the New World in its experimental effects on guinea pigs.[181] Though the results were thus far only temporary, Mooser believed they were sufficient to suggest that the known typhus strains could be traced back to *murine* origins, such as were found in New World typhus.[182] Yet, he was encouraged by his experimental successes to suggest a bolder interpretation: "One could plausibly posit that the virus might also be maintained in rats in the Old World as well. It would be necessary to repeat the experiments conducted in the U.S. and Mexico before declaring that, in the case of European typhus, there exists no murine reservoir outside of humans."[183] All the new evidence of murine typhus in Old World rats appeared to substantiate the interpretation. Further, louse passage might explain the heightened virulence of epidemic typhus.

By 1934, Mooser had moved wholly into the single-typhus camp (called by some French researchers the "*uniciste*" group[184]) and, in so doing, called into question the importance of inapparent infections:

That Old World typhus can be transmitted indefinitely at least in cold countries by the human louse we are not in a position to question. What we do question seriously, however, is the opinion of European workers that this is the only means by which historic typhus is preserved. . . . On account of these experimental results *we question the great importance which Old World investigators give to inapparent infection as a reservoir of the virus during long interepidemic periods.* There is in addition no reason to believe that during long interepidemic periods all cases of typhus should be inapparent. It seems to us more than likely that what is happening in Mexico must happen the world over; i.e., the epidemic adaptation of the original murine virus to the secondary unnatural cycle man-louse-man. . . . there is not a single circumstance which speaks against the hypothesis that the historic typhus of the Old World is also derived from the rat reservoir in nature.[185]

And so, while Nicolle and Zinsser were making a case for calling the agent of New World typhus "*Rickettsia mooseri*" to differentiate it from the Old World *Rickettsia prowazeki* agent, the man after whom the New World strain was to be named was trying to prove that the strains were not so different, after all.

Nicolle had tried to steer Mooser off this path. Obviously, he had failed.[186] Following Mooser's 1932 article, Nicolle responded to his initial set of questions with his own interpretation of the evidence. It was an interpretation that insisted on moving *beyond* the laboratory for confirmation. Mooser's argument rested on the ability of the Old World typhus to produce a New World-type scrotal reaction in guinea pigs inoculated, over time, through a forced rat-flea passage. The successful passage of the Old World virus through rats and fleas in itself, according to Mooser, supported the theory that the rat acted as the natural reservoir for typhus, with unnatural louse passage to humans accentuating the severity and creating "epidemic" typhus. Nicolle responded as he had two decades earlier, when he dismissed Edmond Sergent's claim that he had "demonstrated" the louse transmission of relapsing fever by successfully inoculating experimental animals with crushed lice. Nicolle cautioned against the tendency to overextend laboratory evidence: "the guinea pig is an intruder in the natural history of typhus. It plays only an experimental role. Let us see instead what animals that play an obligatory role in nature show us about . . . typhus."[187]

Field evidence had shown that the rat and the human, on the one hand, and the flea and the louse, on the other, affected the course of typhus in nature. The laboratory had demonstrated that rats and fleas were *capable* of carrying typhus. So were guinea pigs. That did not mean they played any important part in the epidemiology of Old World typhus. The experiments in which Old World mimicked New World typhus could not be sustained outside laboratory conditions. Further, the rat had been shown to react symptomatically with New World typhus—which Nicolle increasingly was referring to as "murine typhus"—but exhibited *only* inapparent infections when inoculated with the Old World strain. To this evidence, Nicolle added epidemiological and clinical distinctions between the two types, as well as their quite different effects on lice. (New World typhus killed lice very rapidly, thereby limiting epidemic spread.)[188] Nicolle now believed that the two typhus varieties shared a common origin, in the distant past; however, "the two types of typhus now have an autonomous existence." For Old World typhus, "the natural reservoir is the human, and its normal agent of propagation the louse. . . . Murine typhus is an endemic disease of rats in the New World, in Oceana, and in parts of Asia. It has the rat and the mouse as its reservoir" and was occasionally transmitted to humans by the flea.[189]

Early in 1933, Nicolle expanded his evidence for the differentiation of the two typhus groups (and thereby for the preservation of human reservoirs) to include a more detailed examination of cross-immunity tests. Did the varieties indeed share, in a strict sense, the whole "community of antigens" that earlier tests had suggested? Did their antigenic similarities merit their consideration as one distinct disease? With Laigret, Nicolle had conducted a number of experiments using different samples of both Old and New World typhus. They found that there was indeed a difference in the scope and "activity of their preventive [vaccinating] powers. . . . Once again, even in the study of antigens, one sees differences between the historic and the murine virus. One could say that there is considerable kinship [*grande parenté*], though not formal identity, in the antigenic properties of these viruses." This, in combination with his earlier evidence, brought Nicolle to conclude that "the historic and murine viruses are not identical."[190]

Back in the United States, Zinsser, too, disagreed with Mooser's interpretation of his typhus conversion experiments. In his own conversion experiments, Zinsser had found that the two forms could only be induced to mimic each other *under experimental conditions*. When these conditions were lifted, however, the strains returned to their original form: "no experimental procedure has so far been devised by which a European strain could be made permanently to assume the behavior of a murine strain."[191] Zinsser agreed with Mooser that both strains were of murine origin. It was just that this origin was much more distant than simply the latest long epidemic. A louse-man passage was indeed responsible for converting the murine into the European form, but true European typhus was a fixed variety and did not return to murine form permanently, even after several rat passages. "The slight, but definite differences between the two," concluded Zinsser, "are well established, biologically deep-seated and, therefore, probably of remote origin."[192]

There remained the persistent problem of the interepidemic reservoir of Old World typhus. Nicolle and his supporters believed they had abundant evidence to support their theory that a combination of inapparent and benign infections preserved typhus in humans between epidemic outbreaks. Zinsser still wasn't convinced. Though he admired the concept of inapparent infection, he didn't believe it accounted for the epidemiological facts of typhus. Soon, he would return to those strange typhus cases observed by Nathan Brill almost four decades earlier. The explanations Zinsser found within Brill's disease would challenge Nicolle's inapparent explanation far more fundamentally than did Mooser's theories. That, however, was in 1934. Early in 1932, Nicolle, Zinsser, and Mooser were still on the same side of the typhus debates. And Nicolle had those other, *Parisian* concerns to worry about as well. Indeed, beyond the conceptual salvation of inapparent infection, he had the more practical salvation of the *Maison mère* weighing heavy upon him.

7

Mosaics of Power

Confronting Paris (1931–34)

> Africa is an ultra-province and Paris does not want to be conquered by French of the "second zone"—the colonials.
> —Nicolle to E. Delabarre, 1931
>
> I believe in an eternal equilibrium.
> —Nicolle to Charles Geniaux, 1928

At the same time that Nicolle was being invited to Mexico to provide his expertise on typhus to the growing international discussion on the disease's contested identity, he was being summoned to return to Paris. The summons was, in part, a sign that Paris was finally giving Nicolle the acclaim he had long sought. Yet, the call came not from the *Maison mère*, but from the Collège de France. Moreover, the Collège wanted him for the Chair of Experimental Medicine.[1] The position, established a century earlier by François Magendie, had been made still more famous by his student and successor, Claude Bernard, and had continued to be the province of physiology, not bacteriology, right up until 1931. In other words, just as he was attempting to determine the nature of experimentation in microbiology, and the extent to which the laboratory spoke to nature, Nicolle was placing himself in a position to challenge the institutional definition of "experimental medicine" in France.[2] All evidence suggests that he was far more interested in challenging the direction of the IP in Paris. By the end of 1933, he would be well positioned to make that challenge.

The Chair of Experimental Medicine

Nicolle knew he was being considered for the Chair of Experimental Medicine at the Collège de France even before he left for his 1931 mission. Only after his return from Mexico that August, however, did he give the matter serious consideration.[3] Although he was well aware of the position's prestige and had been assured that he "would only have to present myself to be appointed," he still hesitated, and turned to Duhamel for advice. Marcelle was now settled in Tunis; he was far from finished with his work there. Moreover, he had become quite attached to his adopted home: if he were to take the position, "Would I have to leave Africa?"[4] Duhamel responded emphatically: "no hesitation is possible. You must accept. . . . I repeat: you must accept."[5]

Nicolle continued to hesitate. There were, in fact, good reasons for his hesitation. His institutional child and legacy, the IPT, was rapidly approaching the goals he had set for it, but had not yet attained them. His signature disease, typhus, was in the midst of redefinition, and he felt he needed to help settle its new identity. The task required active research. However, the previous Chair of Experimental Medicine at the Collège, Jacques-Arsène D'Arsonval, had left the position he had held for thirty-seven years with no affiliated laboratory. Moreover, the Collège appointment itself came with a heavy teaching schedule that threatened to constrain his research time. There was also the more nebulous question of how the post would help him fulfill his lifelong missions. After all, he was sixty-five years old, had recently suffered a severe health crisis, and was beginning to suspect that he might have a finite amount of time to accomplish his larger goals.

In search of certitude, he wrote to Collège administrator (and professor of literature) Joseph Bédier, outlining—at least in part—his concerns and posing questions. Given the state of his own research, the development of his institute, and the absence of laboratory space at the Collège, might he be allowed a reduced teaching load for two years to attend to these important concerns? In fact, the Collège had long been concerned with D'Arsonval's emphasis on teaching to the exclusion of research and would welcome the development of a medical laboratory.[6] Building a new laboratory would take time, further justifying Nicolle's request for a two-year Tunis-Paris joint appointment. His research would have to be conducted in Tunis until his Parisian lab was completed.[7] A cautious Bédier assured Nicolle that such an arrangement was possible if he could guarantee that his Tunis obligations would be fulfilled by December 1933.[8]

Nicolle naturally omitted any mention of his designs for the IPP in his queries to Bédier. Yet, Arnold Netter, one of Nicolle's "*maîtres*" and more vocal champions, had thought of Nicolle for the position precisely because the appointment would allow the colonial Pastorian to return to Paris and effect the kinds of changes at Pasteur's House that no one within its walls seemed willing to make.[9] Netter was himself a Pastorian outsider. A longtime champion of bacteriology and an early advocate for exploration of its clinical significance, Netter was professor *agrégé* at the Paris Faculty of Medicine and an active bacteriological researcher. Indeed, he was even involved with the typhus debates of the 1930s. Eventually, between Netter's conviction that he could indeed revitalize the IPP from the Collège, the Collège's willingness to accommodate his institutional needs, and Duhamel's enthusiastic encouragements, Nicolle began to warm to the idea of accepting the position. He told Mesnil that he sought the Chair "to have an official post in Paris, to be able thereby to help recruit apprentice Pastorians from among the Parisian medical corps by making myself comprehensible to them."[10] It was a reprise of the goals he had stated for the AEEP over a decade earlier. In a letter to Blanc, he was more open about his motives: "I will present my candidacy to the Collège de France without enthusiasm. . . . At the Collège de Fr. I would have a Parisian post with a bit of influence. I would be able to . . . recruit researchers for the *Mère* Dutôt. I would be there should a need arise for me."[11] Nicolle would play the role of the Pasteur Institute's reluctant savior, were he so called.

By the time he decided to "accept" the position, the position could no longer be accepted. It had to be fought for. While Nicolle was considering his options, three serious competitors had emerged: fellow Pastorian Constantin Levaditi; André Tournade, Chair of Physiology at the Faculty of Medicine in Algeria; and Dr. Schaeffer, a student of the Collège's André Meyer. Realizing he was in for a "heated struggle," Nicolle lamented to Vallery-Radot: "Netter, who pressed me into this situation, no longer retains his initial optimism."[12] Three points were raised most frequently against Nicolle's election. First was his age. At sixty-five, would he be effective in his position? Might he not treat it as a titled retirement? The second point was his continued affiliation with the IPT—and, by extension, his continued allegiance to the IPP. Several Collège members wondered whether the lifelong Pastorian could set aside those ties and focus on the needs of the Collège. The former was a valid concern from the outside; the latter, a far greater concern, seen most fully by those on the inside. The third point against Nicolle was that he *was* a Pastorian: a Pastorian who sought to take over the Chair of *Bernard*. Nicolle may have belittled the debate as mere "polemic," but he understood its significance both to the election and to his own disease theories.[13] " 'Pasteurphobia'," he complained, "has been exploited by the supporters of another candidate." His opponents made certain that members of the Collège knew he was a pretender to the throne.[14]

To counter his opponents' objections, Nicolle relied on his friends, his publications, and his considerable persuasive powers.[15] In Paris, men such as Vallery-Radot, Netter, and Duhamel—a good friend of Bédier's—actively lobbied on Nicolle's behalf. From Tunis, Nicolle wrote to each Collège member, enclosing copies of *Naissance, Vie et Mort,* and his Nobel Prize speech.[16] All these efforts, however, could not substitute for a visit to Paris. Nicolle made excuses to avoid the trip,[17] but his friends insisted that it was necessary if he wanted to ensure his victory. Nicolle relented, informing Duhamel: "You have finally convinced me, my friend. Your affectionate insistence has overturned my arguments. How could I not come when you have worked so hard for me?"[18] So Nicolle crossed the sea and politicked in Paris.

The tactics proved effective. Nicolle's accessible science writing, impressive list of novels, and friendship with Duhamel won over many of the literary professors. Despite his age, bacteriological approach, and geographical isolation from Paris, he also won over many of the Collège's scientists. Jean Nageotte, Nicolle's sponsor and spokesperson at the Collège, defended his candidacy before the final vote was taken:

> He has no intention to trespass on the domain of any other establishment, or of anyone here. He will give himself entirely to the Collège, just as he has given himself to the Pasteur Institute of Tunis. Of course, he cannot abandon his institute overnight and will ask for some latitude during the transition period; but this year, if you choose him, he will take possession of the chair.[19]

The final vote was: Nicolle, 19; Tournade, 13; Levaditi, 3; and Schaeffer, 1.[20] A Pastorian had been elected to Bernard's chair. Nicolle was officially appointed to the position on March 17, 1932.

Orchestrating his Introduction

Nicolle finally took the much-anticipated "missionary steamer" north across the Mediterranean in the spring of 1932, to deliver his first lectures as Chair of Experimental Medicine at the Collège de France. It had been nearly three decades since he had taken a similar steamer south, to escape the confines of Rouen society and embark on his missionary quest. In its ultimate ends, that mission had remained unchanged. Yet, the world, and Nicolle, had changed tremendously in thirty years. With those changes, his assessment of the consequences that might follow upon the failure of his missions had gained considerable weight, becoming increasingly grave, and global, as time passed.

Nicolle delivered his introductory lectures that May. In an obvious nod to Bernard, he entitled the series "Introduction to a Career in Experimental Medicine".[21] The five lectures in this series were structured as a kind of overture to the longer course of lectures he had planned for future semesters, setting up in particular the course he intended to present in the autumn of 1932 and the spring of 1933—a reworking of his *NVM* for a more medically interested audience.

In the first lecture, Nicolle outlined his concerns for the future of experimental medicine. These concerns, at least in their more immediate explanations and implications, had not changed much over the years. *French experimental medicine, he explained, was faltering.* This was the fault of monastic old researchers who attempted to impose their Spartan sensibilities on the young and allowed society to believe that brilliant laboratory work would continue, without its financial assistance.[22] The war, of course, had exacerbated these tendencies—first, by killing off many of the young men who would have chosen a laboratory life, and, second, by ensuring that those who remained were far too pragmatic to devote their lives to any endeavor that lacked financial incentives.[23] These difficulties were particularly French: all nations had suffered from the war, but it was France "that suffers the greatest menace." The French menace arose, for medicine, precisely from the combined tendency of the older generation to press its asceticism and that of the younger generation—those who had survived the war—to seek out more profitable career paths. Between them, they threatened to compromise France's future contributions to experimental medicine.

From this point, Nicolle followed the implications of France's apparent abandonment of scientific medicine beyond these more immediate concerns and into a sweeping international vision that he had been developing in the years following World War I. It was a vision that he had laid out in the second volume of his three-part series of biological philosophy: *Biologie de l'Invention* (*Biologie*) had appeared in print just as Nicolle was making preparations for his opening Collège lessons.[24] "Each people," he argued, "has its natural qualities and values. . . . Our talent"—the *French* talent—". . . is the clarity of our spirit, served by an exact language. It is also the originality of a quick intelligence" that, "little inclined to considerations of detail," tended to lead the way to new discoveries. France contributed *genius* to international collaborations. Without French participation in medical research, "human science will suffer."[25] Active French participation was central to the very survival of experimental medicine. To illustrate such French genius, Nicolle turned to one of his favorite examples: himself. *He* had been inspired by his father, his elder brother, and certain of his teachers, to devote himself to the study of medicine. He hoped similarly to inspire his students at the Collège de France.[26]

In his second lecture, Nicolle elaborated on the need for more young medical researchers and expanded upon the importance of science—in particular, of an *"esprit biologique"*—for medicine. This, of course, was the subject of *NVM* and would be the guiding theme of his lectures for the following autumn. Here, however, he touched on the problems of specificity and hinted at the new insights he would soon be providing on this important subject.[27] He devoted his third lecture to genius, following it with two concluding lectures on his own genius: Lecture 4, on inapparent infection;[28] and Lecture 5, on his Nobel Prize–winning typhus work. In private letters, Nicolle defended his tendency to describe genius and creativity with personal examples as doubly necessary: it was his own work that he best knew; and few in France were familiar with a "Tunisian," or "*isolé,*" such as himself.[29]

In addition to lecture preparation, Nicolle's top priority in his new position was to create a research laboratory in Paris.[30] He needed a lab both to continue his typhus research *and* to attract students to his brand of experimental medicine. He also envisioned it to be a physical link between the Collège and the Pasteur Institute, and as a symbolic Parisian power base. Its establishment, however, would be no easy task. Roux, still dominant, was infamous for his reticence to provide much space even for Parisian Pastorians. That spring, Nicolle finally presented his case (or, again, part of it) to the "*Patron.*"[31] The Collège, he explained, had no room, stranding the Nobel Prize–winning researcher in Paris without a lab. In order to continue his internationally important work, and to attract brilliant young medical students to the Pasteur Institute's door, he needed a laboratory. Initially, Roux was noncommittal. Nicolle, awaiting a decision, complained to Duhamel: "A laboratory must be organized as quickly as possible, without which the P.I. of Paris won't aid me in the slightest."[32]

Roux eventually offered Nicolle a place. By October, the laboratory was up and running, with Paul Giroud, his former *boursier* and now trusted colleague, acting as *chef de laboratoire*.[33] The space, however, was quite small: the lab of "6 people, 50 guinea pigs, 20 rats, 2 monkeys," and equipment, was housed in an area, Nicolle told longtime friend Edouard Delabarre, "smaller than your dining room." Indeed, the space was so small that "not only are the animals we are given sick with foreign diseases, but the diseases we inoculate them with are passed among them."[34] It threatened to limit his research even as Roux was pressuring him "to produce immediate results in order to demonstrate my new laboratory's vitality." Nicolle told Vallery-Radot that he planned to ask Roux to grant him more room: "If he opposes the extension, what can I do?" For Nicolle, this laboratory was to act as physical conduit to the reformation of the IPP: "Words, writing are only prefaces. What good are prefatory words without action? It sometimes seems that it would be simpler to reform the whole *maison* than to alter one of its corners."[35] Roux denied the request. By March, Nicolle was so frustrated that he contemplated stopping all work in the lab: Giroud could begin experiments again after Nicolle had left Paris.[36]

Despite logistical trials, Nicolle's laboratory, under Giroud's guidance, productively investigated typhus fever. It was officially titled the "Laboratoire de Médecine Expérimentale du Collège de France"; its letterhead prominently displayed its dual affiliation with the address "Institut Pasteur, 25, rue Dutôt." Zinsser worked there during his Paris visits, including his semester-long stay in 1935. American-born bacteriologist Harry Plotz (Nathan Brill's student) also worked closely with Giroud at the Paris lab. Zinsser brought samples of murine typhus from Mexico and Brill's from the United States; Giroud and Nicolle imported typhus samples from Tunisia; and the Paris lab experimented on them to determine the relation between typhus varieties.[37] Nicolle described the laboratory to his students at the Collège de France:

> The goal of my instruction is to interest you in the future of experimental medicine. . . .
>
> I have at hand the means to carry out this enterprise . . . a laboratory that the Pasteur Institute has placed at my disposal. This laboratory is quite small. Such as it is, it has begun to function and to produce research, thanks to the work of its excellent *chef*, Dr. Paul Giroud. I hope that our installation will develop quickly and that we will soon be able to receive, and work with, the young people who request to do so. . . . In this laboratory . . . I will be at the disposal of those who would like to consult me about problems that interest them, and to guide them, if I am able, in their careers.[38]

Despite its physical constraints, it was a multipurpose laboratory, with grand aspirations.

Life's in the Balance

In the same letter in which he encouraged Nicolle to take the Collège de France appointment, Duhamel expressed similarly passionate conviction about his friend's latest philosophical treatise. In the case of *The Biology of Invention*, however, that conviction was negative: "the tone of your book shocks me. . . . You are at the crossroads of historical essay, philosophical treatise, and personal memoir."[39] Duhamel warned Nicolle not to submit the final manuscript to his publisher until they had discussed it. Without reference to Duhamel's apparently lengthy list of critiques of the *Biologie* proofs, it is unclear whether his charge that the book read in part as "personal memoir" referred solely to Nicolle's inclusion of his own experimental work, or applied as well (or instead) to his more pervasive tendency to draw his picture of "the genius" with the strokes of his own psyche and situation.[40] Nicolle's response suggests that he interpreted the charge as referring exclusively to the former. A strong case for the latter would have taken no psychiatrist to make. Regardless, Nicolle did subsequently rewrite the manuscript, and Duhamel was far more pleased with the results. Even René Vallery-Radot wrote a congratulatory letter: "Your chapters are a stimulus for the spirit of invention. This was Pasteur's word. . . .You have ideas that are similar to his. This is as it should be. These pages will be invaluable to those who walk towards the entrance of the temple. You know how to guide them there."[41]

The second book in his philosophical series, *Biologie* was largely an expression of the new order Nicolle had devised for old certainties that the war had fragmented. In it, he provided a biological explanation for the nature of civilization, the existence of creativity, and the relations between the two. At the heart of his construction was his new deity, "Equilibrium," and its perpetual savior, "The Genius." Like his "mosaic of antigens," "equilibrium" provided a dynamic framework that preserved individuality and accommodated change. The essence of life, he noted, was change; however, that change had to fall within certain limits, or death, not life, would result. Equilibrium, a constant, organic balancing process, was the very basis of life.[42]

"Equilibrium" had become, in varying forms, a popular concept at the time. Nicolle would certainly have acknowledged (were he pressed) the influence of Claude Bernard's famous concept of the *milieu intérieur*: a living organism's internal environment that allowed it to adjust to changes in its external environment.[43] British physiologist Ernest Starling had laid out a system of bodily equilibrium at the start of the twentieth century, directly influencing Walter Cannon in his articulation of "homeostasis."[44] Epidemiologists, too, were devising theories of the rise and fall of epidemics that took equilibrium as an organizing principal.[45] French interwar "holists" (including Duhamel) tended to find the concept quite attractive.[46] In short, it was far from an original concept. Yet, Nicolle's appeal to it—and it to him—was so multidimensional, so central to his efforts to synthesize a new, postwar world view, so revealing of the intersections between, and his urgency toward, his longstanding missions, that it demands consideration. It may be a truism that old scientists often find comfort in synthesizing their science and the world's mysteries as their careers come to an end. Yet, that does not make the analysis of such efforts any less revealing.

In *NVM*, Nicolle had argued that disease was a biological phenomenon, then drew out the consequences of the assertion. In *Biologie*, he emphasized that humanity, in all its misery, glory, and power, was a biological phenomenon, then drew out the consequences of the assertion. Humans, he reminded his readers, were fundamentally biological organisms. Their brains were biological; therefore, their capacities and creations—indeed, their very civilization—were all rooted in nature and tied to nature's shifting balance. This would seem to imply that any configuration or action of human civilization had, by definition, to be "natural." Nicolle, however, believed that the development of *reason* in humans, though originally a product of biology, had so far removed human civilization from nature that it was not *necessarily* in touch with nature. In the disconnection between nature's changing equilibrium and human civilization's apparent progress, pathologies—imbalances—could well result. Once lost, how was balance to be restored? Nicolle believed that this was the function of the *genius*. The genius was an individual with the intuitive power to apprehend immediately any changes in equilibrium, and with the corrective power to restore balance. The genius's corrections were effected by the disequilibrium caused by his creations. In other words, if equilibrium was the principal deity in Nicolle's biological religion, then the genius played the part, not just of *pastor*, but of *savior*.[47]

I do not use the term "religion" rhetorically. Nicolle was a true believer. The genius "leaps forth, bounding onto this virgin domain and, with this mere act, he conquers it. A flash [*Un éclair*]. The problem, until then so obscure that no lamp, with its faint glimmer, could have revealed it, is suddenly flooded with light. One could call it creation."[48] Nicolle's genius was at once the "most talented representative of an immense nation which doubtlessly extends to all men" and its most primitive spirit.[49] He was like our ancestors who lived before the development of reason, and who apprehended nature more directly. Poets most immediately embodied this primitive spirit. Yet scientists, too, relied on intuition; the most creative scientists had poetically gone outside disciplinary definitions to grasp their most significant discoveries. Nicolle illustrated this point not only with the example of Pasteur but also with Lavoisier, Goethe, and even Mendel.[50] Such poetic and scientific deities merited lofty rhetoric: Nicolle described the "dream-state" in which intuition occurred as something akin to a *"state of grace"*.[51] Hence, intuition acted as a kind of naturalistic revelation, more immediate than, but not entirely separate from, reason. One might diagram Nicolle's ideas by starting with a large circle: nature. Within nature are both reason and intuition, which intersect but do not entirely overlap. This diagram also has a third dimension: viewed from its side, it shows intuition as the layer immediately atop nature. Reason is a stratum one more layer removed, constraining and ordering the layer of intuition it covers, almost like a lens bringing into focus intuition's stray analogous perceptions.

Nicolle's ideas on intuition were influenced not only by Duhamel but also by his fellow Nobel Prize winner—also the former teacher of Etienne Burnet—Henri Bergson.[52] Nicolle and Bergson had been in polite correspondence since 1928, when the two were scheduled to appear in Stockholm at the Nobel ceremony.[53] Illness prevented them from meeting, but this introduction placed Bergson on the mailing list for Nicolle's philosophical books, which Bergson praised with diplomatic grace.[54] Nicolle's program drew to a certain extent upon Bergson's notion of intuition grasping the constantly moving duration of a changing reality. Indeed, the mystical rhetoric in which the two men shrouded intuition, and their mutual grounding of intuition in nature, might lead one to assume that Nicolle's ideas were fundamentally Bergsonian. Yet, Nicolle's mystical intuition grasped the moment *in nature*, while Bergson's ultimately grasped the divine. In the final analysis, Nicolle's intuition, despite its rhetoric of dreams and mystical insights, was far more worldly than was Bergson's. As Nicolle himself noted, "I believe that the spirit of invention is a fact of life, a natural phenomenon. To study it, I have used the technique that has helped me figure out other life-related phenomena."[55] That is, he studied it as a *biologist*.

As a biologist, Nicolle saw invention as a natural faculty that functioned in similar fashion to *mutation*.[56] Intuition was a brisk change, a disruption of the established equilibrium. It might bring one closer to the changing harmony of nature than did the slower and more plodding reason; yet it often led to movements away from old harmonies that were jarring. These, however, were precisely the changes needed to restore equilibrium and preserve life. In this way, Nicolle's system relied on the self-correcting nature of science, embodied by equilibrium, and on Darwinian and neo-Lamarckian evolution, to explain the interrelations of nature, the individual, and society.

Given the fundamental significance of creative intuition for restoring equilibrium and thereby ensuring the survival of civilization, it was essential to understand the "rejuvenating" and "revolutionary" giver of creative intuitions, the "genius."[57] Nicolle was convinced that genius could not be "learned." It was a biological faculty, either present or absent at birth.[58] Moreover, it was a rare faculty, protected, he noted in his preface, by a "jealous god." Women and certain races of humanity were incapable of genius, as was anyone born without the faculty. Circumstances of birth, finance, chance; jealous colleagues and shrewish wives[59]—all these had prevented many men gifted with the faculty from realizing their potential. On the other hand, a supportive wife, such as "*notre dame de Pasteur,*"[60] could help fan the flames of genius in those so blessed to be in possession of the faculty. So too could a classical education that avoided early specialization, and the cultivation of a serious hobby (like writing novels and philosophy? one wonders).[61] Genius, Nicolle observed stoically, tended to accompany infirmities and was often expressed in brothers.[62] Moreover, it was a deeply individualistic characteristic. Good collaborators might help lay the groundwork for discovery, but, ultimately, "genius knows no collaborators."[63] Nicolle naturally recounted again the inapparent infection and the Door of the Sadiki discovery narratives.[64] Apparently, both Edmond Sergent and Nicolle's former typhus collaborator Charles Comte took great offense at this final formulation of genius.[65]

Nicolle's "genius," then, was the quintessential individualist. Life was change, variability, and it was the sacred role of the genius to grasp those changes and ensure the proper adaptive movements of human civilization. Like the "mosaic of antigens," "equilibrium" provided a flexible framework that rested on individual adaptations. The organizing metaphor was readily extendable to a model of social order that contained within it dictates on a number of pressing social concerns, all of which were legitimated with natural authority. Nicolle would soon develop this model more fully—largely by bringing together the metaphors of "mosaic" and "equilibrium"; in *Biologie*, however, he laid out its basic formulation.

Nicolle, as we have seen, believed that genius was not only a biological faculty, but a faculty that was the exclusive property of *men* of "certain" races. To his credit, Nicolle did condemn the extreme racist thinking displayed in this era of escalating fascism and Aryan emphasis on purity of blood. In fact, he used his biological system to demonstrate its flaws. Biology was change; it rested on variability and individuality. Anything that bred uniformity—be it the "sterilization" of bloodlines through exclusively internal racial crossing or the mindless embrace of mechanism—was a threat to civilization.[66] (Nicolle himself boasted Italian ancestors.) Did this mean that Nicolle was open to *all* racial mixing? Hardly. There were basic groups of humans, the "black," "yellow," and "white" races, that were well advised to stay with their own kind for the purposes of breeding.[67] Appealing again to his notion of balance, he argued that the mixture of such different bloods would produce a disequilibrium so great that destructive consequences were likely—in particular, "cerebral sterility."[68] Here, then, was where Nicolle drew his line between stasis and change. Biological organisms required certain basic structural components to be viable. Human civilization rested on a strict division of gender roles and a strict separation (at least for breeding purposes) of races. All of life might well be in motion, but group dynamics worked properly only when the component parts remained in their proper spheres.[69] One wonders what Hélène Sparrow, Marthe Conor, and daughter Marcelle thought when they read this.

"Genius," then, was the special faculty of men of European descent. Yet, it was not distributed equally among all Europeans. There was a natural distribution of talents among all peoples—including Europeans—and human civilization would do well to draw upon those talents. Were they to do so, they would produce the most balanced and advanced civilization possible:

> [W]hat will they not be able to accomplish on that day when they are able to work together in peace? The Latin peoples, especially the French, are particularly gifted at clearing new paths. Once discovered, however, they naturally abandon them. The Germans, whose faculties are less vibrant but more meticulous, seize them at this point. They analyze their basis and shore up their weak points. Assured of their solidity, they pass them along to the Anglo-Saxons, who organize their systematic exploitation for the rest of the world.[70]

Part of the danger posed by the direction being taken by the world Nicolle inhabited arose from France's abandonment of its creative capacities, coupled with the rise of the mechanistic Americans, clamoring to take the lead in directing civilization.[71] Indeed, so menacing was the prospect of American sociocultural domination that Nicolle even expressed a new appreciation for conservative forces that resisted innovation: "I was born in a city that, perhaps more than any other in France, conserves the form and the soul of the past. . . . My medical spirit, my reason, once condemned it." Now, however, when he reflected on the development of so many cities whose "houses lack character, with uniform façades, cold walkways, anonymous windows . . . their kitchens, clean like laboratories and their bedrooms indistinguishable from hospital rooms . . . this lack of personality, inseparable from hygiene . . . makes me think." Perhaps Rouen's conservatism had a point: "One cannot make great cuisine in such precision machines."[72]

Nicolle was busy making final revisions of the manuscript that would become *Biologie* in the late summer of 1931 when he submitted his official report on his Mexican mission to France's Minister of Foreign Affairs.[73] In his assessment of Mexican culture, he drew upon the very categories that informed the fears he expressed for the future of civilization in his philosophical treatise. Mexico, he observed approvingly, had been greatly influenced by France: "Our influence predominates in literature, art, and pure science." Yet, this influence was not without a "dangerous rival" in Mexico's northern neighbor. Like Frenchmen drawn toward the lure of material power in the postwar years, young Mexicans were drawn to the "brilliant appearance . . . economic power and . . . wealth" of America.[74] France, Nicolle urged, needed to "persistently oppose the hypocrisy of the United States and its materialistic civilization with the humanitarian ends and ideals of our civilization."[75] His prescription to that end brought together all three of his life missions. Mexican doctors would greatly benefit from either the visit of a well-trained European medical researcher or a brief training session at the Pasteur Institute. Indeed, they might even work for a time at one of the North African Pasteur Institutes, where there existed "conditions very similar to those they find in Mexico."[76] Once medical researchers had been properly trained, they could establish a centralized laboratory at home. The new facility, ideally, would be "a true Mexican Pasteur Institute"—filtered (made virulent?) through a proper French-North African host.[77]

The Forces of Destiny

Nicolle's Collège appointment gained him a number of advantages—among them, the ability to deliver notes on his research to French scientific and medical associations personally. On May 17, 1932, having just arrived in Paris to present his introductory lectures, he delivered the results of his rabies work to the Académie des Sciences. The findings were based on research that he had started nearly a decade earlier, with Etienne Burnet,[78] and concerned nothing short of a challenge to the Pastorian conception of the "virus-vaccine." Pasteur, as we have seen, created his famous rabies vaccine by exposing it (in the form of the dissected spines of infected rabbits) to air. The process attenuated the virus, which eventually attained the state of "fixed virulence" that made it therapeutically viable.[79] As time passed, however, a serious problem had arisen. The fixed virus, which was preserved by repeated rabbit passage, seemed to be gradually losing its "fixed" virulence, leaving vaccines increasingly less effective. Other Pastorians, including Paul Remlinger and Constantin Levaditi, had also studied the problem.[80] Nicolle and Burnet had attempted to restore the vaccinating substance by recreating it—that is, by passing it through dog brains to restore its virulence. In the intervening years, Burnet had left Tunis, but the vaccine substance continued to be passed through dog brains. By the time Nicolle made his 1932 report (now written with Lucien Balozet), the sample had completed over one hundred passages, but had given them results that were the very opposite of what they sought: "Far from increasing its pathogenic power, the inoculations have had the effect of somehow specializing its virulence for the dog's brain, making it lose all ability to confer rabies when it is not in this organ."[81] Later, Nicolle told his Collège audience what he concluded to the Académie: "we return, with something close to certainty, to the belief that Pasteur's transformation of virus into vaccine was *due to a mutation.*"[82] Pasteur's grand triumph had been the result of a happy accident, not the product of scientific intervention.

That autumn, Nicolle presented his first full set of lectures before the Collège. A reworking of *NVM* for a more specialized audience, the lectures would be published in 1933 as *Destin des Maladies Infectieuses* (*Destin*). He brought to his earlier ideas about disease evolution the lessons he had learned from his more recent return to typhus, his mutational conclusions about the rabies vaccine, and his expanded ideas on equilibrium. Moreover, informing his interpretation of disease "destiny" was a conception of "power" that he had long been working to articulate.

The *power* of genius, with its controlled but productive violence, reflected the kind of power that Nicolle held in the highest esteem. It was the "power without violence of symptoms" he had detected in inapparent infection. As he wrote in his 1929 "Letter to the Deaf," "Happy are the weak; for they shall, if they wish, be strong!"[83] The "Letter" was intentionally and explicitly autobiographical. Nicolle saw himself as "weak," in the conventional sense of the word. He suffered from a physical handicap; he lacked physical strength. Yet, there was a different kind of strength—of *power*—that came from recognizing one's ability to change the world without the use of brute force. It was this kind of power that the original Pastorian mission had drawn upon, and that guided fruitful cooperation among international scientists generally.[84] It was, Nicolle believed, the *best* part of France's civilizing mission. It was the best part of France itself. Yet, it was also the part of itself that France had been neglecting, and that the Pastorians had been neglecting, to the world's peril. The resonance of this notion of power, with its necessary connection to "genius," went beyond self and civilization. It even extended to microbiology in a manner that helped complete Nicolle's understanding of disease. For, in *NVM*, "virulence" was the force that adapted the "mosaic of antigens" to an animal host; in *Biologie*, it was the genius who acted to adapt human civilization to an ever-changing natural equilibrium. In *Destin*, Nicolle called upon the ideas of *NVM*, but now brought "equilibrium" to his mosaic. He also brought diversity, hypotheses about structural foundations and the nature of adaptive forces, and he found a way to have his altered conception of "power" acting as directing force. I will start with Nicolle's revised central metaphor, then examine the experiences that helped him shape that revision.

In 1930, Nicolle had appealed to his brother's "mosaic of antigens" to help him explain the nature of pathogenic specificity. He argued, at the time, that the "mosaic" provided answers to a number of intractable questions about disease. By 1933, however, he found the mosaic too limited. What Maurice "did not say, what he perhaps did not see, was how numerous the elements of the mosaic were, and that, among these elements were some that merited the name 'specific,' but were not, themselves, antigens."[85] Nicolle was not entirely happy about calling these component parts "elements." He did not want anything so exclusively material; he sought, instead, a term that did not preclude "an aptitude. I know of no better term," he continued, "than *power*. We may thus say, correcting my brother's expression, that a pathogenic agent is a *mosaic of powers*."[86] The mosaic of powers was composed of a great number of parts, the nature of which—be they force or matter—would become clearer with the progress of scientific knowledge.[87] These parts could accommodate changes from within and without, flexibly withstanding all reasonable challenges to the mosaic's changing *equilibrium* and reestablishing equilibrium with related exterior entities. They could even withstand the loss or gain of a component part.

Nicolle's work on the varieties of typhus informed his expansion of the mosaic metaphor. We have seen that he came to espouse the duality of typhus species, which he did on the basis of no single test but, rather, through layers of evidence, the cumulative effect of which was to suggest strongly that classic and murine typhus were indeed distinct varieties. (Eventually, he decided that the two groups shared a common ancestor from which they had separately evolved, rather than one having evolved from the other.) All the many tests that had been developed to help doctors diagnose a particular disease—cross-immunity tests, agglutination reactions, and the like, all of which he reviewed in *Destin*—had proved inadequate to differentiate classic from murine typhus.[88] In nature, in patients, and even in laboratory animals, the two typhus varieties appeared quite distinct from each other. Yet, most of those antigen-oriented tests had shown them to be identical. Apparently, there was more to pathogenicity, and to pathogenic specificity, than antigens.

This newly diverse microbial mosaic of powers was itself in a kind of equilibrium, which was then adapted to the changing elements of its potential host—otherwise, it would not be a pathogen, but a saprophyte. How was this adaptive balance achieved? In *NVM*, Nicolle vaguely pointed to virulence, but omitted any reference to how this might occur. Now, however, he was convinced that virulence not only was the adaptive power, but that, as such, it directed the very destiny of the pathogenic microbe. Its mechanism was mutation. It will be remembered that Nicolle, who had long been interested in microbial variability, came to think more systematically about microbial *mutation* when Breinl and Weil suggested that rickettsia and Proteus were plausibly related as inframicrobe and microbe of typhus via mutation. By 1927, he was thinking about the divergences between relapsing fever groups as having been effected by mutations. Then, there was his return to typhus: laboratory efforts to *convert* one variety of typhus into the other by animal passage had met with only limited success. Researchers could effect imitation; yet, when laboratory conditions were lifted, the typhus varieties always reverted to type. It appeared that typhus had at some point undergone a mutation in nature that split its trajectory into two groups. Alongside his typhus work, Nicolle had finally brought his extended study of rabies to conclusion. Here, too, laboratory animal passage did not lead to expected results. Time and again, the animal inoculations that were meant to explain observed microbial identities failed to do so. Nicolle was increasingly convinced that microbial conversions previously thought to be the product of gradual adaptation or controlled attenuation were in fact the result of chance mutations. Thus, their results were more durable and far less reproducible than had been predicted.

Nicolle's mutation research encouraged him to think more generally about how changes occurred in organisms, and how those changes were passed on to progeny. To explain the adaptive power of the mosaic of powers, he suggested an interpretation of the mosaic metaphor that drew upon recent advances in genetics.[89] Thomas Hunt Morgan, an American who was almost an exact contemporary of Nicolle, would receive the Nobel Prize in Physiology and Medicine in 1933 for work he had done over the course of two decades, locating inherited characters in the *genes*, which were themselves tied to chromosomes.[90] Yet, in his Nobel speech, Morgan carefully avoided making claims about the precise nature of the gene: some scientists, he noted, still thought of them as hypothetical, while others thought them to be material structures. Regardless, he argued, they served the same purpose.[91]

Nicolle, considering the "powers" of his mosaic, and in particular the locus of virulence, hypothesized that "the specific characters of a pathogenic agent are tied [*liés*] to certain constitutive elements of this entity [*être*]."[92] Microbial mutation would thus play a central role in the "birth" of new diseases:

> One imagines that the brusque acquisition of virulence by a microbe might be linked to the appearance of a new element or a new group of elements in the mosaic. This brusque acquisition would most probably be irreversible. The translation, the repercussions of such a phenomenon in the intimate, elementary constitution of the infinitely small, appears to us as legitimate as changes in chromosomes considered as causes in changes to the properties of superior beings. In the two cases, it is a question of facts of the same order; these facts, in both cases, merit the name, mutation.[93]

In the fine tradition of Pastorians before him, Nicolle pragmatically turned to biology to borrow concepts that might help him illuminate the workings of disease. Theories of mutation and heredity helped him substantiate the viability of his structural rethinking about the pathogenic microbe as a mosaic of powers. Still, he qualified, the nature of this connection between structure and power remained a mystery.[94] It is worth noting that Nicolle's conception of "mutation," which was analogically similar to intuition—and similarly mysterious—acted, in a sense, as a force *spontaneously generating* life's variability. Pouchet had found a place among the Pastorians.

What, then, was the place of virulence within the mosaic of powers, and how did it function? In *NVM,* virulence was the adaptive force, the pathogen's "power," which was somehow separate from its "toxicity." It was also, Nicolle emphasized, of *relative* importance: medical researchers privileged it above other microbial qualities because they were interested in its effects; but virulence was, in the end, simply one of these many properties, one characteristic within a "vast botanical group" of microbes. In *Destin,* he shifted his emphasis: virulence was now *directive*. The "pathogenic action of a microbe or a virus (the word *action* is used here and not the word *power*) is made, at once, of its virulence (pathogenic power) and its *toxic power*," he again stressed. Toxic power was "the ensemble of toxic properties inherent in each type of pathogen."[95] Despite their significance for infectious disease, most toxic substances "play no role in the evolution of disease."[96] Virulence did.

Nicolle had come to think of inframicrobes as entities approximating embodied virulence. After all, there was still no evidence that inframicrobes existed in any form other than pathogenic, and they were so perfectly adapted to their hosts that they could not function outside them. Expanding upon his "great microbial chain of being," Nicolle now had a new perspective on the evolution of inframicrobes. As entities approximating pure "virulence," they would never have come into existence *without* adaptive power—virulence. In this sense, "virulence . . . has guided, does not cease to *guide, the destiny of each microbial species.*"[97] Virulence was no longer a quality that had significance only relative to a medical perspective. To think of it merely as an "accidental fact" whose importance was "commanded by the point of view from which we study them" would be

> . . . a grave error. Pathogenic aptitude, however difficult it may be to localize, even to understand, is the essential character of infectious disease causation. In the most evolved of these agents, in those that have lost all ability to develop outside the organism of superior beings and, often, outside of a single species, pathogenic aptitude dictates [*commande*] the existence of the infinitely small. It fills in them the most prominent function. It merges with [*se confond avec*] their life.[98]

In short, virulence commanded the destiny of infectious disease. It might be one of many possible microbial powers and qualities; however, it was a microbial quality that had the power to direct microbial development.

At the heart of Nicolle's disease model, then, was an understanding of "power" outside "violence."[99] Informed by his disease research, it was also shaped by the values of the old French civilizing mission, which, in its most idealistic (and post-Prussian defeat) expression, sought social transformation without brute force.[100] Nicolle's understanding of power was given further "virulence," if you will, by a metaphor: the mosaic.[101] The mosaic of powers acted to enhance the "window on nature" he had claimed in *NVM*. In *Destin,* he included most of the text of *NVM* and again set his sights on using his discoveries to help show how disease was born, lived, and died, in individual patients, in epidemics, and in disease species. Now, however, the mosaic of powers allowed him to make even more sweeping claims for the importance of virulence. Moreover, like any good metaphor, it gave organizing shape to the many themes in his thinking about civilization (human and disease), missions (the French civilizing mission and the Pastorian mission), and adapting forces (the genius, the virus-vaccine defined through inapparent infection, virulence). In the third book of his trilogy, he would even extend his biologically based mosaic metaphor to explanations of "morality" and conceptions of beauty, goodness, and truth.[102] The mosaic allowed motion yet maintained balance, which was the essential attribute of life: "Rigidity leads to immobility and, in society as in the individual, immobility is death."[103] Nor was this mere theoretical speculation. For, all the while Nicolle was seeking a description of the structural basis of virulent power, he was also seeking power to restructure the IPP. He was now in Paris, which made the task more manageable. Yet, there was a static force, a "creature" that had "placed himself as a barrier on my path."[104] This "creature," rigid and immovable, was Emile Roux.

Deconstructing Roux

Nicolle and Roux had suffered through a tempestuous relationship that would never lose its toxicity and settle into a gentle inapparent infection. In the early years of Nicolle's directorship of the IPT, the two men had enjoyed a respectful relationship as teacher and student. Then, Nicolle started acting less like a dutiful student and more like an independent researcher. He enjoyed laboratory and institutional success, the latter of which was supplemented by a profit-oriented approach to bacteriology that went against the original dictates of the Pastorian mission and the continued expectations of Roux himself. Nevertheless, the two survived further tribulations, including the "tutu"-eliciting critique of 1920.[105] Roux had even supported Nicolle for the Osiris Prize. The pair did not, however, survive geographical proximity. By the spring of 1933, Nicolle had taken to constructing letters in the style of confessional poems (one of which, for its evocative rhetoric, I quote at length), lamenting that the fates had set Emile Roux in the position of Pastorian pope:

> I have collided with the stubbornness of a venerated and spiteful old man. A popular legend has been spun around Roux. It is drawn from numerous elements, a few of which are even true. At its base is the legendary character of the modest and disinterested scientist: a character which barely exists—at least never as simply as it has been represented. More often, this scientist is a conceited monster who envies, even detests all who are more fortunate than he. To this novelesque character is added, in this case, the

undeniable truth that he is the last representative of the historic epoch of
Pasteur. The survivor reaps the benefits. . . . In his youth, he played the part
of a free spirit, independent, mistrustful of academics, even attacking them;
and as soon as was one of them, he became the epitome of them. . . .
Having climbed to the top, he found himself flattered. He seemed to disdain
flattery, which served to increase the ardor of his followers. As their idol, he
made them put up with his ill-nature; indifferent to the suffering of others,
. . . he became authoritarian. He is the head of a private establishment,
without supervision. . . . He favors no one who appears to have any
integrity. He is brutal, and thus appears sincere.[106]

Roux was in a position of power over many; and his human side, protected by myth, was destroying those over whom he ruled. He was "detested by all." His only program was "to avoid all innovation." In essence, Roux was "cowardly and trembling before destiny, but incapable of casting aside the mantle that has been thrown upon his shoulders, which lends him his stature and his glory."[107]

Nicolle adopted the rhetoric of the heretic in his tirade against Roux. The former "Pasteur Alias Murphy" presented his break from the *Patron* as a fall from faith. It was Roux, he noted, who had first led him to the Pastorian faith: "I was touched by his words and these have determined my career." For many years, Nicolle had suppressed his doubts, needing a god, fearing to betray the *Maison mère*. Finally, he abandoned his faith—or, like Don Quixote, he abandoned his illusions: "it cost me much to condemn [the mythic part of Roux], to renounce an illusion, to no longer have a god."[108] This sacred image of Roux was hardly unique to Nicolle. Indeed, in his biography of Roux, Emile Lagrange describes Pasteur's chosen disciple as a "secular saint." The book contains a portrait-caricature of Roux as St. Francis, his sacred head surrounded by a cowl and his feet engulfed in the flaming tongues of the diseases he had trammeled, unscathed.[109]

Over time, and far from Paris, Nicolle had come to have a new faith, believing instead in an "eternal equilibrium," sustained by a "mosaic of powers" that brought all parts into a cooperative collaboration that in turn preserved life's balance. Still, if he had lost faith in Roux, he never wavered in his belief in the goals of the Pastorian mission: "The false saint is unmasked, but the Cause rests sacred." It was this cause—the Pastorian cause—that he thought Roux's rigidity to be fundamentally compromising. Nicolle was finally convinced that he had to take action to save the IP from collapse. Roux

must be made to yield. . . . *If he does not yield, I cannot abandon the cause whose champion I have been made.* . . . Either the cause must triumph or I will make every effort to win ground for it. I am under no delusions about the value of my efforts; whatever happens, I will protect the cause.[110]

And so, in April, Nicolle confronted Roux about the present course and future prospects of Pasteur's institute. He wrote him a letter, "explicit, respectful, and clear," which he had typed by "a discreet person."[111] He had discussed its contents and desired effects with longtime reform partner Vallery-Radot, who had just written an article on Nicolle in the *Revue des Deux Mondes*. Nicolle thanked Vallery-Radot for the article and mused, "I hope that building myself up before public opinion will help me accomplish my task."[112] Unfortunately, the contents of this important letter are unknown.[113] After Nicolle sent it, he lamented, "Epictetus once said: the most desperate contests are the most beautiful. I have no hope."[114] His pessimism was confirmed. A late-April meeting with Roux, who, by then, had received the letter, was anticlimactic: "I expect nothing from him."[115]

Many years earlier, just after the end of World War I, Calmette, newly taking up his position as Roux's assistant director, had complained to a sympathetic Nicolle that the "*Patron*" had no desire to share any of his power over the *Maison mère* and its numerous international extensions. It had been Nicolle's mission, and Calmette's job, to persuade Roux to hand over some of his control. By 1933, there was no evidence that they had made any progress toward this end. Of course, their unspoken power struggle over Roux's eventual succession did not encourage their collaborative efforts. Increasingly from 1930, however, Nicolle and Calmette found a new mutual understanding, brought about by vaccine production and a number of tragic deaths in the German town of Lübeck.

The "C" in the famous tuberculosis vaccine BCG stands for "Calmette." Based on a tuberculosis strain of reduced virulence, it had been used successfully for several years when, in 1929, a batch shipped to Lübeck led to the rapid death or illness of a majority of the 251 infants to whom it had been administered. A thorough investigation soon cleared Calmette and his colleagues of any responsibility: the sample they sent had been contaminated at a lab in Germany.[116] After the crisis, Calmette confided in a once-again sympathetic Nicolle: "You have understood the state of my soul in the wake of this catastrophe."[117] Nicolle supported Calmette not only with letters of encouragement, but with active campaigns on his (and his vaccine's) behalf. In his international travels, Nicolle presented the facts of the case to concerned doctors and medical researchers; he integrated the BCG example into his concepts of disease evolution;[118] and he and his colleagues not only continued to distribute the vaccine in Tunisia—they even went on a publicity campaign. Béchir

Dinguizli, Adrien Loir's former protégé, was tasked with speaking to the "indigenous public."[119] Tragedy had brought Calmette and Nicolle to a place of mutual support. Finally, in 1933, the "obstacle" that had hindered the progress of their planned Pastorian reforms was removed in the only way possible: Emile Roux died on November 3. It is unknown whether Calmette and Nicolle would have collaborated thereafter to achieve their long-standing mission, or whether they would have returned to their old rivalry. For not even exoneration from any wrongdoing over the BCG affair was enough to resuscitate Calmette's deflated spirits. He complained to Nicolle, "The filthy history of Lübeck has made me ill!"[120] Calmette died a week before Roux.[121] "The Pasteur Institute was decapitated";[122] its future was uncertain. Nicolle now faced his last and best chance to fulfill his missions.

Beheaded

What would he do? Rumors proliferated in the heated Parisian environment; Nicolle, then in Tunis, received conspiratorial letters from his friends. Arnold Netter, so crucial to Nicolle's campaign for the Collège position, wrote: "I see that the possibilities I had imagined when bringing you into the Collège are coming to pass. I believe your chances are great."[123] Nicolle's Paris-based assistant, Paul Giroud, wrote: "The whole institute awaits your return."[124] Nicolle, however, remained in Tunis, where he would stay, he told his friends, until he was called to Paris. He told Duhamel that he had "no ambition" to be appointed director: the institute's reorganization would be "a formidable task." If asked, however, "I would respond to the call."[125] Nicolle's Christlike rhetoric reveals his mind-set: the missionary would give himself up in a final gesture of self-sacrifice, if indeed he were asked to save the Pasteur Institute. As he wrote that January in the *Mercure de France*, "To save what is essential, it is often necessary to sacrifice much."[126] His posture may have been that of reluctant savior, but this was, in fact, the moment for which he had been preparing for at least two decades.

In Paris, Vallery-Radot was busily attempting to increase his own influence over the institute's Administrative Council.[127] The council, presided over by Alfred Lacroix, had, until Roux's death, been acting largely as an extension of Roux's will. It was now in a position to shape the institute's future. Opposing Vallery-Radot on the council, however, was its vice president, Louis Vaillard. Vaillard, a longtime friend and collaborator of Roux's, sought to protect the *Patron*'s vision and memory. Among the rumors circulating in Paris was one that Roux had made a dying request of Vaillard: he must oppose Nicolle's candidacy for the directorship.[128] At the council meeting following the deaths of Roux and Calmette, Lacroix proposed that they not rush into naming a successor but, first, take a "moral, scientific, and material inventory" of the Pasteur Institute in order better to decide its future.[129] Louis Martin would act as interim director, but power would rest with the council, which would meet frequently to oversee any problems that might arise. Both Vallery-Radot and Vaillard supported the president's proposal.[130] From it arose the Lacroix Commission, with Lacroix as its president, Vaillard its vice president, and Vallery-Radot its secretary. Vallery-Radot kept his Tunisian coconspirator informed, describing the commission as an effort "to make a complete study of the I.P. and its needs."[131]

By December, Nicolle had become perceptibly anxious about the institute's future and his potential role in shaping it. During the council's inquiry into the institute's status, it had summoned him to present his views, which Nicolle considered "an initial move toward me."[132] Nicolle returned to Paris in December to fulfill his Collège obligations and await further word from the Pastorian commission. Yet by late January, nothing had happened. Convinced that the council's hesitancy belied its inherent weakness and inability to effect meaningful change, he took action. Again, Nicolle turned to the French press, using as his vehicle the Parisian interdisciplinary weekly the *Nouvelles Littéraires* (*NL*). Initially, he sent his text to Duhamel and Vallery-Radot for revisions, explaining his motivations for writing it with the rhetoric of midwifery: he hoped his drastic actions would "give birth to" a director who would do the least damage.[133] The article itself appeared in the February 3, 1934, number. Its title alone could hardly have failed to attract attention: "An Hour with Doctor Charles Nicolle (Professor at the Collège de France; Nobel Prize Laureate, 1928): The Pasteur Institute's Destitution: A Cry of Alarm."[134] A sketch of Nicolle seated, paper in hand, concern and determination on his face, fills the center of the page. To heighten the article's dramatic effect, the *NL* presented it in the form of an interview with one Fréderic Lefèvre, whom Nicolle, in fact, had never met.[135] Moreover, the paper highlighted his most inflammatory statements with boldface type; some were even gathered together in separate boxes.[136] The substance of the "interview" opened with praise of the Collège de France, launched swiftly into an attack on Roux's direction of the Pasteur Institute, then concluded with a laudatory review of Nicolle's work in Tunis. Its effect was to highlight how Nicolle's own work served as a positive model for the ailing Parisian institute's reform.

"One must say what one feels," wrote Nicolle, "even at the risk of criticism." Nicolle was indeed criticized by fellow Pastorians for his charge that

Roux, their heroic and recently deceased leader, "did not direct the Pasteur Institute well."[137] What followed was a direct statement of the private Pastorian critique of Roux, made dramatically public: "[Roux] did not see, while hidden in his voluntary isolation, that society had changed around him and that the kind of old-fashioned scientist he so admired existed only in museums." Consequently, the once-great Pasteur Institute was largely "staffed by useless and lazy functionaries on perpetual vacation."[138] So far was it removed from the needs of society (out of balance, one might say) that "there could be no other solution than a total transformation." The Administrative Council had taken the right step in forming a commission to study the institute's needs; still, directed by outsiders to the Pastorian world, the council members, talented as they were, risked "being tempted to listen to those who, in good faith, believe there is no crisis; that, sooner or later, everything will simply work itself out." If they listened to these conservative arguments, "the death of the Pasteur Institute would be the fatal result" of their inaction.

Nicolle's solution to the "crisis" took on a familiar form. He asserted that only a sweeping reorganization, stemming from a fundamental reconsideration of its place in society, would allow the Pasteur Institute to survive. If, however, the center did not reorient itself, "French microbiology would not die" immediately: "Like Athens, which long ago found refuge in its ships, [the Institute] would survive in its *filials*." The analogy would have made a distinct impression on the classically trained readers of the *NL*. Nicolle was referring to the famous strategy of Themistocles in 480 B.C., when the Athenians, threatened by Persian attack, fled in ships. To save their society, the citizens of Athens had to leave their city.[139] The filial institutes were the ships bearing the Pastorians to outlying destinations, where their doctrines would survive, if temporarily. Eventually, a strong leader would have to emerge to bind them together. If such a leader did not arise, the *filials* would eventually disintegrate in their isolation.

Nicolle's argument was clear: Emile Roux had not adapted his institute to twentieth-century medicine and society. This adaptation had to be accomplished immediately, by embracing the financial, medical, and international resources already available to it, but as yet unexploited by it. The Pasteur Institute had to reconstitute its cosmos. It had to have a strong center, firmly rooted in medical research and profiting from this research through vaccine sales; it had to foster medical alliances and colonial exchange. It had to discover the "organizing and active will" to generate profit and form beneficial links to resources it currently lacked. Only in this way would it attract the talented young researchers and financial support it needed to carry out its international mission.

His critique articulated, Nicolle turned to his own accomplishments in Tunis, providing a none-too-subtle example of exactly how he had implemented this model in his own medical universe. The rhetorical parallels between his story of Paris's current crisis and Tunis's past condition are striking:

> When I arrived [at the Tunis institute] . . . I found it in a state of ruin. Within a few years, I successfully got it on its feet by winning the confidence of the medical community and making of them a rich resource. The budget increased by almost two million francs in the past twenty-five years and the staff has gone from four to more than forty. Our institute, which is a State establishment, is in charge of numerous public services: rabies treatment . . . bacteriological and chemical tests; general vaccine production. . . . Still, our principal interest is not in this industrial production, although it is both indispensable and beneficial, but in original scientific research.

The Tunis institute was, in Nicolle's formulation, the center of an active organization profiting from its industrial and medical alliances. Its means were adjusted to the needs of twentieth-century society so as to preserve Pasteur's universal missionary end. The Pasteur Institute of Tunis, developed in a French protectorate, was set forth as the model on which to restructure the Pastorian core.[140]

Nicolle had thrown down the gauntlet.

Le Temps

Just before his *Nouvelle Littéraire* article appeared in print, Nicolle saw another of his articles published in a major French journal. The *Mercure de France* included his discussion of the current economic depression in its January 1934 number.[141] It seems an odd subject for Nicolle to have been writing on in a public forum. In fact, the article itself was a fitting summary of the myriad assumptions that underlay his devotion to the Pastorian mission and his designs for its future. Here, Nicolle brought his perfected mosaic metaphor into the service of an ideal social equilibrium. "The existence of human societies is a symbiosis," he argued.[142] The best of all possible worlds would be arranged as a collaborative mosaic of states:

> The evolution of history teaches that the great States owe their equilibrium to their progressive extension. Is there a nation made of more diverse elements than ours? Is there one that shows a more perfect cohesion, a better

understanding between compatriots? There only will be, only can be, peace and equilibrium by a union of smaller states with each other, creating a *mosaic of neighbors,* or, if they are isolated, by their adjunction to larger states. This would be a free union, *a free grafting* which alone can lead to mutual understanding, the abandonment of individual conceits and of historic or ethnic prejudices, the forgetting of reciprocal wrongs and the awareness of the need for a common economy.[143]

The root of the world's current problems, he argued, was that it was not thus arranged. Long frustrated with the way that Paris ignored everything that lay outside Paris, and the way Emile Roux had ignored everything that lay outside his own self-myth, Nicolle truly believed that the lack of balanced exchange was threatening the future of civilization: "To exchange, to circulate all the resources that nature offers them, to increase the volume of these resources, is the only way to assure proper [social] equilibrium."[144] And so, with the future of the IPP uncertain, Nicolle railed more generally against the dangers of social "rigidity":

> Some revolutions are useful. The worst may be necessary. When a machine is rusty or a mechanic foolish, egotistical, or impotent, one must change the former, cast out the latter. The process will only be brutal if it meets with resistance. The vital resistances alone must be conserved. . . . To save the essential, it is often necessary to sacrifice much.[145]

The line between his critique of the current social disequilibrium, and of the dangers of the IPP following its past trajectory into the future, blurred. If anyone had doubts about the connections between Nicolle's realms of conviction, those doubts would have been dispelled with the *NL* article, which appeared shortly thereafter.

Reaction to the *NL* article was fierce: "one might even say that it caused a scandal."[146] Those for and against Nicolle's message shared a common interpretation of its intent, reading Nicolle's motivation for writing to be the procurement of the vacant directorship. Even his closest friends read it as such.[147] Indeed, the article's inflammatory content, its self-promoting structure, and Nicolle's own ambitions, would support this idea. Yet his letters denied it: "Far from being a proclamation of my candidacy, this brutal assessment of the I.P. of Paris signified my complete divorce from its problems."[148] By February 1934, it appears that Nicolle had indeed abandoned the personal dimension of his mission. His article and the correspondence surrounding it suggest that, having abandoned all hope of procuring the directorship, he was finally able to speak his mind. This was the same man whose veiled attack on Roux's directorship in the 1920 *Le Temps* article provoked outrage—a man with sufficient cultural and rhetorical sensitivity to know that a public polemic of this type would win him few friends. The article did not come from the pen of a candidate, but from a man conceding the battle—though not the war.

The consequences of Nicolle's actions continued to play out over the next few months. Several Pastorians, including Félix Mesnil, cut off all correspondence for weeks or even months.[149] Many told him gently that they agreed with what he had said, but not with how he had said it.[150] Even Vallery-Radot, whom Nicolle had provided with a manuscript copy for revision before taking the article to the press, was inexplicably upset.[151] In Paris more generally, Nicolle's attack provoked just the response he expected: hostile silence. At the same time, it revealed the cleavage between the Parisian center and its overseas periphery: "The interview enraged almost all the Parisian Pastorians (though not the tropical ones)."[152] Duhamel also assured Nicolle, though perhaps in a somewhat biased interpretation, that his article favorably impressed "French medical circles" outside the IPP.[153] From Nicolle's perspective, the Parisian center was impenetrable. By early March, he was fairly certain that his final effort to effect change would not succeed. He and Paul Remlinger predicted (accurately) that Louis Martin and Gaston Ramon would be appointed to the vacant positions. Neither of the North African Pastorians had much faith in their administrative abilities.[154]

In mid-May, convinced that Martin's election was inevitable, Nicolle conceded defeat. "I wonder," he wrote to Vallery-Radot, "how Martin can accept such a challenge. He doesn't understand it." In a rare unguarded moment concerning his aspirations, Nicolle continued: "I would have given myself wholly—though with no delusions about my powers—to serve the cause that I have been called to." Finally, speculating about the forces that had shaped the outcome of the elections and, consequently, the future of the Pasteur Institute, he speculated: "I don't think that R[oux] ever charged V[aillard] to veto my involvement as Vaillard claimed he did. V's dishonesty has saved me from servitude."[155]

Shortly thereafter, Nicolle enjoyed one last glimmer of hope. The IPP appointed him to its new Conseil Scientifique, which was to act in tandem with the Administrative Council to advise the chosen director on the institute's scientific administration.[156] Nicolle hoped he might persuade his colleagues on the council to support certain reforms:

> [I]f it is decided to divide the colonial institutes into sectors, might I not be given the Mediterranean sector—that is, the *IP*'s of Algiers, Casablanca,

Tangiers, Tunis, Athens, and the smaller establishments such as Marseilles (antirabies I[nstitute]), Beirut, the Suez Canal, Istanbul, etc.? Naturally, I would not encroach upon the power of the local directors; I would merely make certain that their interests were represented to the Council.[157]

His plans to direct the Parisian institute having been thwarted, he might still become Emperor of the Mediterranean Pasteur Institutes and thus gain enough influence to effect at least limited change. Still, his optimism was tempered by long experience: "I am under no illusions," he wrote to Edouard Delabarre. "It is easy to push aside an African when the meetings are held in Paris."[158]

His fears were soon confirmed. In June, Nicolle complained to Duhamel: "The Institut Pasteur's Scientific Council, of which I am a member, has met without me. The meeting was chaotic. I am increasingly convinced that nothing will come of its efforts."[159] He had sent his suggestions about the institute's scientific direction to this meeting, knowing that nothing would be done with them.[160] Throughout the summer and into the fall of 1934, he struggled to persuade the council to meet during his visits to Paris: to little avail. Annoyed, he commented that his ideas were "too bold for such mollusks."[161] By February 1935, Nicolle's resignation was complete: "I do not believe that the Scientific Council will serve any useful purpose."[162] His window of opportunity to transform the *Maison mère* had closed.

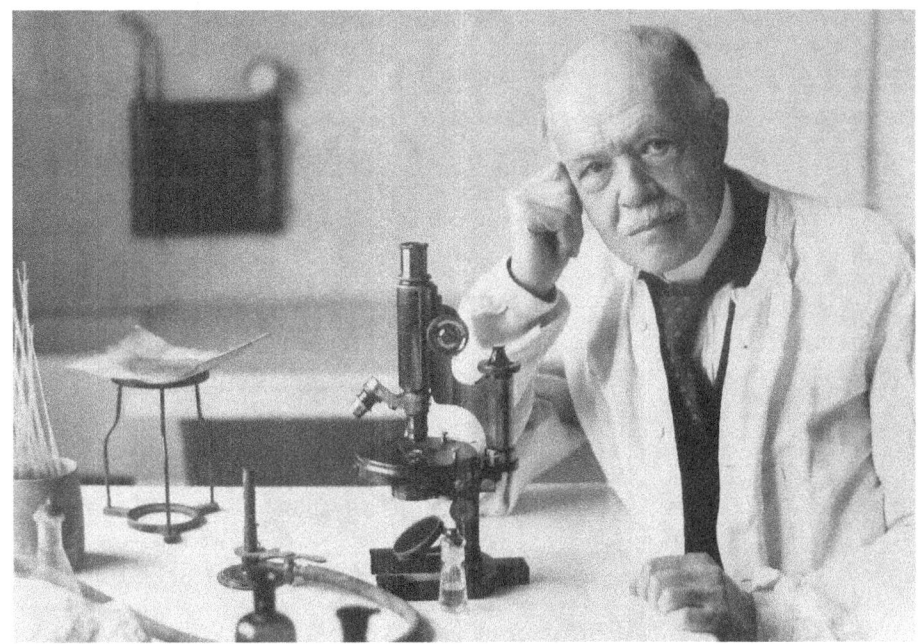

Fig. 1 Nicolle at his microscope.

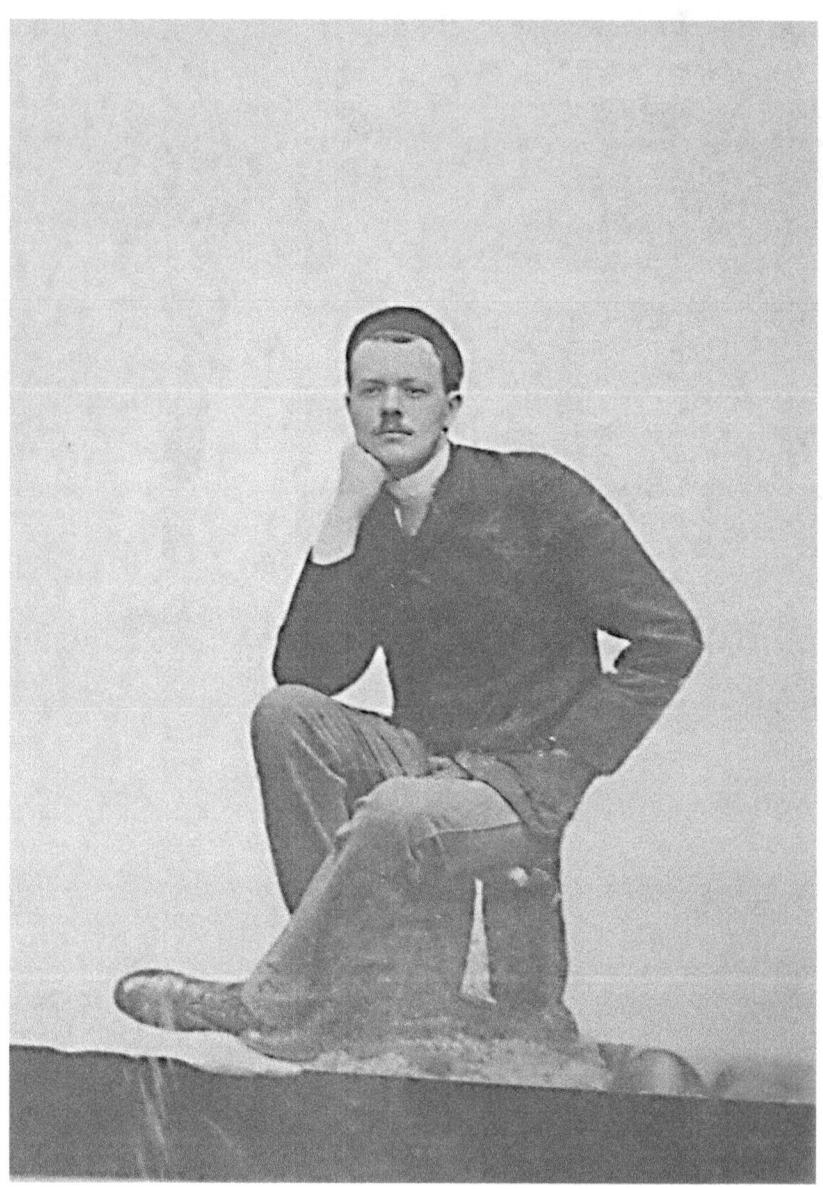

Fig. 2 Young Nicolle.

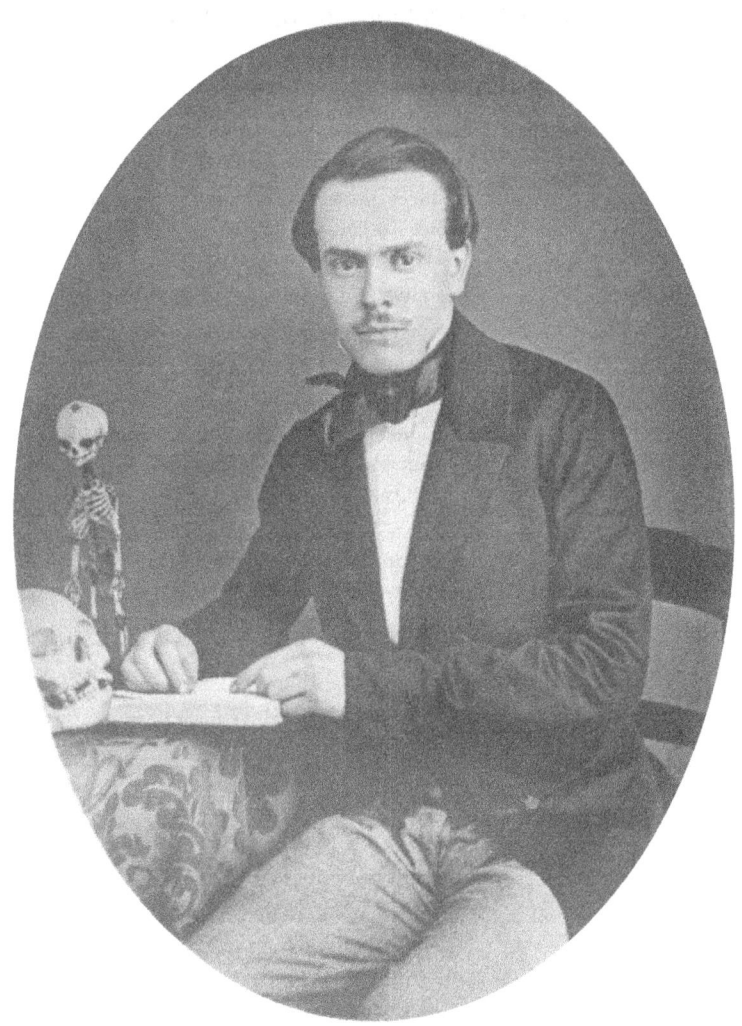

Fig. 3 Dr. Eugène Nicolle.

COURS LIBRE DE MICROBIOLOGIE DU Dr C. NICOLLE

PROGRAMME DU COURS :

Lundi	21 Mai . .	Les microbes — Les fermentations — Classification des microbes — Les bactéries.
Mardi	22 — . .	Cultures pures — Génération spontanée — Stérilisation par la chaleur — Pommes de terre.
Mercredi	23 — . .	Les milieux de culture — Bouillon.
Jeudi	24 — . .	Pléomorphisme des bactéries — Gélatine.
Vendredi	25 — . .	Stérilisation par filtration — Agar.
Samedi	26 — . .	Milieux naturellement stériles — Séparation des microbes — Conditions de développement des microbes dans les milieux de culture.
Lundi	28 — . .	Examen des microbes sans coloration — Microbes colorés et fluorescents — Bacille pyocyanique.
Mardi	29 — . .	Matières colorantes — Méthodes de coloration.
Mercredi	30 — . .	Microbes du sol.
Jeudi	31 — . .	Microbes de l'eau.
Vendredi	1er Juin . .	Microbes de l'air — Microbes lumineux.
Samedi	2 — . .	Pratique des inoculations expérimentales.
Mardi	5 — . .	Charbon.
Mercredi	6 — . .	Choléra des poules — Rouget du porc.
Jeudi	7 — . .	Vaccination du choléra des poules, du charbon et du rouget.
Vendredi	8 — . .	Suppuration — Staphylocoque — Tétragène — Gonocoque — Bacille du chancre mou.
Samedi	9 — . .	Rage.
Lundi et mardi	11 et 12 *juin*.	Fièvre typhoïde — Bacille typhique — Bactérium coli — Psittacose — Fièvre récurrente.
Mercredi	13 *juin* . .	Pneumocoque — Méningite cérébrospinale épidémique — Bacille de Friedlander et microbes voisins.

Fig. 4 Schedule for Nicolle's Microbiology Course, Rouen.

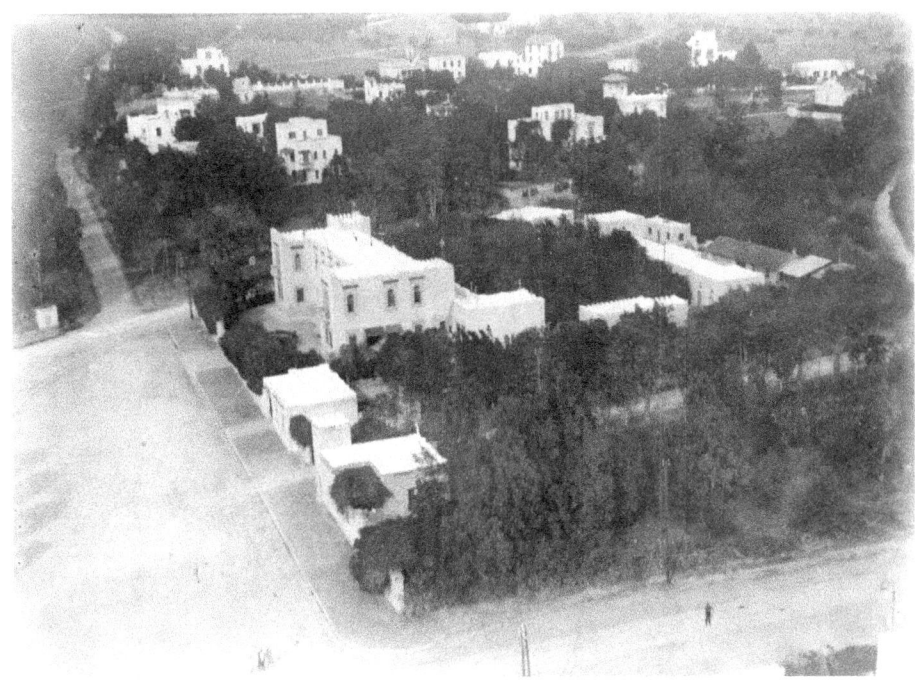

Fig. 5 The Pasteur Institute of Tunis.

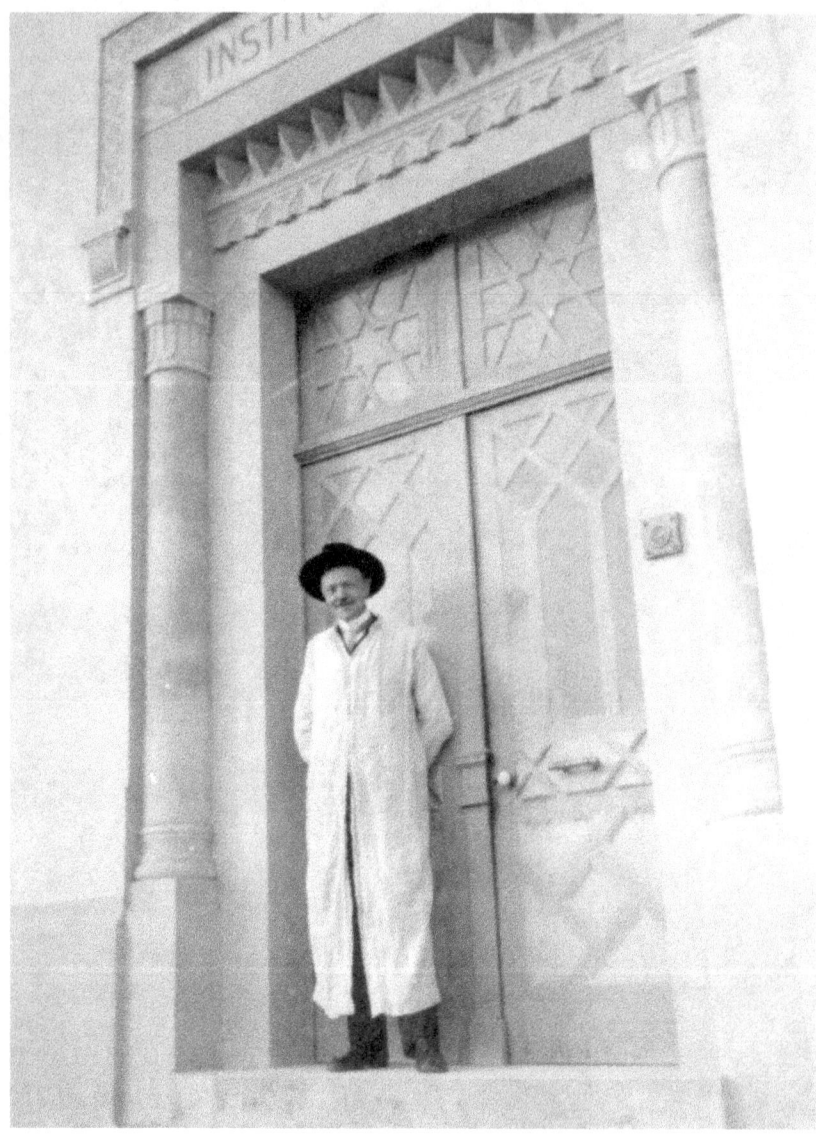
Fig. 6 Nicolle before the Door of his Institute, ca. 1909.

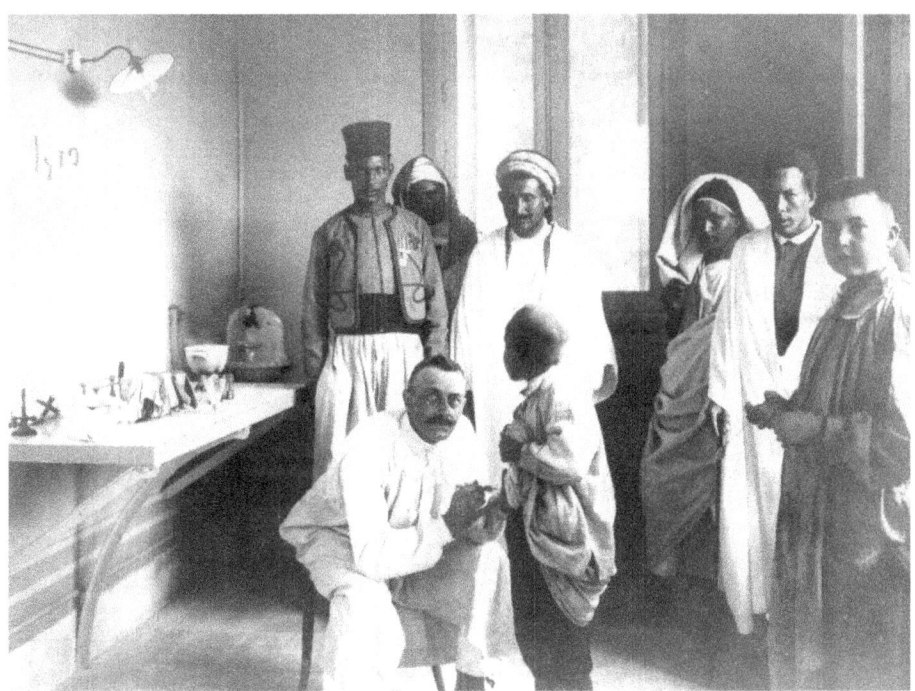

Fig. 7 Alfred Conor Administering Vaccines at the IPT.

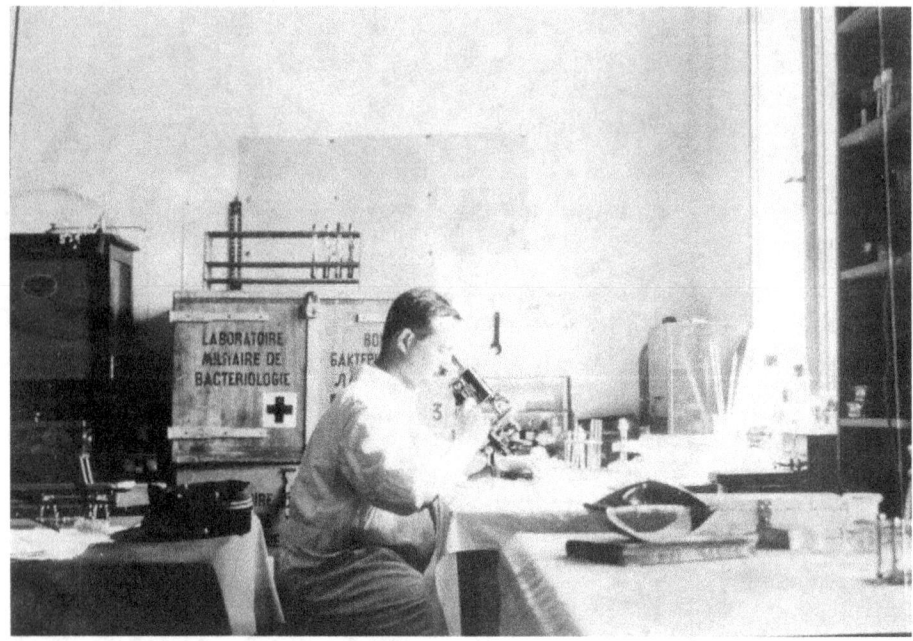

Fig. 8 Georges Blanc in Serbia, World War I.

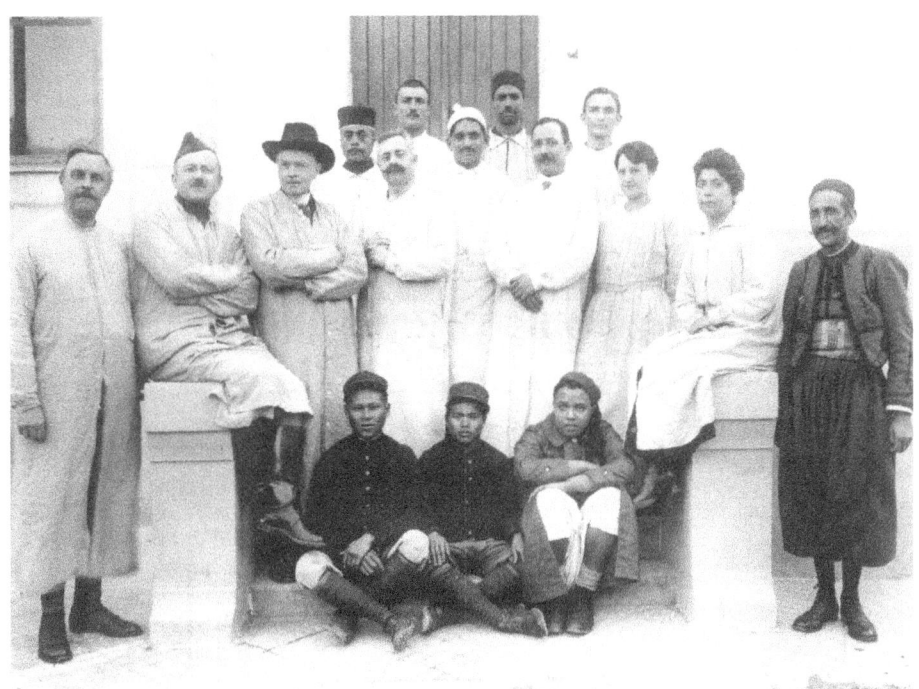

Fig. 9 Personnel of the IPT, World War I. Habib is standing at far right. Nicolle is in the middle row, third from the left.

Algeria. Institut Pasteur.

ARCHIVÉS
DES
INSTITUTS PASTEUR
DE L'AFRIQUE DU NORD

Tome 1 — Année 1921

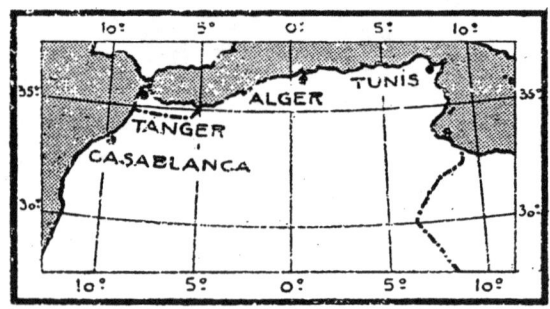

PUBLICATION TRIMESTRIELLE
ÉDITÉE ALTERNATIVEMENT
PAR

L'INSTITUT PASTEUR D'ALGÉRIE | **L'INSTITUT PASTEUR DE TUNIS**
(Fascicules I et III de chaque tome) | (Fascicules II et IV de chaque tome)

Cette publication fait suite aux *Archives de l'Institut Pasteur de Tunis* fondées en 1906

Fig. 10 The *AIPAN*.

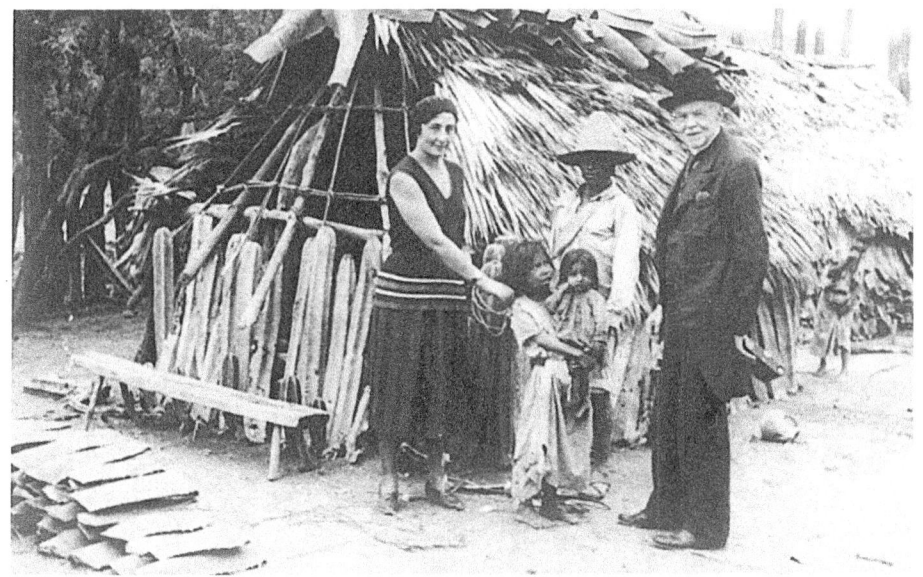

Fig. 11 Nicolle and Hélène Sparrow in Mexico, 1931.

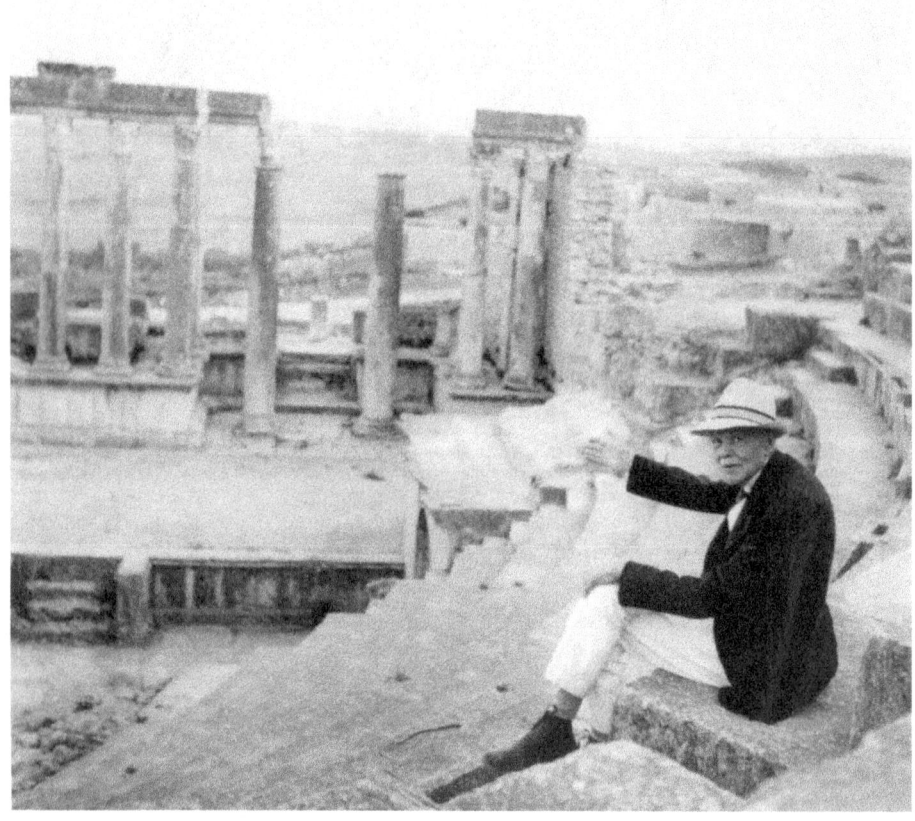

Fig. 12 Nicolle and the Ruins in Dougga (Credit: Paul Giroud).

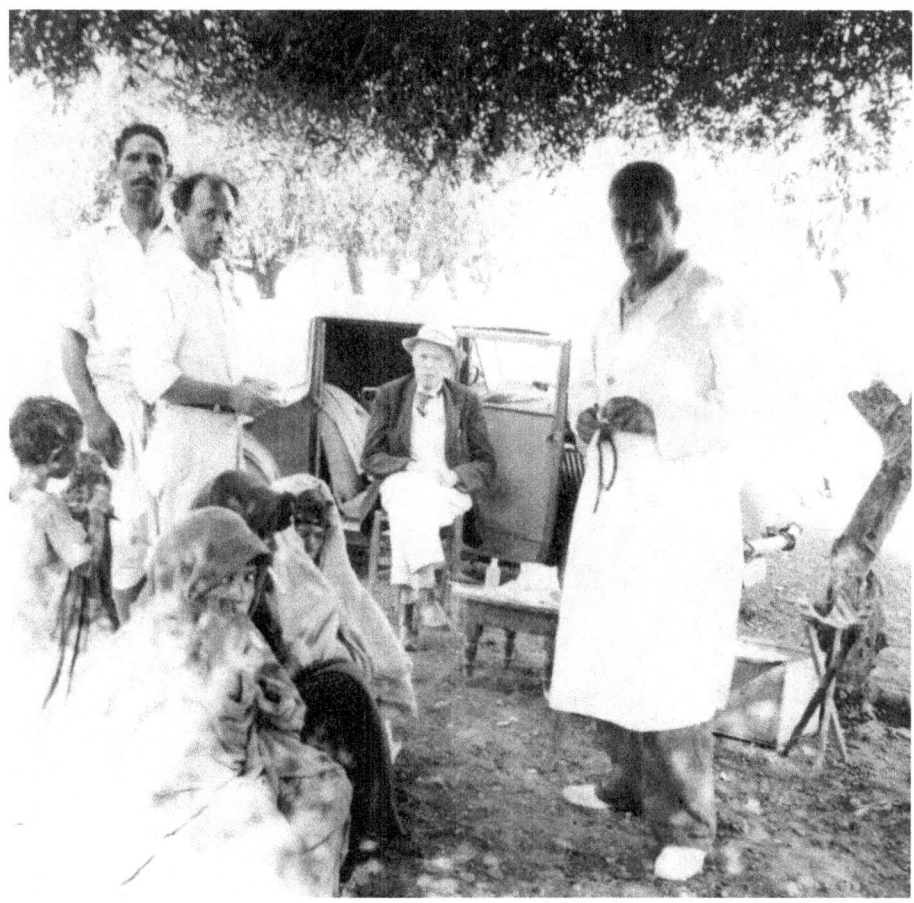

Fig. 13 Nicolle in the Bled, Tunisia (Credit: Paul Giroud).

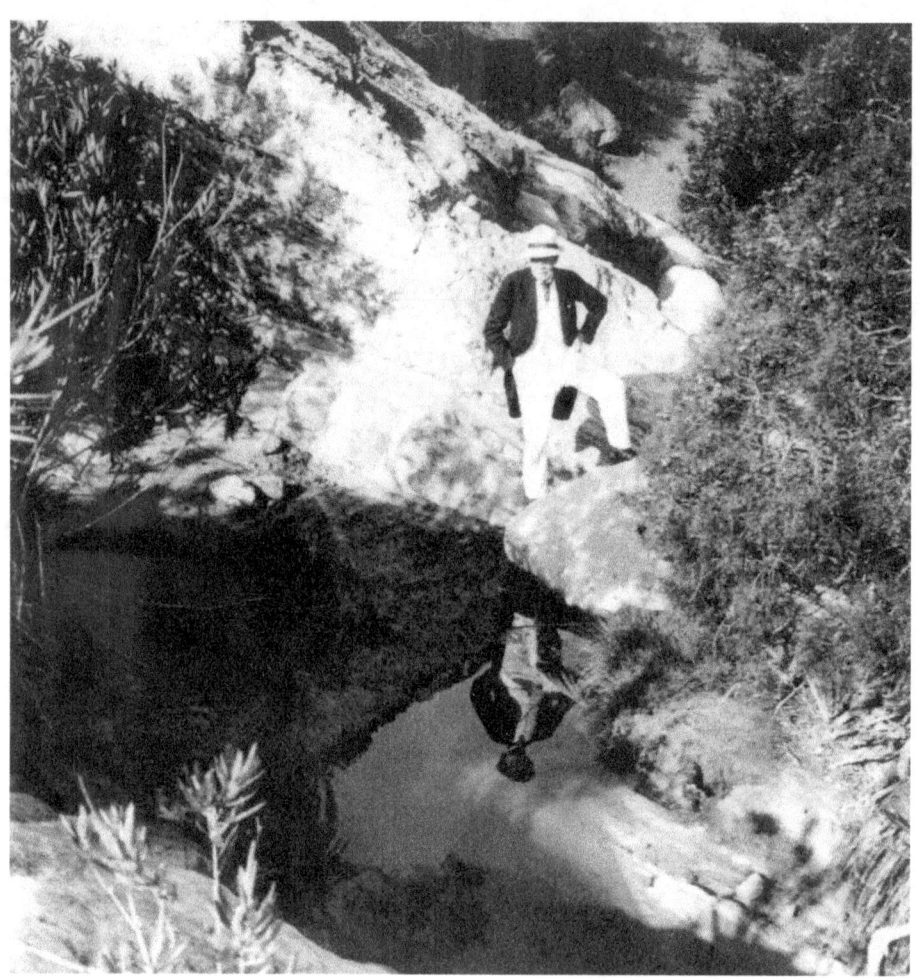

Fig. 14 Nicolle, Reflecting (Credit: Paul Giroud).

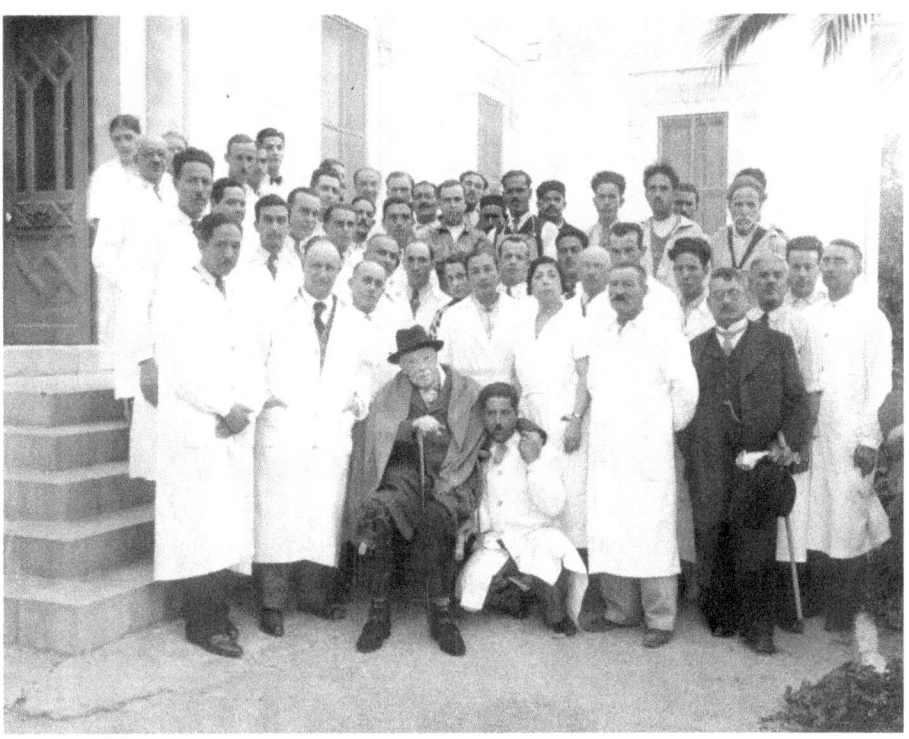

Fig. 15 Personnel of the IPT, ca. 1935.

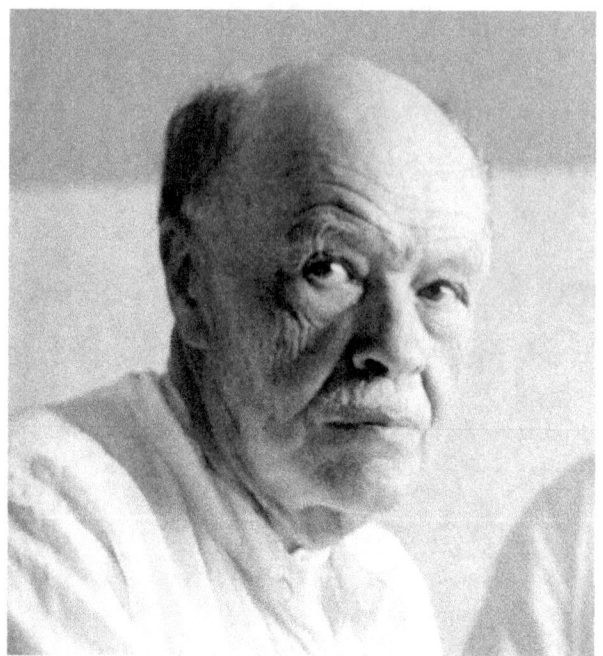

Fig. 16 Nicolle (Credit: Paul Giroud).

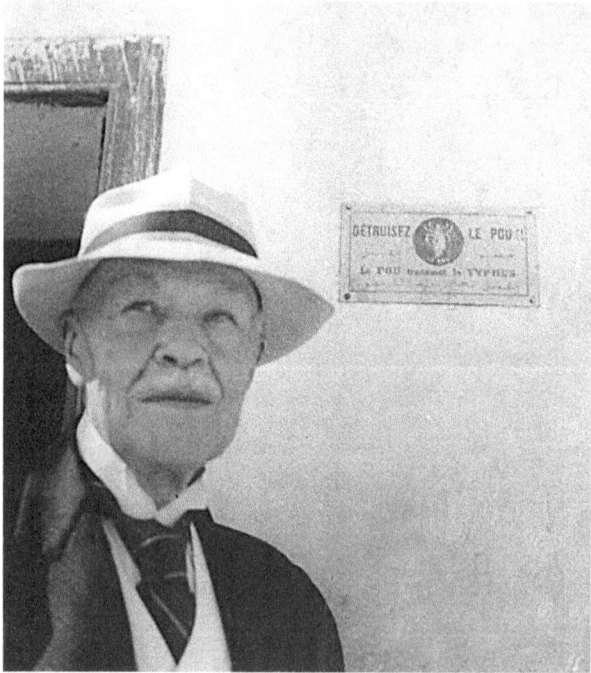

Fig. 17 Nicolle standing before a warning sign (in French): "Destroy the louse! The louse transmits typhus." (Credit: Paul Giroud).

Part Five

Denouement

Between the idea
And the reality
Between the motion
And the act
Falls the Shadow
> *For Thine is the Kingdom*

Between the conception
And the creation
Between the emotion
And the response
Falls the Shadow
> *Life is very long*

Between the desire
And the spasm
Between the potency
And the existence
Between the essence
And the descent
Falls the Shadow
> *For Thine is the Kingdom*

For Thine is
Life is
For Thine is the

This is the way the world ends
This is the way the world ends
This is the way the world ends
Not with a bang but a whimper.

—T. S. Eliot, "The Hollow Men," 1925

8

AT HOME WITH MY SHADOWS

Patrie de Nomade

> *Patrie de nomade.* Nowhere to feel at home with my shadows.
> —Nicolle, *Mémoires*

In 1934, Nicolle published the final book in his biological/philosophical trilogy. *La Nature: Conception et Morale Biologique* [*Nature*] opens with the author's personal invitation to the reader to accompany him in his narrative explorations. More specifically, he summons the reader to join him at a window, looking out over "nature": "We approach the window. I open it. Reader, you lean on the sill next to me."[1] Outside, the garden is coming to life; "beyond it, the sea gently stirs up its pebbles." Inspired by the scene, Nicolle proclaims, " 'Nature is beautiful.' You add, 'She is caring [*aimant*].' " Nicolle and his reader return to the window in winter. The cold wind chills them. "Now invisible, the roaring sea hurls its waves." The garden is in ruins. "I say, 'Truly nature is ugly.' You add, 'Worse, she is cruel to all living things.' "[2] How, then, does one reconcile these contradictory observations, made of the same place, if in different times? "Beauty and benevolence; the ugliness and evil that we define as their opposites, are but the sentiments with which we clothe nature. Intelligence, absurdity: it is our human judgment that so labels it. Nature is neither beautiful nor ugly, neither good nor bad. It does not know reason or illogic. It is."[3] It is from this "nature" that Nicolle, in the book *Nature*, seeks to explain human civilization. What, within such an animate but deanthropomorphized nature, could possibly give rise to logic and intuition, to perceptions of beauty, goodness, and truth, or to the visceral *need* for justice to prevail?[4]

Three decades earlier, Nicolle had believed that human civilization could *master* nature. He had embraced the Baconian dream of a world in which knowledge, properly obtained, conferred such power. This dream not only gave force to his ideas of what might be achieved; it also helped propel both Pastorian and French civilizing missions.[5] Long wary of reason detached from empirical observation, after World War I, Nicolle increasingly saw limitations in the power of scientific reasoning as well. Eventually, he emphasized the role of "intuition" in his formulation and added "equilibrium" to give it vital flexibility. This was his vision in *Biologie*. By the time *Nature* appeared, even this vision had paled. In fact, Nicolle wrote the bulk of *Nature* in 1931, just as he was finishing final revisions on *Biologie*. However, he continued to tinker with *Nature* well into 1934.[6] By that time, his pessimism cast a long shadow over any traces of earlier optimism. Equilibrium was a pendulum; and, for each oscillation toward apparent progress, there was a counteroscillation. He drew evidence for his despair from the world around him—in particular, from examples that were generally thought to demonstrate the progress of civilization.[7]

What benefits did modern civilization confer? Such advances as charity, equality, hygiene, public works, technology, efficiency—these come to mind. Yet, each example contained its own counterexample. Humanity's humane impulse to protect its weak, Nicolle observed (in mildly eugenic tones), precisely preserved the weak and allowed them to weaken society.[8] Democracy stopped the pendulum of politics "midway between despotism and anarchy," opening a path for the abuses of politicians, the weakening of government, and the eventual emergence of a dictator.[9] Then, there was technology. Irrigation opened new territories for cultivation, agricultural and cultural, but also brought with it mosquitoes, which in turn brought in diseases such as malaria. Hygiene worked to control these diseases but constantly faced resistance from "the apathy of indigenous peoples, the carelessness of colonials, skepticism," on the one hand; and from the vastness of nature on the other.[10] Indeed, the control of typhus, which in theory appeared quite achievable, had not been achieved: "the total suppression of the louse is not a question of hygiene, it is a question of civilization."[11] The division of labor permitted industrial advances, but also destroyed individuality, "reducing humans to the rank of machine parts."[12] It was a host of technological developments, moreover, that had not only facilitated the escalation of the last world war, but would ensure that the next one "will afflict above all the non-combatant population. Civilization will destroy itself by the monstrous development of its power."[13] It was even the case that too much erudition killed creativity.[14] In sum, "weighing the pro and the con—not the good and the evil, which are arbitrary points of view—we realize only that life changes, it never gains. *There is no progress.*"[15]

In this frame of mind, Nicolle returned to the themes with which he was struggling in 1915, when he wrote "Souvenir."[16] I have suggested that, in its structure, themes, and questions, "Souvenir" paralleled Fyodor Dostoevsky's earlier reworking of the Garden of Eden story, "The Dream of a Ridiculous Man." In *Nature*, Nicolle returned to these themes in a manner still more strikingly similar to Dostoevsky's.[17] To make his point about the illusory nature of civilization's progress, he offered a thought-experiment, which followed after a rhetorical presentation of the advantages of present-day civilization over the past. Was there "on the whole, for humans in our current civilization," he challenged his reader, "any advantage over the human brutes from which they descended"?[18] Certainly, today's civilized humans lived longer and more *convenient* lives. They had lost physical strength, but they enjoyed a more fully developed brain: "It is to this monstrous development that members of our civilization owe their superiority. . . . Intelligence alone conducts the marvelous destiny of humanity." It was clearly true that "the development of our intelligence has better informed us of the conditions of life; it has made this life more rational, more logical, for us; it has apparently suppressed many external miseries, it has given us new joys."[19] Yet. . . .

The "Dream"-like question followed: "But is man happier?" The question set up Nicolle's thought experiment: "Let us suppose that one of our primitive ancestors reappeared among us and compared his life, hard but simple, with our easier but much more complicated existence. He would find no advantage to our lives." Indeed, he would soon "ask to return to his cave, sure to savor there the blessings that civilization keeps from us"—blessings that "all beings, besides ourselves and our social animals, savor: the relaxation of repose after needs are met." The civilized are "slaves to the disciplined life that they have made" and "know only one joy: to have these chains, for a time, removed." Even then, "they are vexed by troubles. The civilized existence is one of ceaseless work. The pleasures that we have added are fatigue, complications, or depravities."[20] Nicolle might well have been addressing the citizens of Dostoevsky's fallen world of innocence, who were chanting:

> "We may be deceitful, wicked and unjust, we know it and we grieve over it. . . . But we have science, and by the means of it we shall find the truth and we shall arrive at it consciously. Knowledge is higher than feeling, the consciousness of life is higher than life. Science will give us wisdom, wisdom

will reveal the laws, and the knowledge of the laws of happiness is higher than happiness."[21]

Nicolle had fallen from his faith in the power of science over nature—and over *human* nature.

Civilization would not, however, improve its lot by returning to some primitive state. Nicolle was too familiar with examples of the devastating power of nature left wholly unchecked—particularly in its epidemic forces—to advocate such a solution. Besides, he noted, the tendency to look to the past for utopian solutions suffered from the same logical flaw as did looking to the future: it was motivated by an illusory search for a "golden age." If golden ages did exist, he suggested in a rare moment of guarded optimism, they existed only in the time in which one lived: "if we knew how to savor it."[22] Ultimately, our only choice was to continue on, and to encourage the work of the "geniuses" who had the power to restore harmony between human civilization and nature. Geniuses, however, had their own limitations. They, too, were informed by the social assumptions of their day; they effected their reforms through destructive disequilibria—and they were not always right. One senses in *Nature* Nicolle's increasing awareness of the burdens, the futility even, of genius, and the transient value of his accomplishments:[23] "We evolve constantly. We appear to advance toward a goal. We do not progress. The goal, the ends, are illusions."[24] There was only the struggle. The man who had finally been thwarted in his long efforts to achieve his intertwined missions again quoted Epictetus: " 'the most hopeless struggles are the most beautiful.' "[25]

The Specter of Typhus

1934 was not wholly bleak: during the summer (before Nicolle felt that the IPP's Scientific Council had fully betrayed its mission), Jean Laigret was conducting the dramatic yellow fever vaccine trials that Nicolle believed demonstrated the ability of inapparent infections to act as virus-vaccines. Yet, at the same time, the epidemiological component of his vision—the part that he claimed offered insight into the workings of nature itself—was facing mounting opposition: "we question the great importance which Old World investigators give to inapparent infection as a reservoir," Herman Mooser reported.[26] Another attack struck still closer to home.

In 1934, Hans Zinsser's *Rats, Lice, and History* appeared in serial form in the *Atlantic Monthly*. (It was published as a book in 1935.) The study's casual interdisciplinary eloquence and wit made it an instant classic. It also effaced much of the remaining debate over the unity or plurality of typhus. "There are . . . two distinct types of true typhus virus," Zinsser noted with assurance.[27] In addition to dedicating the book to Nicolle, Zinsser drew reverent attention to Nicolle's typhus contributions on a number of occasions.[28] He made special mention of inapparent infection. The concept, Zinsser observed, "is beginning to possess an importance of the first order in epidemiological reasoning in many fields." Then, however, he finished his sentence: "other than that of typhus fever."[29] He based his assertion on his own recent examination of Nathan Brill's mysterious sufferers of mild typhus. From this study, "a partial answer—in our view a complete one"—to the persistent question of the interepidemic reservoir of classic typhus had emerged[30]—and it had nothing to do with inapparent infection.

In 1933–34, Zinsser compiled records of more than five hundred cases of Brill's disease that had been observed in Boston and New York. (Many of these case notes had been taken by Nathan Brill himself.) Zinsser was inspired to undertake the study because there was "no precise information concerning the manner in which the European disease is kept alive in the often prolonged periods between epidemic outbreaks." What about inapparent infections? Without mentioning either the term or Nicolle, Zinsser dismissed their explanatory value: "For want of a better explanation . . . it has been tentatively assumed that the European disease may be kept going either by the existence of human carriers or by the persistence of a constant trickle of mild and unrecognized cases. Neither of these views, however, is based on more than a desire to explain a situation for which no accurate experimental data are available."[31] Zinsser collaborated with colleagues in New York, including a statistician, to analyze the Brill's data.[32] The study indicated that nearly 98 percent of the patients had been born in Europe (including Russia).[33] Eliminating the possibility of contact or louse transmission among them, Zinsser concluded "that these cases were, almost all of them, recrudescences of infections acquired in childhood in the native heaths of classical typhus, and that the classical European typhus can maintain itself in human reservoirs indefinitely without the intervention of extraneous animal vectors."[34]

From their correspondence, it is clear that Nicolle agreed with Zinsser's interpretation of the *etiology* of Brill's disease—soon rechristened "Brill-Zinsser disease." He even published an early version of the study in his own *Archives* that July, and he himself corrected his American colleague's French.[35] In the article's conclusion, however, Zinsser did not draw out the obvious implications his interpretation had for the future fate of inapparent infection: "In our opinion, there is only one explanation for the conservation and propagation of the virus of Brill's disease—and, by extension, for classic typhus: a human reservoir."[36] Others, however, would quickly make the connections. Brill-Zinsser disease, *not* inapparent infection, explained the persistence of typhus between epidemic outbreaks. It is unlikely that Nicolle missed the study's epidemiological significance—though, soon quite ill, he may have appreciated his friend's reserve. When Nicolle's illness reached a particularly ominous crisis in the spring of 1935, Zinsser, then working in Giroud's Paris laboratory, came to visit him. Marcelle Nicolle had been distracting her ailing "Papa" shortly before Zinsser's arrival by reading him the newly published *Rats, Lice, and History*.[37]

It was Nicolle's heart that was, once again, troubling him. This time, however, his cardiac crises were brought on by an infection. Early in September 1934, Nicolle was stricken by a disease that he and his colleagues believed to be *fièvre boutonneuse*. As a consequence of this misdiagnosis and an apparently rapid recovery, Nicolle did not take sufficient rest.[38] His tachycardia soon returned in dramatic fashion, along with a number of other symptoms. Eventually, it became clear that he had in fact contracted murine typhus while working on the disease. Nicolle made the unfortunate event part of an article, "Murine Typhus Contracted during Research," that he published in the *AIPT*. Among the six cases discussed, he calmly described the attack on "Doctor N., 67 years old, French, tachycardic; vaccinated one year previously with the Weigl vaccine."[39] Over the next year and a half, Nicolle's health steadily declined. He continued to work, but he had lost almost everything he believed in. His personal and professional missions had failed; the future of civilization looked grim. Nicolle's actions make it clear that he once again felt as if he had been cast adrift. Once again, he would turn to Tunisia.

Remissions

Despite his rejection by the *Maison mère*, Nicolle was still Chair of Experimental Medicine at the Collège de France. For many others, the position would have been the culmination of a career, but to Nicolle, it was principally a means to a now-failed end. This is evident in his reactions in the wake of Pastorian developments and in the ease with which he abandoned the post when the opportunity presented itself. Indeed, shortly after he failed to gain the IPP directorship, Nicolle asked Vallery-Radot, "What good will it do to persist in my work at the Collège de France?"[40] Just as his illness struck that September, he again wrote to Vallery-Radot, "It is only so as not to abandon our common goal that I have not resigned my post at the Collège de France, where I am wasting my time and compromising my health."[41] Soon, he would concede that no true change would come to the IPP, regardless of his actions. It was thus time to leave his Paris post, and his illness provided him with the opportunity for a diplomatic exit. Eventually, another friend of Duhamel's, surgeon René Leriche, was named Nicolle's replacement.[42]

His missions and his Parisian obligations at an end, Nicolle was left with himself—the self he had become. Contained within this identity were his friends, and his "children": Marcelle and Pierre, his disease concepts, his writings, his institute. He counted on his friends to help ensure the future of these diverse children. Nicolle made Duhamel, with his children, his literary executor; he knew well that the Duhamels and Vallery-Radot would watch over Marcelle and Pierre. As for his institute, he had worked for years to provide for its survival after him. All was in order, except the director's position. Though there is evidence that a number of Nicolle's collaborators believed the position would be theirs, Nicolle came to a decision that pleased him.[43] Reconciled to the fact that Georges Blanc would not return, he turned to another former collaborator. Initially through his wife, Lydia, Etienne Burnet had enjoyed a warm reconciliation with Nicolle in the 1930s.[44] The IPP honored Nicolle's wishes, appointing Burnet his successor. Blanc, who may not have wished to take over Nicolle's institute, did gladly carry forth his mentor's disease concepts and methodological commitments, as would any number of former collaborators.[45]

In 1935, Nicolle personally revisited a few of his intellectual children: inapparent infection and (if "his" only by adoption) inframicrobes. He continued to argue that the former both explained the birth and death of diseases and, through transformation into vaccines, promised to control the effects of those diseases.[46] The latter merited special consideration. Returning to his 1902 paper on variability in agglutinating properties of microbes, Nicolle grappled with the developments concerning inframicrobes and mutation in the intervening years. Now convinced that mutations were largely *inherited*, he remained committed to his belief that *infra*-microbes were living entities that had evolved from microbes.[47] If he learned of Wendell Stanley's crystallization of tobacco mosaic virus that year, it is unclear whether the news affected his interpretation.

Yet, even with all the time he devoted to science in the last months of his life, Nicolle had become convinced that the knowledge produced by science was of limited value. In March 1935, in the space of ten days, Nicolle composed all but the conclusion of his final book, *La Destinée Humaine*.[48] Presented as "a companion to *La Nature*," the book completed his trajectory into the abyss.[49] It illustrated "the evolution" of Nicolle's thoughts since his earlier philosophical work, with an emphasis on the limits of human reason. Reason, Nicolle wrote, was a valuable instrument but, even in its intuitive form, was limited by physiological constraints. It might clarify our understanding of the world, but it could never fully explain the world.[50] Human destiny moved us not toward intellect, but toward faith. And in the end, it was faith that he sought. Nicolle may have had his friends and his assorted children, but he had no place that gave him solace—and he desperately sought such a place: "The reformer, his obligations to society having been fulfilled, reflects on the melancholy of all human endings, and seeks to lose himself in the sweet and tender images that have consoled so many before him."[51]

In his autobiography, Duhamel later reflected on his friend's spiritual conversion. It was a phenomenon he had seen before:

> the irrational nearly always takes its revenge towards the close of these learned lives . . . for the illustrious Charles Richet spiritualism represented the revenge of the irrational.
>
> Subsequently I have seen that revenge operate in quite another fashion on minds of high quality. Some idea of this may be gained by reading the last works of Charles Nicolle and of M. Cuénot. The final utterances of Henri Bergson made me aware of an altogether similar evolution. If a date must be assigned to this tendency of certain minds, I would place it after 1930. . . . [It reflects] the efforts of a lofty mind to reconcile the rational and the revealed.[52]

At the end of his life, Nicolle, an agnostic since adolescence, saw his religious skepticism disappear. His religious rhetoric lost its rhetorical status and became the foundation of his intellectual and spiritual convictions. On one level, he replaced his fervor for Pastorian reform with a passion for religion: the missionary looked for redemption. Consulting a Jesuit priest, he learned that his desire for faith permitted him to reenter the Church.[53] Nicolle, then in France, formally embraced Catholicism on August 10, 1935.[54] From that day until his death, he awaited a moment of grace that would reveal the truth of his faith to him. If such a revelation came, however, he did not write of it.

Nor did his embrace of faith seem to bring Nicolle the peace—the sense of place—he longed for. Shortly after her father's conversion, Marcelle, who dutifully tended to her father during his illness, wrote to Duhamel: "For the past dozen days Papa has had the fervent desire to return by plane to Tunis in order, he says, to end his days at home, in his beloved institute."[55] Once he had returned to Tunisia, Nicolle himself was more blunt: "I have returned to exile so as not to die in France."[56]

Denouement

Nicolle returned one last time to Tunisia's shores—to set his affairs in order and, ultimately, to die. He addressed heartfelt letters to many of his friends, often enclosing, or promising, some memento: photographs, sculptures, paintings. He put his voluminous correspondence in order.[57] The self-proclaimed nomad, the *isolé*, then attempted to find a final resting place that would allow him to be at peace. He chose a location that, symbolically marked, reconciled the often-conflicting parts of himself: Pastorian, provincial, colonial, "Tunisian":

> I wish to be buried in the vestibule of the Pasteur Institute [of Tunis], where the mosaic of the dog is located. On my stone, I would like my name: Charles Nicolle; the date and place of my birth (Rouen); the date of my death; the dates of my directorship; and nothing else. . . . I leave the construction of the stone itself to M. Edouard Delabarre. . . . I would like the design to be that of two branches: apple and olive.[58]

Nicolle's tombstone brought together the symbols of Normandy and Tunisia, located in a true House of Pasteur—a house that had been made also in his own image. Moreover, having arranged for his body to remain in Tunis, Nicolle decided to leave the body of his work to Rouen.

Nicolle had long referred to himself as a "Tunisian Pastorian." On February 1, 1936, he wrote his final letter to Georges Duhamel: "My friend, I write to you on the banks of Carthage, between the ruins of the ancient baths and the sea." He was concerned that Duhamel knew his wishes for his final book manuscripts and understood "my spiritual evolution." In particular, there was the manuscript that he had written much earlier but that had yet to find a publisher: "Mon Camarade Habib." His closing thought to Duhamel—a postscript—read, "I would very much like to see Habib appear before I die."[59] This wish would not be fulfilled. Habib's memory continued to haunt Nicolle, a symbolic combination of his youth, his Tunisian identity, and his communion with Duhamel. In the codicil to his will, he made provisions for Habib's family.[60]

Nicolle spent many of his last days at the seaside: in Carthage, in Hammamet. There, he dictated the final passages of his memoir and wrote a final letter to Pasteur Vallery-Radot. In the letter, he reflected on his own father's death: "I can say that I have never been consoled." With his "tender heart," this "student of Pouchet" had given up his own professional aspirations to ensure the security of his family, conferring upon his eldest son "the mission that he could not himself undertake." Eugène Nicolle had died at the age of fifty-one, "worn away . . . by professional fatigue"; he did not live to "see the success of his sons."[61] His middle son—whose successes he did not fully foresee—died on February 28, 1936, at the age of seventy. He was buried, as he wished, behind the doors of what was then the entrance to his institute.

In a part of his memoir that he had written earlier, Charles Nicolle had grappled with his constant feelings of placelessness. It was there that he reflected on his lifelong relationship with the sea, remembering in particular his childhood vacations with his father:

> Yes, you are most certainly my *patrie*, my little *patrie*, the mantle of my soul; dear little fishing port where the wind of the open sea, of carefree days, freed and broadened my spirit so that I could begin to think. Little port of fishermen, welcome your child, who returns to you.[62]

Reflections

"The work of the extension of civilization—that is to say, the work of colonization," Nicolle asserted in his 1934 lectures at the Collège de France, "includes a medical component. This component part is so closely tied to the whole that it appears difficult to consider it separately." Nicolle thus dedicated one entire lesson before his Collège audience to "the responsibilities of medicine in the work of the extension of civilization."[63] By this time, however, he was no uncritical advocate of colonial expansion: indeed, he included consecutive sections on the "harmful consequences of the colonial enterprise" on both colonized and colonizers.[64] With colonialism, as with so many other aspects of his life, Nicolle preserved faith in long-standing convictions by redefining them in accordance with his own experiences and inclinations. The "colonialism" he advocated in the end was a colonialism grounded in education and medicine, which conferred "benefits to all humanity [*la communauté des hommes*]." These benefits—seen clearly, he noted in some detail, in the work of "France in Africa"—alone "legitimated" the colonial project.[65] Ultimately, Nicolle envisioned a world that preserved "the diversity of the intellectual qualities of all races." Such diversity would even extend to an international cooperation between national laboratories, which would in turn ensure the continued vitality of science. "The defense and cultivation of diverse natural types of human intelligence is thus a duty to those of us whose mission it is to ensure the future of our science."[66]

The historical assessment of the West's nineteenth-century colonial project was long consistent with Nicolle's own views. Even after World War II, in the wake of decolonization, medicine enjoyed a relatively protected status as one of the true "benefits" the West had conferred upon the world. In our own decolonized and postmodern world, however, most of the trappings of colonialism have (at least externally) been stripped away, by historians, cultural critics, and the citizens of countries once colonized. Medicine has not retained its privileged status. In Tunisia, the names of most of the streets and buildings that were once French have been changed to reflect the country's history *outside* the Protectorate. Yet, the Avenue Charles Nicolle, a main road that passes by one side of the IPT, has retained its name. As a former city official explained: "Charles Nicolle was not just for France. He was for all humanity."[67] Moreover, the Pasteur Institute of Tunis continues to celebrate the contributions of its formative French director, even under the direction of Tunisian scientists. Former director Amor Chadli, a great admirer of Charles Nicolle, authored a number of articles and organized several official gatherings in tribute to his illustrious French predecessor. Under director Koussay Dellagi, the centennial of the institute's foundation was celebrated in grand fashion. Anne Marie Moulin spoke on "Charles Nicolle, Tunisian Scientist."[68] And Nicolle's tomb at the IPT remains in place.

Historians are wise to treat their historical "actor's categories" with suspicion. Such categories, before they can be critically understood, must be broken apart, deconstructed, and reconstructed in the light of a host of sociocultural considerations. The case of Charles Nicolle, however, suggests that such reconstructions, while of central importance, do not wholly account for the trajectories of history. Nicolle's vision of an internationally cooperative science rising above nationalistic differences, though hardly unique to him, cannot be simply reduced to self-interest and social contingencies—even if these did inform it. For, this vision—*Nicolle's* vision, derivative or not—continues to have a tangible effect on the social structures—indeed, the medical identity—of France's former protectorate.

When I first started this project, many years ago, I was fascinated with "interwar" literature. It was filled with the ambiguities that emerged from the fragmentation of traditional certainties; and I, younger then, found that it appealed to that poetic angst one has time to feed when one has few other responsibilities (though I must confess that I still find it appealing). I was also interested in the intersections of science and the humanities, as well as the construction of disease concepts. And so, I looked for a fitting interwar project. When I read Hans Zinsser's classic "biography" of typhus, *Rats, Lice, and History*, I thought I'd found my subject. There was typhus, there was war, and there was the larger-than-life, interdisciplinary persona of Hans Zinsser himself. A trip to the Countway Library at Harvard's Medical School, where Zinsser had been a professor, brought me into contact with the encyclopedic and helpful Richard Wolfe, who gently informed me that little remained of Zinsser's private papers. As I had also been intrigued by Zinsser's dedication of the book to the similarly multitalented Charles Nicolle, I asked about the existence of what Zinsser had described as a monthly correspondence the two had carried on from the late 1920s until Nicolle's death. These letters were reported to have ranged in subject from literature and philosophy to immunology and bacterial mutation, making them perfect for my purposes. Wolfe, to assist me in locating the correspondence, put me in touch with several of Zinsser's former collaborators, and a series of exchanges made clear that there had indeed been a significant correspondence. Shortly after Nicolle's death, Zinsser was having it translated (both men wrote in French), with the thought of having it published. Zinsser died before completing the project. The correspondence, which remained in the Zinsser family, had last been seen in a living room filing cabinet in the 1950s. One of Zinsser's former collaborators, Dr. Morris Shaffer, wrote to me in 1992:

> In May 1991 during a visit to Boston I had the opportunity to meet . . . two of the other old-timers who had been associated with Dr. Z. in his last months. . . . In this encounter we talked about the fate of the missing correspondence but came up with no conclusions or promising leads. It is still hard for me to understand what transpired in the matter as Dr. Zinsser was clearly anxious to have the correspondence made available so that others might utilize it in future.[69]

What remained was a mere handful of Zinsser's letters in the Nicolle collection in Rouen. And so, I turned to Charles Nicolle. Nicolle turned out to be a very different character than his friend Zinsser—so different, in fact, that I almost changed topics again.

In recent years, it has been fashionable for historians to approach the materials of history as "discourse." This approach has produced tremendous insights into how certain groups came to subjugate other groups (women, minorities, the poor).[70] Colonialism's medical history has provided a fertile field for such inquiry, *particularly because* medicine was so long held to be one of the few positive contributions made by colonizers to the colonized.[71] Charles Nicolle provides plenty of evidence to substantiate such historical critiques. His negative views of women alone were enough to give me pause. Yet, in a sense, these aspects of Nicolle, though important to who he was and how he thought, were not a very interesting piece of the story I was beginning to see. This was, in part, because they were just *so* typical of his time. There was little here that had not been treated by other historians before, on other subjects, and with more skill and substance than anything I might put together on Nicolle. But the story I was beginning to see, one that lay principally outside this particular style of historical inquiry, was not entirely evident to me, even after I had finished the project. I set it aside. When I returned to it again after nearly a decade, that story was more evident. Shortly after I finished writing it, I learned that the Zinsser-Nicolle correspondence had materialized at Harvard. I consulted it with some trepidation. Soon, however, I was relieved: the letters were interesting, but not quite as revelatory as I had anticipated.[72] Reading them, I realized that the story I had already told went beyond the personalities and contributions of either man—even as vital as those personalities, and as important as those contributions, had been.

At the heart of this story is the nexus of "microbiologist" and "mission." Both contained elements at once personal, professional, and more broadly social; within their interrelation was also a far more general story about the ways in which individuals have attempted to find—or create—meaning in a fragmented, modern world. The mission itself was a powerful metaphor. It resonated with traditional religious convictions and substantiated more immediate historical impulses; it served as a locus for the existential struggle between individual and society (a struggle that in turn reconstituted the identity of both individual and society).[73] In its Pastorian manifestation, it informed Nicolle's initial microbiological project, sent him to Tunisia, and encouraged him to select an emblematic disease. As he applied that mission to his chosen disease—typhus—and his new colonial home—Tunisia—Nicolle found, over time, that his mission changed how he perceived himself on a number of levels. Moreover, he came to believe that the mission had to be refashioned to survive in changing times—particularly, in times that had been irrevocably altered by world war. It had to be cast more broadly, made more flexible. If it was to remain viable, it had to encourage reciprocal exchanges, acknowledge the importance of financial gain, and accept the evolution of infectious diseases. In other words, Pastorian "missionaries" needed to embrace the categories established by Pasteur's own life and works, and altered by the varied contingencies of society, to save Pasteur's mission. At the same time, Nicolle had become convinced that the Pastorian mission, as defined in Paris by Emile Roux, was instead growing narrower and less flexible. From the tensions between Pasteur's "original" mission, Nicolle's personal reconstitution of its contents, and the mission as articulated at the *Maison mère*, Nicolle's own missionary inclinations deepened. His perception of his missionary duties in turn shaped his actions. And, as we have seen, his actions had consequences for Pastorian medicine, in France and in its colonies. If those consequences were in part reactionary, their impact, and their impetus, were not forgotten. Nicolle may have felt in the end that he had failed because he never secured Paris's blessings. Yet, to this day, his challenge is remembered there, in both its wisdom and its folly.[74]

Perhaps Nicolle should have been aware that the view of the morally elevated scientist on which his revised faith in science rested was, at best, a shaky foundation. The IPP's treatment of him during the politicking of 1933–34 made him painfully aware that he had built his new model Pastorism on swampland. If not even such scientists could put aside their differences for the sake of saving the "mission"—both Pastorian and civilizing—what hope was there for humanity at large? Here, too, lay a contradiction. Emile Lagrange, Roux's biographer, devoted a section of his biography to Nicolle and his efforts to procure the director's position in Paris. Lagrange certainly had his biases. Yet, one cannot help but find a certain plausibility in his assertion that Nicolle, as director of the IPP, would have been a "possible dictator, not to mention a probable tyrant."[75]

Charles Nicolle was a man of contradictions, constantly struggling to reconcile apparent opposites; the "creations" that arose out of these struggles were not always positive. On more than one occasion, he stated baldly, as biological facts, inflammatory statements that his own life contradicted. His ideal woman, for example, was someone who stayed at home and attended to the moral upbringing of her children and the needs of her husband. Perhaps his own wife, Alice, fell short in some of these areas: yet, she was certainly far closer to this stated ideal than were Nicolle's fascinating and talented mistresses, Marthe Conor and Hélène Sparrow. Along these same lines, he argued that the dire state of the global economy in the 1930s was greatly the result of all those women who, ignoring their biologically determined roles as conservers of hearth and home, remained in the working world after World War I. (It was this very "conservative," life-preserving, nature that Nicolle believed prevented women from becoming geniuses.) Again, his two mistresses were by all accounts brilliant and dynamic women, active in the working world. Additionally, there were Nicolle's "factual" assertions about national tendencies toward genius. The French, of course, were civilization's current font of discovery. Yet, this biological "fact" came from a man who claimed that "all nationalistic fanfare is a call to war" and who enjoyed greater status among his international colleagues—with whom he collaborated—than he did in France.[76] The conservative "facts" that Nicolle upheld, and that were contradicted by his own life, acted as the fixed skeleton in the otherwise dynamic physiology of his mosaic of powers. They were, in a sense, the conservative elements of his own upbringing that he had long struggled to reconcile with his more liberal tendencies. As he grew older and more disheartened with the world, he leaned increasingly on these traditional structures: though still principally when it suited his purposes.

These contradictions between actions and ideals did not, however, prevent Nicolle from facing much of the changing nature of knowledge and society in the postwar world directly. He clung to his faith in a Pastorian mission that had been carefully adapted (by his genius, he would claim) to those changing circumstances. He embraced the unfolding complexity of a world at once shattered and more fully revealed, and attempted to create of these parts something new and meaningful: a mosaic that rested on an equilibrium based on adaptive intervention rather than on brute force. I believe he was aided in his efforts by the fact that some of the most influential people in his later life—Georges Blanc, Marthe Conor, Pasteur Vallery-Radot, and Georges Duhamel—were all a generation *younger* than he was. As they were all roughly of the generation most directly affected by the world war, they brought a different perspective to the postwar world. Nevertheless, they were perhaps young enough at the time to preserve more faith that things could indeed change for the better. It was this group of friends who most vocally encouraged Nicolle to take the actions necessary to fulfill his missions. It was they who encouraged his writing, aided him in finding acclaim, helped him see the significance of his conceptual innovations, encouraged him to *act* to become the new Pasteur.

Charles Nicolle was an important microbiologist who practiced his science in a French colonial outpost, at a time when that science existed in a kind of no-man's-land between Golden Ages. From within the uncertainty of his time and the distance of his place, he was able to envision an uncertain future of emerging diseases, medical limitations, and global science. If Nicolle did not live to see the next medical Golden Age, he did contribute toward its establishment. For a time, the "Door of the Sadiki" opened onto a world that listened to his ideas and followed his work. It opened onto resources that encouraged him to conceive of a "mosaic of powers" resting on "virulence" without "toxicity"—on power without violence. The mosaic was Nicolle's answer to the fragmentation of his era. It gave him an outlet for his faith. Yet, in the end, it was not generally accepted as a solution to any of the problems to which he had applied it. Nor were the revised components of his Pastorian mission gratefully embraced. The *next* postwar generation of medical researchers themselves borrowed elements from Nicolle and his colleagues— once again, one might argue, mosaic-like—and enjoyed a sense of conceptual stability that their predecessors had lacked. Indeed, once the tangible accomplishments of biomedicine were secured, they acted to obscure the very work that created them. Eras of certainty are far easier to grasp than are times of complexity and contradiction, even if certainty often emerges from apparent chaos.

Nicolle himself observed that the "genius" belongs as much to his own time as to the time the products of his invention would create. Born four years before the Third Republic was established, he died four years before the Third Republic heard its death knell. Charles Nicolle was, in many ways, a man of his times.

Appendix A

Vaccines and Analyses at the Pasteur Institute of Tunis

Year	Rabies**	Smallpox	Analyses†
1905	306	47,007	1,246
1906	489	88,940	1,825
1907	293	307,360	2,746
1908	374	86,283	3,506
1909	340	101,163	7,223
1910	409	127,820	4,755
1911	296	156,339	5,997
1912	370	154,772	3,353
1913	351	142,660	3,530
1914	380	222,658	4,080
1915	420	123,350	4,194
1916	632	245,872	4,048
1917	761	121,403	5,822
1918	785	84,874	8,456
1919	853	125,102	8,225
1920	780*	192,445*	9,269*
1921	909	189,310	13,091
1922	855	165,050	11,097
1923	836	244,233	13,571
1924	1,166	371,832	14,984

Year	Rabies**	Smallpox	Analyses†
1925	934	1,207,994***	20,058
1926	789	592,130	22,651
1927	855	554,690	21,293
1928	829	655,881	25,338
1929	1,382	768,882	23,199
1930	1,345	1,058,346	27,603
1931	1,152	792,247	33,610
1932	1,150	561,375	41,076
1933	1,208	616,104	54,785
1934	1,222	644,230	54,285
1935	1,237	793,895	55,361

Sources: All statistics compiled from Nicolle's report, "Fonctionnement des Services de l'Institut Pasteur," published annually in the *AIPT,* except *, published in the *AIPAN.*

**Rabies statistics refer to the number of individuals treated, rather than the number of inoculations given.

***In the wake of a smallpox epidemic, the Pasteur Institute increased its vaccine production, and the Tunisian government decided to make vaccination and revaccination law. The Tunis institute profited well from this decision. See "Fonctionnement . . . 1925," *AIPT* 15 (1926): 184.

†Numbers do not include military analyses.

APPENDIX B

Personnel at the Pasteur Institute of Tunis, 1903–35

DIRECTEUR:
Charles Nicolle, 1903–[36]

DIRECTEUR ADJOINT:
Étienne Burnet, 1927–28

SOUS-DIRECTEUR:
Alfred Conor, 1909–14
Étienne Burnet, 1920–26
Charles Anderson, 1929–35
Lucien Balozet, 1931–35

CHEF(S) DE LABORATOIRE:*
Charles Comte, 1906–9
Albert Husson, 1906–8 (malaria service)
Ludovic Blaizot, 1910–21
Georges Blanc, 1913–20
Jean Bance, 1914–35

---

*The *chef de laboratoire* position could be divided to include one assistant director. The numbers here include assistant directors.

Charles Lebailly, 1917–18**
Louis Caillon, 1917–18**
Paul Durand, 1923–33
J. Colas-Belcour, 1928–30
Jean Laigret, 1931–35
Hélène Sparrow, 1933–35
Roger Durand, 1934
Pierre Nicolle, 1935

CHEF(S) DE LABORATOIRE, ADJOINT:
Gaston Catouillard, 1909–12, 1924–26
? Prevel, 1910

ASSISTANT:
Gaston Catouillard, 1913–23

PRÉPARATEURS:
Gaston Catouillard, 1906–8
? Boselli, 1906–8
Joseph Chaltiel, 1910–18
Alfred Jannot, 1912–18 (died in World War I)
? Loiselier, 1914–18, 1922–23
Mlle. Huret, 1924–35
Henri Roussel, 1925–35
Camille Disdier, 1925–35
René Lafont, 1925–35
Roger Chene, 1928, 1931–35
Salah Ounais, 1931–35
Jean Moulin, 1931–35
Magid Rahal, 1931–35
Georges Carre, 1934–35

AIDES-PRÉPARATEURS:
Chaltiel was the *aide-préparateur* during 1906–8; in 1909, he was joined in this position by Jannot. From 1909, the position was vacant, until five people—including Lafond, Roussel, and Huret, who later became *préparateurs* and remained at the Institute throughout Nicolle's tenure—were hired to fill the position. The number of *aide-préparateurs* varied between four and six in the years 1919–35.

**Lebailly and Caillon were appointed, by ministerial decree, to this position temporarily, when all three of Nicolle's regular *chefs* were called to army service.

NOTES

Prelude

1. Charles Nicolle, *Responsabilités* I, 7. For more on the historiography of the themes informing this "Prelude," please see my "Introduction." All translations are my own unless otherwise noted.
2. L. Bertholon, "Mentalitè Française et Colonisation Tunisienne," *Revue Tunisienne* 8 (1901): 379–406, 399–400. Emphasis in original.
3. Nicolle, *Responsabilités* I, 7–8.
4. Stephen J. Rogers, unpublished note, 1983.

Introduction

1. For more on sources written by and relating to Nicolle, see my "Bibliographic Note" at the end of this book. For general, book-length biographies, Maurice Huet, *Le Pommier et l'Olivier: Charles Nicolle, une Biographie (1866–1936)* (Paris: Sauramps Médical, 1995), and Germaine Lot, *Charles Nicolle et la Biologie Conquérante* (Paris: Editions Seghers, 1961).
2. Nicolle's later return to Paris, to take up his position as Chair of Experimental Medicine at the Collège de France from 1932, did not entail a full-time residence: he remained director of the Pasteur Institute of Tunis and continued to call Tunis, not Paris, his home.
3. I make this claim for the Parisian centralization of science despite Mary Jo Nye's excellent argument for the importance of science in the French provinces: Nicolle was far from exceptional in his concern with acceptance by *Parisian* scientific circles, above all else. See Mary Jo Nye, *Science in the Provinces: Scientific Communities and Provincial Leadership in*

France, 1860–1930 (Berkeley: University of California Press, 1986). At the same time, I would qualify that the relationship between "metropole" and "province," like that between metropole and colony, was far more dynamic and complex than traditional sources tended to suggest. Nicolle's story will offer instances of both relationships. The word *metropole*, currently popular among English-speaking academics and derided by some as jargon, was indeed used by the historical French actors of this period, including Nicolle.

4. The start of the Third Republic is often dated from September 1870; however, it did not become a stable general government until May 1871, after the end of the Franco-Prussian War and the conclusion of the bloody Paris Commune. That said, it was unclear through the 1870s whether the republic would stand, or whether a constitutional monarchy would instead rule.

5. Nicolle, "Mémoires," 4, Archives Départementales de la Seine-Maritime (ASM), Rouen, France, fonds Charles Nicolle, ASM 146 J 13. See my "Bibliographic Note" for further information on the ASM. This is a typed transcription of memoirs Nicolle dictated later in life. He began them around 1928, when he was suffering greatly from a cardiac condition, then set them aside until the mid-1930s, taking them up again during a later illness. He never made it, chronologically, up to his arrival in Tunisia, or even to his time at the IPP: just days before he died, Nicolle dictated his final entry, on his days as a medical student in Paris. Any material taken from the main section (1928) is simply labeled "Mémoires." Other sections, which are repaginated, contain a year reference.

6. For an introduction to nationalism, see Eric Hobsbawm, *The Age of Empire, 1875–1914* (New York: Vintage Books, 1989) and Ernest Gellner, *Nations and Nationalism* (Ithaca, NY: Cornell University Press, 1983).

7. The younger Napoleon, of course, ruled over both the (brief) Second Republic as Louis Napoleon and the Second Empire as Napoleon III. The Third Republic was established after the Prussian Army captured the emperor, who, upon being released, fled to England.

8. Eugene Weber, *Peasants into Frenchmen: The Modernization of Rural France, 1870–1914* (Stanford, CA: Stanford University Press, 1979).

9. There are numerous collections of Auguste Comte's writings, including e-texts of the three-volume collection translated and edited by Harriet Martineau, *The Positive Philosophy of Auguste Comte* (Batoche Books, 2000) (originally London: George Bell and Sons, 1896), available at http://socserv2.mcmaster.ca/~econ/ugcm/3ll3/comte/index.html. See also Andrew Wernick, *Auguste Comte and the Religion of Humanity: The Post-Theistic Program of French Social Theory* (Cambridge: Cambridge University Press, 2001). It should be noted that many early Catholic and conservative opponents of the Republic also appealed to positivism. See Michael Sutton, *Nationalism, Positivism and Catholicism: The Politics of Charles Maurras and French Catholics, 1890–1914* (Cambridge: Cambridge University Press, 2002) and, for an overview, Martha Hanna, "Introduction" and "Chapter One: The Discord of the Elders," in her *The Mobilization of Intellect: French Scholars and Writers during the Great War* (Cambridge, MA: Harvard University Press, 1996).

10. Harry Paul, *From Knowledge to Power: The Rise of the Science Empire in France, 1860–1939* (Cambridge: Cambridge University Press, 1985). Paul also discusses positivism.

11. A general overview of the Scramble for Africa is in Thomas Parkenham, *The Scramble for Africa: The White Man's Conquest of the Dark Continent from 1876 to 1912* (New

York: Random House, 1991). The existence of a distinct "scramble" has more recently been called into question by many historians.

12. "By the early twentieth century, Britain, France, Germany, Italy, Belgium, the Netherlands, Denmark, Spain, and Portugal together held sway over almost 84 percent of the earth's surface." Alice L. Conklin and Ian Christopher Fletcher, "Introduction," *European Imperialism, 1830–1930: Climax and Contradiction,* eds. Conklin and Fletcher (Boston: Houghton Mifflin, 1999), 1–9, 1. Conklin and Fletcher have produced a compilation of texts, both primary and secondary, that serve as an excellent introduction to this particular period of imperial expansion.

13. It was Napoleon III who brought Cochin-China and Cambodia under France's control. On colonialism in the French Third Republic, a classic is Henri Brunschwig, *French Colonialism, 1871–1914: Myths and Realities* (New York: Frederick A. Praeger, 1966). For a thought-provoking take on the French colonial project in West Africa, see Conklin, *A Mission to Civilize: The Republican Idea of Empire in France and West Africa, 1895–1930* (Stanford, CA: Stanford University Press, 1997).

14. I will discuss the establishment of the Tunisian Protectorate in more detail in Chapter 1. For an overview of nineteenth- and twentieth-century Tunisian history, see Kenneth J. Perkins, *A History of Modern Tunisia* (Cambridge: Cambridge University Press, 2004).

15. Brunchwig is particularly critical of the economic aspects of French colonialism: "it cannot be denied that, if nationalism had not coloured the whole of this period, it would in the long run have been impossible for a small group of profiteers to insist on the carrying out of a policy which enormously increased the budget." Brunchwig, *French Colonialism,* 151. Of course, later in the French colonial project, access to Moroccan ports became an increasingly important motive, particularly as Europe looked set to go to war. For more on the connections between French humiliation over Prussian defeat and its rising nationalism and colonialism, see Conklin, *A Mission to Civilize,* esp. 11–13.

16. A good sense of these forces, and the concerns and needs that shaped them into nationalist identities, is Benedict Anderson, *Imagined Communities: Reflections on the Origin and Spread of Nationalism,* rev. ed. (London: Verso Press, 1993).

17. For a French example, see Robert Gildea, *The Past in French History* (New Haven: Yale University Press, 1994).

18. Conklin, *Mission to Civilize,* 1. Though Conklin does not necessarily brand the civilizing mission a "metaphor," her description of its functions supports the label.

19. Conklin, *Mission to Civilize,* 5–6.

20. Herman Lebovics, *True France: The Wars over Cultural Identity, 1900–1945* (Ithaca, NY: Cornell University Press, 1994).

21. I am referring to Daniel R. Headrick, *The Tools of Empire: Technology and European Imperialism in the Nineteenth Century* (New York: Oxford University Press, 1981). Medicine, bringing, as it did, hygiene and improved health to many colonies, perhaps resisted this judgment longer than did science and technology. On medicine more specifically, see the influential collections of David Arnold, ed., *Imperial Medicine and Indigenous Societies: Disease, Medicine, and Empire in the Nineteenth and Twentieth Centuries* (Manchester: Manchester University Press, 1988), and Roy MacLeod and Milton Lewis, eds., *Disease, Medicine, and Empire: Perspectives on Western Medicine and the Experience of European Expansion*

(London: Routledge, 1988). Arnold gives an overview of the subject in "Medicine and Colonialism," in *Companion Encyclopedia of the History of Medicine,* eds. W. F. Bynum and Roy Porter, 2 vols. (London: Routledge, 1993), 2: 1393–1416. See also *Isis* 96 (March 2005), esp. Michael A. Osborne, "Science and the French Empire" (80–87).

22. There are hundreds of sources on Louis Pasteur. Among them, see Gerald Geison, "Pasteur," in *Dictionary of Scientific Biography,* ed. Charles Coulston Gillispie, 16 vols. (New York: Scribner and Sons, 1972), 10: 350–416, and his *The Private Science of Louis Pasteur* (Princeton: Princeton University Press, 1995); Patrice Debré, *Louis Pasteur,* trans. Elborg Forster (Baltimore: Johns Hopkins University Press, 1998); Bruno Latour, *Pasteur: Une Science, un Style, un Siècle* (Paris: Perrin, Pasteur Institute, 1994). There is also the classic study, published originally in 1900 and subsequently printed in numerous editions and translations, by René Vallery-Radot, *La Vie de Pasteur* (Paris: E. Flammarion, 1900). The twenty-sixth edition, for example, appeared in 1924.

23. Pasteur's early speculations in this direction encouraged Britain's Joseph Lister to advocate the use of carbolic acid to prevent surgery-related infections.

24. Latour, *The Pasteurization of France,* trans. Alan Sheridan and John Law (Cambridge, MA: Harvard University Press, 1988), 89. Technically, Pasteur's development of a vaccine against chicken cholera (1880) preceded his anthrax demonstration; however, Pouilly-le-Fort is the grand display that captured public imagination.

25. Anne Marie Moulin, "La Métaphore Vaccine: De l'Inoculation à la Vaccinologie," *History and Philosophy of the Life Sciences* 14 (1992): 271–97. Moulin demonstrates how Pasteur appropriated the term *vaccine*—and its associated legacy—from Jenner and smallpox.

26. In this public experiment, Pasteur and his colleagues inoculated half the gathered animals with an attenuated form of anthrax. A few weeks later, they gave them a second, stronger dose. Finally, after two more weeks, all the animals were given a dose of the highly infectious anthrax bacillus. Dramatically, when the witnesses returned to the field a few days later, all the inoculated animals were alive and well, while all the control animals (our term, not theirs) were either sick or dead. In other words, as Latour shows, Pasteur turned a farm itself into a great public laboratory, to demonstrate the power, and the containment, of microbes.

27. Moulin, "Métaphore Vaccine"; Geison, "Pasteur," 390–406; and J. Andrew Mendelsohn, "'Like All that Lives': Biology, Medicine and Bacteria in the Age of Pasteur and Koch," *History and Philosophy of the Life Sciences* 24 (2002): 3–36.

28. Many have also commented on its dubious ethical status. Among the critics was Nicolle himself, who pointed out in his lectures before the Collège de France in the 1930s that, had Pasteur been a doctor instead of a chemist by training, he never would have asked his collaborators to inoculate the boy, regardless of his condition. See also Geison, "Pasteur, Roux, and Rabies: Scientific *versus* Clinical Mentalities," *JHM* 45 (1990): 341–65.

29. Moulin, "Bacteriological Research and Medical Practice in and out of the Pastorian School," in *French Medical Culture in the Nineteenth Century,* eds. Mordechai Feingold and Anne La Berge, 327–49 (Atlanta: Rodopi, 1994).

30. Moulin, "Patriarchal Science: The Network of the Overseas Pasteur Institutes," in *Science and Empires: Historical Studies about Scientific Development and European Expansion,* eds. Patrick Petitjean, Catherine Jami, and Anne Marie Moulin, 307–22 (Dordrecht:

Kluwer, 1992), 313. For a history of the Pasteur Institute's early decades, Albert Delaunay, *L'Institut Pasteur des Origines à Aujourd'hui* (Paris: France-Empire, 1962).

31. It is hard to overstate the extent to which Catholic values, structures, and practices informed the metaphors of "Pastorism" in general, and the "Pastorian mission" in particular. Fortunately, medical historian and practitioner Anne Marie Moulin has carefully laid out the taxonomy of the early Pastorians and their organizations. The term *Pastorian* itself was in use as early as the 1890s. On the place of the Pasteur Institute within (or outside) traditional Parisian medical and academic circles, see her "Bacteriological Research and Medical Practice." On the institute's international expansion and its reliance on Catholic structures and rhetoric, see idem., "Patriarchal Science": "this group exemplified many characteristics not only of a doctrinal school, but of a monastic order" (308). She expands upon this argument, and discusses the Pasteur Institute's "scientific empire," in "The Pasteur Institute's International Network: Scientific Innovations and French Tropisms," in *Transnational Intellectual Networks: Forms of Academic Knowledge and the Search for Cultural Identities,* eds. Christophe Charle, Jurgen Schriewer, and Peter Wagner, 135–64 (Frankfurt: Campus Verlag, 2004). (It is here that she cites Pasteur's "apocryphal injunction to 'Go and Teach all Nations!' " [136].") For further substantiation of the importance of religious structures in Pastorian tradition, see Lorraine Ward, "The Cult of Relics: Pasteur Material at the Science Museum," *Medical History* 38 (1994): 52–72.

32. The 1844 Patent Act, for example, forbade medical patenting "on the grounds that it was immoral to allow monopolies to develop in this field." Michael Robson, "The French Pharmaceutical Industry, 1919–1939," in *Pill Peddlers: Essays on the History of the Pharmaceutical Industry,* ed. Jonathan Liebenau (Madison, WI: American Institute of the History of Pharmacy, 1990), 107–22, 108.

33. Moulin, "The Pasteur Institute and the Logic of Non-Profit," unpublished paper delivered at the Third International Conference of Research on Voluntary and Non Profit Organizations, Indiana University Center on Philanthropy, 1992. Moulin develops her discussion of the Pasteur Institute's financial and business interests with Annick Guénel in "L'Institut Pasteur et la Naissance de l'Industrie de la Santé," in *La Philosophie du Remède,* ed. Jean-Claude Beaune, 91–109 (Seyssel: Champ Vallon, 1993). Eugen Weber notes a general French contempt for "business" and "profit" in French society. Eugen Weber, *The Hollow Years: France in the 1930s* (New York: Norton, 1994), 51. On the French approach to profit, see Edward C. Carter, Robert Forster, and Joseph N. Moody, eds., *Enterprise and Entrepreneurs in Nineteenth- and Twentieth-Century France* (Baltimore: Johns Hopkins University Press, 1976).

34. Pasteur was well aware of the need for profit; however, he was also brilliant at gauging the needs and values of society, shaping his approaches to ensure maximum success. (This Pasteur is evident not only in Geison's work, but even in Paul de Kruif's.) Nicolle differed from Pasteur in this sense: though generally good at reading social cues, Nicolle would sometimes press his agenda beyond social acceptability, as we shall see.

35. Moulin, "The Pasteur Institute and the Logic of Non-Profit," 3, 5. In particular, she discusses the meaning of "foundation" in France.

36. Ibid. It also constrained the development of the French pharmaceutical industry more generally. The institute's profit structure is also discussed by Jonathan Liebenau and Michael Robson, "L'Institut Pasteur et l'Industrie Pharmaceutique," in *L'Institut Pasteur: Contributions à Son Histoire,* ed. Michel Morange, 52–61 (Paris: Editions la Découverte, 1991).

37. For the American perspective on this "gospel," see Nancy Tomes, *The Gospel of Germs: Men, Women, and the Microbe in American Life* (Cambridge, MA: Harvard University Press, 1998). The Pastorians' colonial project was described directly by one of its central figures: Albert Calmette, *Les Missions Scientifique de l'Institut Pasteur et l'Expansion Coloniale de la France* (Paris, 1923).

38. On "tropical" medicine and its qualifications, see Moulin, "Tropical without the Tropics: The Turning-Point of Pastorian Medicine in North Africa," in *Warm Climates and Western Medicine: The Emergence of Tropical Medicine, 1500–1900*, ed. David Arnold, 160–80 (Amsterdam: Clio Medica, 1996). For an excellent study of conceptions of disease causation in India before the "germ theory," see Mark Harrison, *Climates and Constitutions: Health, Race, Environment, and British Imperialism in India, 1600–1850* (New Delhi: Oxford University Press, 1999).

39. On the health of Western soldiers and settlers in the colonies, see Philip D. Curtin, *Death by Migration: Europe's Encounter with the Tropical World in the Nineteenth Century* (Cambridge: Cambridge University Press, 1989), and, more recently, his *Disease and Empire: The Health of European Troops in the Conquest of Africa* (Cambridge: Cambridge University Press, 1998). The impulse to expand medicine and hygiene to the colonies was by no means limited to Pastorians: even if the Pastorians had their own approach to the problems of tropical medicine. See Mark Harrison, *Public Health in British India: Anglo-American Preventive Medicine, 1859–1914* (Cambridge: Cambridge University Press, 1994); Helen Power, "The Calcutta School of Tropical Medicine: Institutionalizing Medical Research in the Periphery," *Medical History* 40 (1996): 197–214; Ahmed Awad Abdel-Hameed, "The Wellcome Tropical Research Laboratories in Khartoum (1903–1934): An Experiment in Development," *Medical History* 41 (1997): 30–58. Striking parallels exist between the plans and inclinations of Nicolle and Britain's Andrew Balfour, who was in Khartoum. See Andrew Balfour, "Introduction," *First Report of the Wellcome Research Laboratories at the Gordon Memorial College, Khartoum* (Khartoum: Department of Education, Sudan Government, 1904). See also E. M. Tansey and Rosemary C. E. Milligan, "The Early History of the Wellcome Research Laboratories, 1894–1914," in Liebenau, *Pill Peddlers*, 91–106, esp. 102–3.

40. *L'Institut Pasteur: Cinquantenaire de la Fondation* (Paris: J. Demoulin, 1939) includes a review of the overseas institutes. For more detail, see Moulin, "Patriarchal Science." Moulin carefully demonstrates the extent to which the Pastorian project was, and was not, tied to French colonialism.

41. Annick Guénel, "The Creation of the First Overseas Pasteur Institute, or the Beginning of Albert Calmette's Pastorian Career," *Medical History* 43 (1999): 1–25.

42. *L'Institut Pasteur: Cinquantenaire*. Additionally, Moulin has prepared a chronological list of institutions bearing the name Pasteur.

43. Moulin, "Les Instituts Pasteur de la Méditerranée Arabe: Une Religion Scientifique en Pays d'Islam," in *Santé, Médecine et Société dans le Monde Arabe*, ed. Elisabeth Longuenesse, 129–64 (Paris: Editions l'Harmattan, 1995), 134.

44. Moulin, "Patriarchal Science," 317.

45. For example, Nicolle referred to a speech he gave for the centenary of Pasteur's birth as a "Midnight Mass" in a letter to Georges Blanc, March 27, 1923, ASM 146 J 24. The brothers Sergent erected what was essentially a shrine to Pasteur at the Pasteur Institute of Algeria. More contemporary commentary has been provided by Moulin, "Patriarchal

Science," and Ilana Lowy, "From Guinea Pigs to Man: The Development of Haffkine's Anticholera Vaccine," *JHM* 47 (1992): 270–309.

46. As Warwick Anderson sagely comments about otherwise excellent new studies that claim to bring something "new" to scholarship by examining such core/periphery dynamics: "all of these books . . . challenge the old-fashioned notion that British culture—including medical and scientific culture—simply diffused from London and Liverpool to the distant outposts of empire. Of course, one has to go back to the 1960s to find anyone who actually believed this. For decades now, convention has demanded interactive studies that look for evidence of reciprocity and exchange between 'center' and 'periphery.' " Warwick Anderson, "How's the Empire? An Essay Review," *JHM* 58 (2003): 459–65, 462. For studies and other considerations of this dynamic, Ann Laura Stoler and Frederick Cooper, "Between Metropole and Colony: Rethinking a Research Agenda," in *Tensions of Empire: Colonial Cultures in a Bourgeois World*, eds. Frederick Cooper and Ann Laura Stoler (Berkeley: University of California Press, 1997), 1–56; Douglas M. Haynes, *Imperial Medicine: Patrick Manson and the Conquest of Tropical Disease* (Philadelphia: University of Pennsylvania Press, 2001); Paolo Palladino and Michael Worboys, "Science and Imperialism," *Isis* 84 (1993): 91–102; David Wade Chambers, "Does Distance Tyrannize Science?" in *International Science and National Scientific Identity: Australia between Britain and America,* eds. R. W. Home and Sally Gregory Kohlstedt, 19–38 (Dordrecht, Holland: Klewer, 1991); Richard Drayton, *Nature's Government: Science, Imperial Britain, and the 'Improvement' of the World* (New Haven: Yale University Press, 2000).

47. Several years ago, David Wade Chambers called upon the "history of colonial science" to ". . . account for the putting into place of this infrastructure (journals, museums, libraries, laboratories, societies, invisible colleges, funding bodies, educational institutions and, of course, people and ideas)." Nicolle's case offers precisely such information about the establishment of Western medicine in Tunisia. Chambers, "Does Distance Tyrannize Science?," 33.

48. "As always, the ultraprovincial, infraparisian that I am is unaware of anything." Nicolle to Félix Mesnil, October 21, 1931, Archives de l'Institut Pasteur (AIP), Paris, France. AIP FR IP NCP.11.

49. "Despite my age, I was not one of [Pasteur's] direct disciples; I was the student of these students." Nicolle, "Discours de M. Nicolle: Inauguration d'un Buste de Pasteur à l'Institut Pasteur de Tunis," *Revue Tunisien des Sciences Médicales* 17 (1923): 264–66, 265. Moulin also makes this point in her article, "Charles Nicolle, Savant Tunisien," *AIPT* 71 (1994): 355–70.

50. Claire Salomon-Bayet, ed., *Pasteur et la Révolution Pastorienne* (Paris: Payot, 1986).

51. See the "Introduction" to the English translation of Emile Duclaux, *Pasteur: The History of a Mind,* trans. Erwin F. Smith and Florence Hedges (Philadelphia: W. B. Saunders, 1920; Metuchen, NJ: Scarecrow Reprint Corporation, 1973). The reprinted edition is a direct reproduction of the 1920 edition, with the addition of a forward by René Dubos.

52. I have called attention to the term *microbiology* because it was used in two senses. First, it represents (yet again) the French–German antagonisms: the French preferred "microbiology"; the Germans, "bacteriology." Second, for Nicolle, it represented a broader application of microbial research beyond medicine proper—for example, to agriculture and industry.

53. Duclaux, *Pasteur: Histoire d'un Esprit* (Sceaux: Charaire, 1896); René Vallery-Radot, *Vie de Pasteur* (1900).

54. Pauline Mazumdar makes this argument in her *Species and Specificity: An Interpretation of the History of Immunology* (Cambridge: Cambridge University Press, 1995), 73. This should not be taken to mean that Duclaux was a believer in the fixity of microbes—to the contrary. See Chapter 6.

55. On Koch, William Coleman, "Koch's Comma Bacillus: The First Year," *BHM* 61 (1987): 315–42; J. Andrew Mendelsohn, "Cultures of Bacteriology" (Ph.D. dissertation, Princeton University, 1996). Also, K. Codell Carter, "The Development of Pasteur's Concept of Disease Causation and the Emergence of Specific Causes in Nineteenth-Century Medicine," *BHM* 65 (1991): 528–48, and his *The Rise of Causal Concepts of Disease: Case Histories* (Aldershot, England: Ashgate, 2003). For a classic overview of bacteriology's early decades, see William Bulloch, *The History of Bacteriology* (London: Oxford University Press, 1938). Also, Patrick Collard, *The Development of Microbiology* (Cambridge: Cambridge University Press, 1976).

56. On the variety of germ theories being posited, see Michael Worboys, *Spreading Germs: Disease Theories and Medical Practice in Britain, 1865–1900* (Cambridge: Cambridge University Press, 2000). For a reconsideration of just how "specific" the early research of Pasteur, Koch, and their followers really was, see Mendelsohn, "'Like All That Lives'"; Olga Amsterdamska, "Medical and Biological Constraints: Early Research on Variation in Bacteriology," *Social Studies of Science* 17 (1987): 657–87.

57. J. Henry Dible, *Recent Advances in Bacteriology and the Study of the Infections*, 2nd ed. (London: J. & A. Church, 1932). Dible provides excellent reviews of many topics then current in bacteriological research, often including historical background, assessment of debated topics, and bibliographic references at the end of each chapter.

58. Emile Lagrange, *Monsieur Roux* (Bruxelles: Goemaere [1954?]). Roux was one of Nicolle's great foils. It is unfortunate that so little of their direct correspondence remains.

59. As we shall see, Nicolle defined science, "properly" performed, as a Baconian rather than Cartesian venture. This put him at odds with many of his fellow French citizens—though not, it seems, with his fellow French microbiologists. See Chapters 2 and 4.

60. Hanna, *Mobilization of Intellect*, on the growing suspicion of science after World War I.

61. Georges Duhamel, *Civilization, 1914–1917,* trans. E. S. Brooks (New York: The Century Co., 1919).

62. Eugen Weber opens the first chapter of his book on this period in French history with the statement, "The 1930s begin in August of 1914." Weber, *The Hollow Years,* 11. Striking insight into the force with which World War I reshaped individual and cultural identities is Paul Fussell, *The Great War and Modern Memory* (New York: Oxford University Press, 1989).

63. Garland E. Allen, "Naturalists and Experimentalists: The Genotype and the Phenotype," in *Studies in the History of Biology,* eds. William Coleman and Camille Limoges, 179–209 (Baltimore: Johns Hopkins University Press, 1979).

64. Daniel J. Kevles and Gerald L. Geison, "The Experimental Life Sciences in the Twentieth Century," *Osiris* 10 (1995): 97–121. Kevles and Geison argue that the increasingly experimental approach to biology "led to the emergence of new disciplines such as embryology, cytology, endocrinology, the reproductive sciences, and genetics, which rapidly took on lives of their own, independent of evolutionary debates, and produced a wide range of conceptual and utilitarian triumphs" (97).

65. T. J. Horder, J. A. Witkowski, and C. C. Wylie, eds., *A History of Embryology* (Cambridge: Cambridge University Press, 1985, 1986); and Viktor Hamburger, "Wilhelm Roux: Visionary with a Blind Spot," *Journal of the History of Biology* 30 (1997): 229–38.

66. Garland E. Allen, *Life Sciences in the Twentieth Century* (Cambridge: Cambridge University Press, 1978); Peter J. Bowler, *The Mendelian Revolution: The Emergence of Hereditarian Concepts in Modern Science and Society* (London: Athlone Press, 1989).

67. Conklin, *A Mission to Civilize*, esp. Chapter 7. Nicolle, too, would become far more concerned about questions of race after the war. For a broad overview on ideas of race, including the rise of "scientific racism," see Ivan Hannaford, *Race: The History of an Idea in the West* (Baltimore: Johns Hopkins University Press, 1996). Like so many other trends, from epidemiology and evolution to bacteriology and genetics, the French adopted scientific racism in a fashion that was distinctive. French adherence to scientific racism was less absolute than elsewhere. Michael A. Osborne and Richard F. Fogarty, "Views from the Periphery: Discourses of Race and Place in French Military Medicine," *History and Philosophy of the Life Sciences* 25 (2003): 363–89. For more on scientific racism and its cultural progeny, eugenics, see Kevles, *In the Name of Eugenics: Genetics and the Uses of Human Heredity* (New York: Knopf, 1985). On French eugenics in particular, see William H. Snyder, *Quality and Quantity: The Quest for Biological Regeneration in Twentieth-Century France*, new ed. (Cambridge: Cambridge University Press, 2002). See also the formative text on constructions of the "other": Edward W. Said, *Orientalism* (London: Routledge and Kegan Paul, 1978).

68. The classic study of typhus, which pays careful attention to the long relationship of typhus and war, is Hans Zinsser, *Rats, Lice, and History: The Biography of a Bacillus* (Boston: Little, Brown, 1934, 1935).

69. Bacteriology's most evident failure came as the war was ending: the infamous influenza pandemic of 1918–19 offered a bleak assessment of the new medical science's very real limitations.

70. Nicolle was an early supporter of the theory that the causal agent of the influenza pandemic was a filterable virus. At the time, filterable viruses were also called "ultramicrobes" (Nicolle insisted on referring to them as "inframicrobes"). The filterable viruses played an important part in Nicolle's research and his ultimate conception of disease evolution, and will thus be discussed, periodically, throughout this book.

71. Arthur Silverstein, *A History of Immunology* (San Diego: Academic Press, 1989); Moulin, *La Dernière Langage de la Médecine: Histoire de l'Immunologie de Pasteur au Sida* (Paris: Presses Universitaires de France, 1991).

72. Mendelsohn, "Cultures of Bacteriology."

73. Nicolle's term, in French, was *infections inapparents*. A literal translation—"unapparent infections"—lacks grace and does not make up for that deficit by bringing more clarity to the term. It is perhaps closest to today's "subclinical infection." However, it was not yet that, and calling it "subclinical" would encourage readers to make inappropriate assumptions about its nature. I have thus chosen to preserve "inapparent infection."

74. Mazumdar, *Species and Specificity*, on transformism.

75. Amsterdamska, "Medical and Biological Constraints"; Ludwig Fleck, *Genesis and Development of a Scientific Fact*, eds. Thaddeus J. Trenn and Robert K. Merton, trans. Fred Bradley and Thaddeus J. Trenn (Chicago: University of Chicago Press, 1979).

76. There were in the meanwhile developments in the inoculation of hormones, such as insulin. Michael Bliss, *The Discovery of Insulin* (Chicago: University of Chicago Press, 1982).

77. See this book's opening quotation for Nicolle on "Golden Ages." Also, see Chapter 8.

78. The few historians who have worked on this transitional period in the history of bacteriology have suggested that later biomedical successes made this period somehow uninteresting for historical study. See, for example, Robert E. Kohler, "Bacterial Physiology: The Medical Context," *BHM* 59 (1985): 54–74. Kohler argues that "the discovery of bacterial genetics shifted attention away from physiological complexities to cleaner problems of gene mapping and gene expression. The widespread use of antibiotics after 1945 swept away the rationale for investigating the complex physiology of the host-parasite relationship." Within this shift, the "theory of the origin and physiology of parasitism was forgotten. Only the bare facts of bacterial nutrition remained" (74). Similarly, Amsterdamska notes that "arguments about whether or not bacteria undergo numerous cyclic changes of form and function played a significant role in pre–World War II investigations of bacterial variation—but although articles on bacterial variation dating from the period in question run into the hundreds, postwar developments in microbial genetics, biochemistry, and molecular biology have made almost all this earlier work on variation appear scientifically irrelevant and historically invisible. Historians tend to examine prewar bacteriology looking for the precursors and forerunners of the postwar revolution in biological research; and since postwar bacterial genetics and biochemistry are not the direct progeny of this investigative tradition, this entire area of prewar bacteriology has often been simply dismissed." Amsterdamska, "Stabilizing Instability: The Controversy over Cyclogenic Theories of Bacterial Variation during the Interwar Period," *Journal of the History of Biology* 24 (1991): 191–222, 191.

79. Nicolle, *NVM* (1930), revised and expanded as *Destin* (1933).

80. "Species" is even too absolute a word. By the end, Nicolle preferred to call similar individuals "groups."

81. Warwick Anderson, "Natural Histories of Infectious Disease: Ecological Vision in Twentieth-Century Biomedical Science," *Osiris* 19 (2004): 39–61; and, in the same volume—an indication of the rising interest in the subject—Helen Tilley, "Ecologies of Complexity: Tropical Environments, African Trypanosomiasis, and the Science of Disease Control in British Colonial Africa, 1900–1940," *Osiris* 19 (2004): 21–38. Nicolle's place in the context of this largely Anglo-American work still needs to be clarified.

82. Nicolle to Georges Duhamel, May 13, 1923, AIP FR IP NCP.8–10.

83. Books warning of the dangers of emergent diseases and of antibiotic resistance have proliferated since the 1980s. See, for example, Laurie Garrett, *The Coming Plague: Newly Emerging Diseases in a World Out of Balance* (New York: Farrar, Straus and Giroux, 1994); Stuart B. Levy, *The Antibiotic Paradox: How the Misuse of Antibiotics Destroys their Curative Powers*, 2nd ed. (Cambridge, MA: Perseus, 2002).

84. Thomas Soderqvist, "Existential Projects and Existential Choice in Science: Science Biography as an Edifying Genre," in *Telling Lives in Science: Essays on Scientific Biography*, eds. Michael Shortland and Richard Yeo, 45–84 (Cambridge: Cambridge University Press, 1996).

85. Literally, "homeland of the nomad." Nicolle, "Mémoires," 88, ASM 146 J 13.

Chapter 1

1. Although, technically, Nicolle was overlooking the Gulf of Tunis—an arm of the Mediterranean—he generally referred to the water surrounding Tunisia as "the sea." I shall do the same. Many of his visitors and collaborators commented on Nicolle's love for Sidi Bou Saïd and the sea. The author of his obituary in the *Archives de l'Institut Pasteur de Tunis* even noted: "Charles Nicolle loved to meet with his collaborators. . . . In the summer, dinner would be taken by the sea, at Sidi Bou Saïd. On grand occasions, the whole of the Institute was invited." "Charles Nicolle (1866–1936)," *AIPT* 25 (1936): 201–7, 204. Tourists have subsequently discovered the charms of Sidi Bou Saïd, disrupting its tranquility; however, it remains a lovely place.

2. Perhaps there was something about the isolation of French colonials in North Africa, about the nearness of the Mediterranean drawing constant attention to the distance between its coasts, that encouraged seaside introspection. Albert Camus, born in Algeria in 1913, would scatter the image of the sea through many of his works. Indeed, Germaine Lot dedicates the biography *Charles Nicolle* to "*la solaire mémoire d'Albert Camus, d'Afrique.*"

3. Nicolle soon began referring to himself and his colleagues at the Pasteur Institute of Tunis as "Tunisians." It was an identity he would wrestle with and redefine for the rest of his life (Moulin, "Charles Nicolle, Savant Tunisien"). He would only in some sense make peace with it while making plans for his own burial. See Chapter 8.

4. Moulin, "Pasteur Institute's International Network."

5. See, for example, William C. Summers, *Félix d'Herelle and the Origins of Molecular Biology* (New Haven: Yale University Press, 1999), 120. D'Herelle spent several months at Nicolle's institute in 1915, studying locusts (43). It would be interesting to learn more about how the two men, who obviously shared a number of character traits and scientific inclinations, got along.

6. The basic facts of Nicolle's early years have been recounted in numerous books and articles. In addition to Huet, *Pommier*, and Germaine Lot, *Charles Nicolle*, see Paul Giroud, "Eloge: Charles Nicolle (1866–1936)," *Bulletin de l'Académie Nationale de Médecine* 45 (1961): 714–22; Amor Chadli, "Charles Nicolle et les Acquis de sa Pensée Scientifique," *AIPT* 63 (1986): 3–14; Yoelli Meir, "Charles Nicolle and the Frontiers of Medicine," *New England Journal of Medicine* 276 (1967): 670–75; Etienne Burnet, "Charles Nicolle," *AIPT* 43 (1966): 91–97; Félix Mesnil, "Notice Nécrologique sur M. Charles Nicolle," *Bulletin de l'Académie de Médecine* 115 (1936): 541–49; Andre Prévost-Barancy, "Charles Nicolle" [thesis conducted under Pasteur Vallery-Radot] (Paris: R. Foulon, 1950); Moulin, "Charles Nicolle, Savant Tunisien"; Marcelle Nicolle, "Charles Nicolle: 1866–1936," *Femmes Médecins* 11 (1966): 289–310; Pierre Nicolle, "La Vie et la Personnalité de Charles Nicolle," *Annales d'Hygiène de Langue Française* 3 (1967): 87–91.

7. Indeed, Nicolle appears to have drawn from his mother (and from Mme. Pasteur) his ideal of the "true and best" nature of "woman" as moral nurturer, teacher, and supporter (but never genius), in contrast to the more common "woman as distracting and destructive she-wolf." See Chapter 7.

8. Nicolle, "Mémoires," 43, 48.

9. In 1883, for example, Nicolle won the Lycée Corneille's medal for the "Premier Prix d'Histoire Ancienne de la Classe de Rhétorique."

10. "In school, I was one of those of whom it is said, He will succeed, if he wants to." Nicolle, "Lettre aux Sourds" (1929), 1, ASM 146 J 87. This short article was published both in a journal and as a separate pamphlet.

11. Nicolle, "Mémoires (1936)," 3. These disinclinations remained with Nicolle and were evident throughout his life. In particular, his correspondents frequently complained of his illegible letters (a complaint with which I deeply sympathized).

12. Nicolle, "Mémoires," 101. The family went to Bayeux, near Caen, and spent time at the fishing port, Port-en-Bessin.

13. Nicolle, "Mémoires," 20.

14. Although medical education had begun to be reformed, most French medical schools in the provinces were limited to teaching the first two years only. Thereafter, students seeking to qualify in medicine had to finish their studies at one of the few sanctioned, complete medical schools: such as in Paris. George Weisz, "Reform and Conflict in French Medical Education, 1870–1914," in *The Organization of Science and Technology in France, 1808–1914,* eds. Robert Fox and George Weisz (Cambridge: Cambridge University Press, 1980), 61–94.

15. Lot, *Charles Nicolle,* 21. Nicolle was in Gombault's lab. Nicolle would call upon his Faculté de Médicine connections throughout his life.

16. Nicolle, "Lettre aux Sourds" (1929), 2. Moulin notes that most Pastorians "did not follow the 'royal path of the *internat*'"—distinguishing Nicolle from many of his colleagues. Moulin, "Bacteriological Research," 339.

17. For more details on the Pasteur Institute of Paris in its early incarnation, see the Introduction.

18. Basic details of Eugène Nicolle's life and work may be found in Jules Roger, *Les Médecins Normands du XIIe au XIXe Siècle: Biographie et Bibliographie* (Paris: G. Steinheil, 1890), 358–59.

19. This case was most famously made by Latour in his *Pasteurization of France*. A recent study of medicine in Rouen during Nicolle's lifetime uses the dichotomy between "conservative" clinicians and "progressive" bacteriologists (or bacteriologically sympathetic) quite strictly as its fundamental analytical framework. See Melanie Mataud and Pierre-Albert Martin, *La Médecine Rouennaise à l'époque de Charles Nicolle, de la Fin du XIXeme Siècle aux Années 1930* (Editions Bertout, 2003). On the other hand, it should also be noted that Eugène Nicolle taught public courses in hygiene. Latour demonstrates how hygienists precisely helped extend Pasteur's doctrines—whether they understood his theories (Andrew Mendelsohn's argument) or not. Mendelsohn, "'Like All That Lives,'" 9–10.

20. Robert Fox, "The *Savant* Confronts His Peers: Scientific Societies in France, 1815–1914," in Fox and Weisz, *Organization of Science and Technology,* 241–82.

21. Pouchet was Chair of Natural History from the very opening of Rouen's École Préparatoire des Sciences et des Arts in 1855. A number of similar schools in other provincial French cities opened at the same time, as part of the ongoing efforts to reform the educational system. Fox and Weisz, "Introduction: The Institutional Basis of French Science in the Nineteenth Century," in Fox and Weisz, *Organization of Science and Technology,* 1–28, 6 note "c." Archival information on the establishment and functioning of Rouen's *Ecole Préparatoire* may be found in ASM 1 T 0683—0684—0685.

22. Nicolle would reject the extreme forms of transformism, even as he embraced microbial mutation. See Chapter 7. John Farley and Gerald L. Geison, "Science, Politics and

Spontaneous Generation in Nineteenth-Century France: The Pasteur–Pouchet Debate," *BHM* 48 (1974): 161–98. Farley and Geison stress the efforts of both Pasteur and Pouchet to avoid the appearance that they were questioning religion in the conservative Second Empire. For a challenge to Farley and Geison's interpretation of Pasteur's "science," see Nils Roll-Hansen, "Experimental Method and Spontaneous Generation: The Controversy between Pasteur and Pouchet, 1859–64," *JHM* 34 (1979): 273–92. Nicolle, in his personal collection of papers, kept a copy of the 1907 article "Un Débat Scientifique: Pouchet et Pasteur," by Georges Pemetier. Nicolle also commented on the debate in his biographical portrait of brother Maurice—and even noted Pouchet's influence not only on his father, but on Maurice as well. Nicolle, *Maurice Nicolle* (Tunis: Imprimerie J. Aloccio, 1935), 3–4. Apparently, it was Pouchet's example that made Eugène Nicolle dream of a life of scientific research for his eldest son: something he wished he had been able to do himself (4).

23. Pouchet died in 1872.

24. Charles Nicolle deified Pasteur despite—or, perhaps, because of—having met the Master only once. See Chapter 4. A historian with more psychological training might be able to comment further on the fact that both Nicolle's own father and his chosen intellectual/spiritual father were "absentee" fathers who devoted their lives to their work: and that Nicolle himself would often be absent to his own children. As for the significance of the Nicolle *père*–Pouchet/Pasteur connections, little more may be said without knowing quite a bit more about Eugène Nicolle than is contained in standard sources.

25. One might, using terminology more common today, characterize Nicolle's approach as "ecological." Warwick Anderson, "Natural Histories." (I am not the first to suggest this; however, I would not quite go so far in my claims as Professor H. Harant, author of "Charles Nicolle, 'Inventeur' de l'Ecologie Médicale," *AIPT* 43 [1966]: 323–30.) See Chapter 6. For connections between ecology and imperialism, Tilley, "Ecologies of Complexity"; and Peder Anker, *Imperial Ecology: Environmental Order in the British Empire, 1895–1945* (Cambridge, MA: Harvard University Press, 2001). On France and evolutionary theory more specifically, Yvette Conry, *L'Introduction du Darwinisme en France au dix-neuvième siecle* (Paris: J. Vrin, 1974).

26. For a reverent review of Roux's life and work, see Lagrange, *Monsieur Roux*. On the relations between Roux and Nicolle, see my "Prophet for Profit in French North Africa: Charles Nicolle and the Pasteur Institute of Tunis, 1903–1936," *BHM* 71 (1997): 583–622.

27. On Metchnikoff, see Alfred I. Tauber and Leon Chernyak, *Metchnikoff and the Origins of Immunology: From Metaphor to Theory* (New York: Oxford University Press, 1991).

28. Assessing the Darwinian versus Lamarckian inclinations of Pastorians tends to drag one down thorny paths earlier traveled by historians attempting to determine, for example, whether scientific ideas were "mechanistic" or "vitalistic." Moulin has argued that the early Pastorians were more Lamarckian; Mendelsohn has challenged her interpretations and has further argued that the Pastorian interest in variable virulence was closely connected to ideas of evolution of species. Most historical accounts, however, agree that the Pastorians were, first and foremost, pragmatic. Theories and techniques were introduced as they helped Pastorians solve the medical problems at hand. Evolutionary theory was rarely applied in a systematic fashion. This is where men such as Metchnikoff and, later, Nicolle, differed from their colleagues. They were far more consciously using evolutionary ideas as means to understand the development of biological functions—and, for Nicolle, of disease itself.

29. In 1908, Metchnikoff was awarded a Nobel Prize for his work on immunology. He shared the award with the author of a rival immunological theory, Paul Erlich. On Metchnikoff's evolutionary inclinations and his struggles with the Darwinian "struggle for existence," see Daniel P. Todes, *Darwin without Malthus: The Struggle for Existence in Russian Evolutionary Thought* (NewYork: Oxford University Press, 1989), 82–103.

30. Nicolle later took great pleasure in emphasizing the contrasting natures of his two pastorian mentors. See, for example, Nicolle, "Première Leçon," *Introduction à la Carrière de la Médecine Expérimentale* (Tunis: Maison Tunisienne de l'Edition, 1981), 38–39.

31. The title of Nicolle's laboratory project comes from Pierre Nicolle, "Charles Nicolle, Homme de Caractère," *Précis Analytique des Travaux de l'Académie des Sciences, Belles-Lettres et Arts de Rouen* (Fécamp: L. Durand et Fils, 1967), 23–32, 28.

32. A fixed salary, even a small one, helped research-oriented practitioners set aside time out of their clinical day for lab work.

33. They started the lab in 1886–87. Nicolle outlined his experiences in Rouen in an unpublished and undated series of notes, entitled "Chronologie de mon Passage au Laboratoire de Bactériologie de l'Ecole de Médecine de Rouen" ["Chronologie"]. The chronology details his first years in Rouen, then provides brief annual summaries through 1902. ASM 146 J 56, folder "Vie Professionnelle/Lutte Antivénérienne." See also Mataud and Martin, *Médecine Rouennaise,* 50.

34. The false membrane was not always present, but the disease could be fatal, nonetheless.

35. Yersin is best known for his work on bubonic plague. See Henri H. Mollaret and Jacqueline Brossollet, *Alexandre Yersin, le Vainqueur de la Peste* (Paris: Fayard, 1985). Yersin left Paris for Saigon soon after this work was complete, in 1890.

36. Lagrange, *Monsieur Roux*, 113–24. Paul de Kruif presents the French/German diphtheria research in his inimitable—or, more accurately, much imitated—style in the chapter "Roux and Behring" in his *Microbe Hunters* (San Diego: Harvest/HBJ, 1926, 1954).

37. The congress took place in Budapest that summer.

38. Nicolle, "Chronologie," 3–4.

39. Nicolle, "Immunisation d'un Cheval contre la Diphtérie," *Bulletin de la Société de Médecine de Rouen* (1895). I have been unable to obtain a copy of this article (as well as a couple other early articles) and do not know its page range. The reference is from the published Nicolle bibliography.

40. Nicolle, "Réflexions sur Cinq Années de Pratique de Laboratoire," *La Normandie Médicale* 16 (1899): 409–26, 411. In the first three months of 1894, 76 cases of diphtheria had been treated "conventionally," and 55 percent of the children died. During the first three months of 1895, however, the Pastorian treatment brought the mortality rate for that year's 129 cases down to 27 percent.

41. Huet, *Pommier*, 31.

42. Given the Catholic structure of the IPP, one cannot help but wonder whether Charles chose the name "Pierre" for symbolic reasons.

43. Nicolle, "Réflexions" (1899), 423.

44. Nicolle gave numbers of students for each *Cours,* and number of lectures for the *Grand Cours,* in his "Chronologie." Lecture notes from a few of his classes have survived. All may be found in ASM 146 J 56.

45. G. F. I. Widal and A. Sicard, "Recherches de la Réaction Agglutinante dans le Sang et le Sérum Desséchés des Typhiques et dans la Sérosité des Vésicatoires," *Bulletin des Membres de la Société des Médecins des Hôpitaux de Paris* 13 (1896): 681–82. Fernand Widal was born in Algeria, the son of an army surgeon. Roughly Nicolle's contemporary, he went to Paris to study medicine in 1884 and remained in Paris for the duration of his successful career. He died in 1929.

46. Widal's innovation was to take the known laboratory phenomenon of agglutination and determine its clinical application for typhoid diagnosis. Priority disputes naturally followed.

47. Nicolle and A. Halipré, "Sérodiagnostic de la Fièvre Typhoïde. Modification du Procède Widal; Examen de Trois Cas," *La Normandie Médicale* (July 15, 1896). On Nicolle's practical applications and modifications of the Widal test, see Mataud and Martin, *Médecine Rouennaise*, 70; and Mesnil, "Notice Nécrologique."

48. Nicolle received this appointment along with his loyal collaborators, including A. Halipré, who coauthored a number of Nicolle's early articles. Mataud and Martin, *Médecine Rouennaise*, 70.

49. Nicolle, "Recherches sur la Substance Agglutinée," *AIP* 12 (1898): 161; idem., "La Réaction Agglutinante dans les Cultures Filtrées," *CRSB* 50 (1898): 477.

50. Nicolle and M. Trenel, "Recherches sur le Phénomène de l'Agglutination: Variabilité de l'Aptitude Agglutinative et la Fonction Agglutinogène; Leurs Relations entre Elles; Leurs Rapports avec la Mobilité des Microbes," *AIP* 16 (1902): 562–86. In this work, Nicolle was at the cutting edge of investigations into bacterial variation. At the same time, he was following in the (fledgling) tradition of IPP director Duclaux, whose 1898 bacteriology textbook abounded in considerations of bacterial physiology and variability. Duclaux, *Traité de Microbiologie*, 4 vols. (Paris: Masson et Cie., 1898), for example, Chapter 15, "Changements Morphologiques sous l'Influence du Milieu," 1: 250–63. See also William C. Summers, "From Culture as Organism to Organism as Cell: Historical Origins of Bacterial Genetics," *Journal of the History of Biology* 24 (1991): 171–90, 176 (on Nicolle). On early questions of variation generally, Olga Amsterdamska, "Medical and Biological Constraints." Nicolle continued his investigations on the nature and applications of agglutination into his early years in Tunis; he then left them aside, returning to them at the very end of his life. The broader natural history interests that motivated the work, however, continued to inform his research throughout his career. I will discuss some of the particulars of this early work throughout this book, in connection with closer examinations of Nicolle's efforts to bring a biological perspective to bear on understandings of infectious disease.

51. Nicolle, "Reproduction Expérimentale du Chancre Mou Chez le Singe," *Comptes Rendus, XIIIe Congres Internat de Médecine, 1900* (Paris: 1901): 48–50.

52. Nicolle, "Réflexions" (1899), 412–13.

53. Ibid., 426. Emphasis added.

54. Nye, *Science in the Provinces*.

55. This was particularly the case from April 1895, when a law was passed limiting antitoxin production to the IPP. Mataud and Martin, *Médecine Rouennaise*, 58–59.

56. Huet, *Pommier*, 33; Mataud and Martin, *Médecine Rouennaise*, 61–63.

57. Mataud and Martin, *Médecine Rouennaise*, 63.

58. This strategy is hardly unique to Nicolle, or to his fellow Pastorians, who also made use of it on a number of occasions. Nicolle would again use it, more than once, in Tunisia. See Nicolle, "Chronologie," 6.

59. Brunon appears to have opposed Nicolle even before being appointed director of the medical school. Mataud and Martin, *Médecine Rouennaise*, 58.

60. Marthe Conor to Pierre Nicolle, July 18, 1963, ASM 146 J 39.

61. On "clans," see Marthe Conor to Pierre Nicolle, ibid. Conor referred to Nicolle's group as the "clan Charles." Conor's father, Georges Bugnot, was also a physician in Rouen. He did not speak to his daughter about Brunon, but he did take his family, when ill, to visit Dr. Halipré, Nicolle's close colleague—and, occasionally, to Nicolle himself. The "clan" formulation also appears in many of the biographical pieces on Nicolle. It was made public at the time by the fact that Rouen's two newspapers took opposing sides on all issues that divided the clans. (Mataud and Martin give excellent examples of this partisan reporting.) I will not repeat here the many historical analyses that have concerned themselves with the clinic–lab split in medicine during this period. Although there is much evidence that this split existed, and had real force, there is also evidence that a more complex story exists than the one traditionally told, where Nicolle is simply the "hero."

62. Nicolle, "Chronologie," 5.

63. This was "Le Chronique de Maître Heurtebise." M. Conor to P. Nicolle, July 18, 1963, ASM 146 J 39. Conor described this story as "the key to what transpired between Brunon," Nicolle, and his friends. Huet, *Pommier,* summarizes the events nicely, integrating Nicolle's literary reconstructions into the story where possible (Chapter 1).

64. A rhetorical formulation borrowed, with appropriate alterations, from Richard M. Burian, Jean Gayon, and Doris Zallen, "The Singular Fate of Genetics in the History of French Biology, 1900–1940," *Journal of the History of Biology* 21 (1988): 357–402, 358.

65. Regardless of how one assesses the value of his project, one must acknowledge that Nicolle's zeal might well have been as off-putting to his project's detractors as it was imperative for his eventual successes.

66. Moulin, "Pasteur Institute and Non-Profit."

67. Nicolle's 1894 appointment had been as médecin adjoint at the Hôpitaux de Rouen. There were then two hospitals in Rouen: the Hospice Général and the Hôtel Dieu. For more on the hospitals and their division of medical labor, see Mataud and Martin, *Médecine Rouennaise,* 29.

68. The Rouen collection contains scattered documents in Nicolle's file about his attempts to control syphilis. Nicolle, true to the spirit of bourgeois reform at the time, was also actively working for the temperance movement. Nicolle, "Lutte Antivénérienne Rouen," ASM 146 J 56. On stigmas attached to syphilis (primarily in the American context), see Allan M. Brandt, *No Magic Bullet: A Social History of Venereal Disease in the United States since 1880,* expanded edition (New York: Oxford University Press, 1987). On the Third Republic and social reform, see Sanford Elwitt, *The Third Republic Defended: Bourgeois Reform in France, 1880–1914* (Baton Rouge: Louisiana State University Press, 1986), and, for public health, Martha Lee Hildreth, *Doctors, Bureaucrats, and Public Health in France, 1888–1902* (New York: Garland, 1986).

69. Though Nicolle's associated "Chronologie" contains the supporting documentation and makes clear the timeline, Pierre Nicolle's article brings the events to life and sets them in some context. P. Nicolle, "Charles Nicolle: Homme de Caractère."

70. Mataud and Martin, *Médecine Rouennaise*, 91–92.

71. Ibid., 92. Mataud and Martin also believe that this was the final, deciding event in Nicolle's departure from Rouen.

72. Nicolle, "Chronologie," 13. By "laboratory," I mean, of course, his methods and research plans, not his beakers and assistants—though, as we shall see, he did gather up a number of colleagues from Normandy while in Tunisia.

73. Only in the late 1920s did Nicolle's references to Rouen grow more sympathetic. Interestingly, this sympathy accompanied Nicolle's renewed appreciation for traditional aesthetic choices over a "democratizing" hygienic similarity. See Chapter 7. Pierre Nicolle said that his father "exhibited an evil temperament" toward the French bourgeoisie because of his Rouen experiences: although they "could have financially sustained his efforts to create a center of medical study and education in Rouen, they instead turned a deaf ear to his repeated requests." P. Nicolle, "Les Premières Années de Charles Nicolle à la Direction de l'Institut Pasteur de Tunis," 31. This is a small, bound booklet, with no publication details, that expands upon articles Pierre Nicolle wrote in 1975–76. It gathers together excerpts from Nicolle's correspondence and a number of photographs.

74. Autobiography was one of Nicolle's favored motivational tools from the mid-1920s on, as will be evident in later chapters.

75. Nicolle, "Lettre aux Sourds" (1929), 3. "Isolation," too, would come to be a dominant trope in Nicolle's portrayals of his life in Tunisia.

76. Charles Rosenberg has rightly insisted that oppositional categories, though rarely extant in life, are useful analytic tools for the historian. Charles Rosenberg, "Explaining Epidemics," in *Explaining Epidemics and other Studies in the History of Medicine,* ed. Charles Rosenberg (Cambridge: Cambridge University Press, 1992), 293–304, 293–94. Latour (*Pasteurization*) has demonstrated this to be the case with his thought-provoking analysis of acceptance and resistance to the Pastorian program. For, next to the hygienists in France, it was the colonial doctors and the colonial Pastorians who most successfully applied Pasteur's teachings. This, he explains, is because they met with no real resistance from preexisting medical institutions. Although there is a relative truth to this assertion, it seems, in and of itself, to fall prey to Pastorian rhetoric.

77. Moulin, "Instituts Pasteur de la Méditerranée Arabe," 134.

78. Nicolle could well have applied this formula to his Rouen years, but he did not. Instead, he tended to use his troubles in Rouen as a way to accentuate his later success in Tunis.

79. On "germ theory" and French colonialism more generally, see my Introduction.

80. As Moulin noted of the Mediterranean Pasteur Institutes, they were "active and conscious instruments of colonial politics." They were not, she continues, wholly reducible to colonialism, as the numbers of noncolonial institutes, and the postindependence survival of others, demonstrate. Moulin, "Instituts Pasteur de la Méditerranée Arabe," 136. For an example of an IP established in the wake of decolonization, see Guillaume LaChenal, "Le Centre Pasteur de Cameroun: Trajectoire Historique, Stratégies et Pratiques de la Science Biomédicale Post-Coloniale (1959–2002)" (Thesis, University of Paris VII, n.d.), and his more recent manuscript, "Franco-African Familiarities: A History of the Pasteur Institute of Cameroon, 1945–2000." See also Jacques Leonard, "Comment Peut-on être Pasteurien?," in Salomon-Bayet, *Pasteur et la Révolution Pastorienne,* 143–79.

81. Guénel, "Creation of the First Overseas Pasteur Institute."

82. On the extension of the IP of Algiers into a true research institution, see Chapter 3. Albert Calmette himself was sent to oversee the transformation from laboratory to research institute. Marie-Paule LaBerge, "Les Instituts Pasteur du Maghreb: La Recherche Scientifique Médicale dans le Cadre de la Politique Coloniale," *Revue Français d'Histoire d'Outre-Mer* 74 (1987): 27–42, 29–31, 35–37.

83. On Maurice Nicolle's tenure in Constantinople, see Moulin, "L'Hygiène dans la Ville: La Médecine Ottoman à l'Heure Pastorienne (1887–1908)," in *Villes Ottomanes à la Fin de l'Empire*, eds. Paul Dumont and François Georgeon, 186–209 (Paris: Editions L'Harmattan, 1992), 199–204.

84. Moulin highlights, with some irony, the resonance of Loir's appointment with Christian teachings in "Patriarchal Science," 313. In her article, it is clear that Loir, though no Nicolle, accomplished more than his successor would have the world believe. For more on the foundation of the Tunis laboratory, as well as on Loir, see Moulin, "L'Apprentissage Pastorien de la Mosaïque Tunisie," in *La Tunisie Mosaïque: Diasporas, Cosmopolitisme, Archéologies de l'Identité*, eds. Jacques Alexandropoulos and Patrick Cabanel, 369–88 (Toulouse: Presses Universitaires du Mirail, 2000), 371–74. See also Adrien Loir, "La Vaccination Obligatoire en Tunisie," *Revue Tunisienne* 4 (1897): 405–15.

85. On French colonial aspirations of the period more generally, see Brunschwig, *French Colonialism*. For closer consideration of the Tunisian case, see Lisa Anderson, *The State and Social Transformation in Tunisia and Libya, 1830–1980* (Princeton: Princeton University Press, 1986).

86. Anderson, *State and Social Transformation*, 65–70. Anderson notes that this project of "defensive modernization" effected dramatic social changes, relying, as it did, on taxes and on bodies to fill the military's growing ranks. Before this time, inhabitants of the countryside, including the nomadic tribes, had lived in relative isolation from the Bey and his government.

87. On the epidemics of the 1860s, see Nancy Gallagher, *Medicine and Power in Tunisia, 1780–1900* (New York: Cambridge University Press, 1983).

88. Anderson notes that there were about eight thousand Europeans in Tunisia in 1834; twelve thousand in the 1860s, and nearly nineteen thousand in 1881. Anderson, *State and Social Transformation*, 100, 104.

89. On Tunisia's relative healthiness in the first decade of the Protectorate, see Bertholon, "Etude Statistique sur la Colonie Française de Tunisie, 1881–1892," *Revue Tunisienne* 1 (1894): 362–78. Typhoid was particularly problematic. Bertholon, who went on to be the first president of the Society of Medical Sciences of Tunis, noted that Tunisia was not as healthy as France, but Tunis was healthier than certain French cities—including Rouen (364). Over all, "Tunisia boasts the privilege, almost alone among our recent acquisitions, of not exposing immigrants to more chances of dying than would a tour of the mother country [*mère patrie*] (365). Bertholon's analysis of the statistics is certainly open to challenge.

90. The main resistance to French control came from the south and lasted about a year. Otherwise, the French appropriation of Tunisia was relatively peaceful, from a military standpoint.

91. Brunschwig, *French Colonialism*, 59–60.

92. Anderson, *State and Social Transformation*, 145–51. Given the realities of the protectorate in Tunisia, when the "Tunisian government" is mentioned by a historical actor or myself, it will be the French government in Tunisia, unless otherwise noted.

93. Many of these new landowners remained in France. Anderson, *State and Social Transformation*, 151–57. This, she explains, was the period of "private colonization" and met with little success. Within a decade, a more active stage of "official" colonization became the rule. See also Perkins, *History of Modern Tunisia*, Chapter 2.

94. On Pasteur's early work, see Geison, "Pasteur," 357–83.

95. Loir's lab produced and administered vaccines and serum to fight rabies, smallpox, and diphtheria; and it conducted medical tests for hospitals, dispensaries, and private patients. In many ways, then, it was reminiscent of Nicolle's laboratory in Rouen. These were not similarities Nicolle would later choose to stress.

96. Gallagher, *Medicine and Power*. See also Mohamed Moncef Zitouna, *La Médecine en Tunisie 1881–1994* (Tunis [?]: Simpact, 1994 [?]). Moulin points out that the Tunisian Sanitary Board followed the establishment of a similar body by Egypt, in reaction to the cholera epidemic in 1831. Moulin, "Instituts Pasteur de la Méditerranée Arabe," 131–32. See also Kmar Annabi-Ben Nefissa, "L'Organisation Sanitaire en Tunisie à la Veille de la Création de l'Institut Pasteur de Tunis," *AIPT* 71 (1994): 345–49.

97. Gallagher, *Medicine and Power*, Chapters 2–4.

98. Described in an anonymous, typed manuscript, "Hygiène Publique," ASM 146 J 57: 1–3. Hand-written corrections of the text and assorted passages suggest that Nicolle may not have been its author (or that he dictated it), and that it was written around the time of his death. Etienne Burnet is a possible author. Unfortunately, the section on the Pasteur Institute of Tunis's interactions with Hygiene was not included ("à rédiger," 30) in this report. The West was quite concerned about the role religious pilgrimages played in spreading infectious disease. See Arnold, *Colonizing the Body: State Medicine and Epidemic Disease in Nineteenth-Century India* (Berkeley: University of California Press, 1993), 184–91.

99. Gallagher, *Medicine and Power*, 92–96. The decree "declared that all persons who had practiced medicine for five years or less in Tunisia had to prove that they had completed at least three years of medical school. Each additional year was equivalent to a year of practice. Indigenous practitioners under sixty years of age who had practiced for at least twenty years were allowed to continue if they had an *ijaza* from the Bey. Indigenous doctors who practiced in towns where there were no licensed doctors were allowed to continue without an *ijaza*, but could not perform surgery" (93). Algeria had a medical school, but Tunisia would remain without its own school until 1964.

100. Zitouna, *Médecine en Tunisie*, 129–30. Zitouna further notes that, as of 1900, the whole of Tunisia had a total of seventy-six licensed doctors, forty-seven of whom were in Tunis, which had an estimated population of 160,000.

101. Zitouna, *Médecine en Tunisie*, 78–82.

102. The French "ambulance" in this case describes a small, mobile medical unit with limited holding and nursing capacities.

103. The hospital took in patients and was inaugurated in 1898. Zitouna, *Médecine en Tunisie*, 90–103.

104. We have seen that Moulin has made restoring Loir's reputation a priority, and others are following her example.

105. Moulin, "L'Apprentissage Pastorien," 371. Moulin stresses Loir's efforts to bring together feuding cultures as she notes the mosaic-like nature of medical relations in Tunis (371–75). The institute was originally called the Association Tunisienne des Lettres, Sciences et Arts.

106. Yves Chatelain, *La Vie Littéraire et Intellectuelle en Tunisie de 1900 à 1937* (Paris: Guenther, 1937), 35–36.

107. Zitouna quotes from the announcement of this separation, described at the time as the " '*grande fille quittant sa mère.*' " The same announcement mentioned Loir's support for the move. The separation, Zitouna explains, was largely a reaction to the portioning of dues. Members paid 18 francs per year, 12 of which went to the Institut de Carthage. What, they asked, might be done with this extra 12 francs per member? Zitouna, *Médecine en Tunisie,* 168.

108. Loir was president in 1900. On the first fifty years of the society, see Raoul Dana, "La Société des Sciences Médicales de Tunisie de 1902 à 1952," in [ed.] Société des Sciences Médicales de Tunisie, *Médecine et Médecins de Tunisie de 1902 à 1952* (Tunis, 1952).

109. On Bechir Dinguizli and his relations with Loir, see Moulin, "Institutes Pasteur de la Méditerranée Arabe," 151–54. She stresses in particular Loir's debt to Dinguizli for his nuanced and culturally aware articles on smallpox—the subject of the latter's thesis—in Tunisia.

110. Moulin notes that certain *colons* opposed the creation of " 'hybrids speaking simian-French' " and, on a more revealing level, of people who " 'understand us better than we understand them.' " Moulin, "Institutes Pasteur de la Méditerranée Arabe," 137.

111. Nicolle subsequently employed some of these individuals and they would, in turn, prove invaluable to him, personally, professionally, and socially. See Chapters 4 and 8.

112. Pierre Nicolle, "Les Premières Années," 6.

113. According to Moulin, Loir left for "personal reasons." Moulin, "Institutes Pasteur de la Méditerranée Arabe," 137. All these changes make "dating" the IPT a challenge. It was founded as a laboratory in 1893; made permanent in 1894; given formal status as an Institute in 1900, welcomed Nicolle as its director in 1903, and inaugurated in its new (and present) location in 1905. Similar difficulties exist when specifying "founding dates" for Algeria and Morocco.

114. Nicolle recounted his institute's creation in his article, "L'Institut Pasteur de Tunis," which appeared in the *AIPT* 1 (1906): 5–34.

115. Mataud and Martin, *Médecine Rouennaise,* 93–94.

116. The Tunisian government's expanded interests in medicine around 1900 also reflect a general shift in French colonial policy. After Africa had been carved up, it became clear that a longer term approach to colonial life had to be embraced; consequently, governments such as Tunisia's began taking a more systematic approach to medicine. Comité d'Histoire du Service de Santé, *Historie de la Médecine aux Armées,* 3 vols. *De la Révolution Française au Conflit Mondial de 1914* (Paris: Charles-Lavauzelle, 1984), 2: 363–65.

117. Albert Calmette to Stephen Pichon, October 8, 1902, ASM 146 J 57.

118. Nicolle to Avice Nicolle, December 28, 1902, in P. Nicolle, "Les Premières Années," 9. The letters themselves are in ASM 146 J. I have used Pierre Nicolle's typed transcriptions of them in this article, where available.

119. P. Nicolle, "Charles Nicolle—Homme de Caractère," 28–29.

120. It is probable that this was R. Guy, author of *L'Architecture Moderne de Style Arabe*, whose interest in traditional forms is noted in Paul Rabinow, *French Modern: Norms and Forms of the Social Environment* (Cambridge, MA: MIT Press, 1989), 311–12. Hubert Lyautey, Governor General of Morocco from 1912 to 1925, also integrated this architecture into his Western restructuring of North African society—or, in Rabinow's eloquent formulation: "Morocco's public buildings would present Moroccan forms in the service of modern norms of technology and administration" (312). The Pasteur Institute of Tunis stands as another example of this mentality.

121. Nicolle to Mme. Avice Nicolle, March 1, 1903, in P. Nicolle, "Les Premières Années," 29.

122. Nicolle to Mme. Avice Nicolle, May 8, 1903, in ibid., 40–43. In the letter, Nicolle quoted at length from the article on Mougeot's visit that appeared in the local paper, *La Dépêche Tunisienne*. The article adopted rhetoric common to descriptions of Pasteur Institutes: the "'eminently humanitarian work,'" success with rabies treatment and various vaccines, and so on.

123. Despite the credit extension, the veterinary services so necessary to vaccine and serum production were not attached to the institute: nor would they be attached for nearly three decades. Instead, Ducloux directed a *service de l'élevage* in the building that housed the first institute.

124. Nicolle to G. Bugnot, February 23, 1903, in P. Nicolle, "Les Premières Années," 25.

125. Pichon was to become France's Ministre des Affaires Etrangères in 1906 and again from 1917 to 1921.

126. The description is from Nicolle, "L'Institut Pasteur de Tunis" (1906): 7–16. The library, which received doctoral theses from several French faculties as well as journals and major publications, was soon expanded in a separate building.

127. Ibid., 16. This tendency went beyond the Pasteur Institutes and into French colonialism in general. See Rabinow, *French Modern*.

128. Nicolle, "L'Institut Pasteur de Tunis" (1906), 6, 17 (the quotation is on page 17). The original institute building contained Ducloux's *service de l'élevage* and an office for the purchase and distribution of vaccines and serum not manufactured in Tunis.

129. Roux to Nicolle, October 2, 1905, ASM 146 J 33. Nicolle frequently lamented the inadequacies of narrow-minded bureaucracy. See, for example, Nicolle to Bugnot, February 23, 1903: "Being immortal by definition, it [bureaucracy] has no concept of time. Now, to me, time is life itself (to the English, money is life); I am angry to waste life marking it" (in P. Nicolle, "Les Premières Années," 25). Order might have been Nicolle's ideal, but order for order's sake was a mentality for which he had little tolerance.

130. Nicolle did, however, find ways to channel his sense of the ironic in a manner that served his purposes, describing the absurdity of the event to Bugnot. Reflecting upon the comic scene, he composed a verse ["'Le Ministre (un ex-morticole), / Me dit: 'Mon vieux Charles Nicolle, / Reçois le Mérite Agricole / —Je lui réponds d'un ton frivole: / J'aime mieux ça que la vérole.'"]. Nicolle to Bugnot, October 30, 1905, in P. Nicolle, "Les Premières Années," 67.

131. Nicolle to Georges Bugnot, February 23, 1903, in ibid., 26.

132. Nicolle to Mme. Avice Nicolle, December 28, 1902, in ibid., 8–10. The parenthetical inserts are Pierre's. Nicolle expressed identical sentiments to longtime friend Bugnot.

133. I am not arguing that the annual reports were fabrications. They did, however, include occasional reconstructions of the past—and, later, publicity moves for the present and future—within otherwise strictly "appropriate" materials. This is certainly neither the first nor the last time a journal editor has taken such liberties (or that an annual report has reflected a political agenda). In a nice historical twist, Loir himself would later contribute to the dismantling of the very carefully constructed myth surrounding Pasteur: Geison, *Private Science*, 274.

134. Nicolle, "L'Institut Pasteur de Tunis" (1906), 18. Emphasis in original.

135. Ibid., 29.

136. Ibid., 32, 34. Nicolle's teaching-oriented criticisms were evidently drawn from his Rouen experience. Ultimately, in Tunis, he would be far less interested in formal medical education than Loir had been, wholly abandoning his predecessor's efforts to create a cadre of professionally trained Tunisians.

137. Nicolle, "La Grande Misère de l'Institut Pasteur: Un Cri d'Alarme," *Les Nouvelles Littéraires*, February 3, 1934.

138. This tended to be the case for medicine in general, not just for Pastorian medicine. David Arnold cites Lyautey, who argued that " 'the [Western] physician alone justifies colonialism.' " Arnold, "Introduction," in *Imperial Medicine*, ed. Arnold, 3.

139. Guènel, "Creation of the First Overseas Pasteur Institute," for the formative example.

140. This free service for the local French and Tunisian hospitals served as both symbolic and pragmatic link of France, French medicine, and Tunisian culture. Nicolle describes the service in his "L'Institut Pasteur de Tunis" (1906), 31.

141. In the first volume (1906) of the *AIPT*, Nicolle noted the institute's link to the city's water supply ("Travaux Scientifiques de l'Institut Pasteur," 71–74) and described its study of the *lac de Tunis* ("Travaux," 74–77).

142. Nicolle himself gave lectures on hygiene to "the Tunisian people" in 1903 and 1905. Nicolle, "L'Institut Pasteur de Tunis" (1906), 34. His talks would have to have been in French.

143. Latour, *Science in Action: How to Follow Scientists and Engineers through Society* (Cambridge, MA: Harvard University Press, 1987). Moulin notes that such adaptation was a point of pride for Pastorians and was, moreover, central to the overall success of their mission. Moulin, "Pasteur Institute's International Network," 163.

144. Nicolle, "L'Institut Pasteur de Tunis" (1906), 33.

145. See Chapter 2.

146. G. Grandsire, "L'Hôpital Sadiki de 1902 à 1915 sous la Direction de Brunswic-le-Bihan," *Tunisie Médicale* 25 (1931): 240–48; Zitouna, *Médecine en Tunisie*, 49, 82–84.

147. Grandsire refers to Comte as "*un de ses* [Brunswic's] *anciens camarades d'études de Paris*" (Grandsire, "L'Hôpital Sadiki," 242). Huet (*Pommier,* 50) claims Comte was at the time the préparateur of "Ch. Marey" at the Collège de France, and that Nicolle knew both Brunswic and Comte earlier. It is possible that Comte worked under *Etienne Jules* Marey, who was at the Collège de France and died in 1903.

148. According to Zitouna, Conseil was "adored by Tunisians, particularly the poor; he lived in their neighborhood and welcomed them all [en foule]." Zitouna, *Médecine en Tunisie*, 51. See also Prévost-Barancy, *Charles Nicolle*, 40.

149. Huet, *Pommier*, 51.

150. The institute's budget reflected its unique status: a civil institution, it received a state subsidy, but, like the Paris institute, it could receive gifts and donations, and was allowed to keep the profits it made from its sale of products and from medical analyses it conducted. By the early 1920s, half of the institute's budget came from sales. Nicolle, *Notice sur l'Institut Pasteur de Tunis* (Tunis: J. Barlier et cie, 1924), 20. In 1921, the institute moved from Agriculture to the Interior. See Chapter 4.

151. Nicolle, "Fonctionnement . . . 1906" (1907), 40.

152. Nicolle, "Fonctionnement . . . 1907" (1908), 38; "Fonctionnement . . . 1908" (1909): 51–52. Husson continued to head the malaria service (aided by Comte) until he retired in 1909. He died shortly thereafter, in 1911. The service continued, though in a greatly diminished capacity, during the war; in January 1924, it was attached, in expanded form, to the *Direction de l'Hygiène*. Nicolle, *Notice* (1924), 15.

153. This was a small epidemic—only thirteen cases were diagnosed that year.

154. Nicolle himself set the scene—in the third person: on November 21, 1909, a sailor was admitted to a Tunisian infirmary. Because his symptoms were suspicious, Nicolle was called to examine him. "The Director of the Pasteur Institute . . . went immediately to the sick person and confirmed that same day a diagnosis of plague." Nicolle, "Fonctionnement . . . 1907" (1908), 41. Who says bacteriologists don't make house calls?

155. Ibid.

156. F.-J. Guégan, "La Station Sanitaire de La Goulette: Son Fonctionnement pendant la Dernière Campagne Anticholérique," *AIPT* 7 (1912): 53–60, 59.

157. A. Guégan, "L'Evolution de l'Assistance Médicale en Tunisie," *Tunisie Médicale* 3 (1913): 150–53, 153.

158. Appearing in the *Bulletin Officiel Municipal de la Ville de Tunis*, Conseil's report of about one hundred pages was by far the longest single *Bulletin* document of the year. The next longest report in the 1913 *Bulletin*, for example, is the five-page budget report.

159. Ernest Conseil, "Rapport du Chef du Bureau d'Hygiène, 1910," *Bulletin Officiel Municipal de la Ville de Tunis* 3 (1911): 91–166, 166. We will return to this important assertion in Chapter 2.

160. Conseil, "Rapport du Chef du Bureau d'Hygiène de Tunis pour l'Année 1909," *Bulletin Officiel Municipal de la Ville de Tunis* 2 (1910): 125–96, 195.

161. Nicolle, "Fonctionnement . . . 1910" (1911), 159.

162. Numerous articles on Nicolle's scientific discoveries can be found throughout later volumes of the *AIPT*. See, for example, M. F. Kennou, "Propos sur Toxoplasma gondii," 63 (1986): 123–32; R. Nataf, "Charles Nicolle et les Maladies Oculaires Transmissibles," 43 (1966): 449–53; André Eyquem and Jacqueline de Saint Martin, "Hommage à Charles Nicolle: Naissance, Éclipse et Résurgence du Concept et des Maladies par Auto-immunisation," 64 (1987): 5–14; Pierre Nicolle, "Alphonse Laveran et Charles Nicolle," 88 (1981): 265–79.

163. Nicolle, "Les Nouvelles Acquisitions sur le Typhus Exanthématique," *Tunisie Médicale* 1 (1911): 3–9, 4. See Chapter 2.

164. Nicolle, "Culture du Parasite du Bouton d'Orient," *CRAS* 146 (1908): 842–43; idem., "Sur un Protozoaire Nouveau du Gondi," *CRAS* 148 (1909): 369–72. Nicolle did not follow this disease's path in any detail. Its significance—which has heightened with the AIDS epidemic—was not realized for fifty years. M. F. Kennou, "Propos sur *Toxoplasma gondii*." See also Moulin, "Historical Introduction: The Institut Pasteur's Contribution," *Research in Immunology* 144 (1993): 8–13. Nicolle's role in research on toxoplasmosis is discussed on pages 9–10.

165. Abram S. Benenson, ed., *Control of Communicable Diseases in Man*, 14th ed. (Washington, DC: American Public Health Association, 1985), 209.

166. Lot, *Charles Nicolle*, 31–32. "NNN" takes liberties with the name of its second contributor, McNeal, in its acronymic formulation.

167. Although Calmette was technically in Lille at this time, I include him among the "Parisian Pastorians" because, in practice, he was an integral part of the IPP's relations with its colonial institutes and labs.

168. Roux to Nicolle, August 4, 1909, ASM 146 J 33. Roux wrote in the postscript to this letter, "I forgot to tell you that the Academy of Sciences has awarded you the Montyon Prize . . . for your work on Kala-Azar. Laveran made the report to the Commission on which I sat. There was no discussion, everyone just agreed." Laveran's presentation underscores the fact that the Pastorian network helped Roux, Calmette, and Mesnil carry out their colonial endeavors.

169. Stephane Kraxner, archivist of the IPP, is currently teasing out the much-neglected Mesnil's role in coordinating the overseas Pasteur Institutes. For information on Mesnil (1868–1938) and a growing number of Pastorians, see the "Biographical" section of the AIP's invaluable Web site: www.pasteur.fr/infosci/archives/f-bio.html

170. See the description of then-director of the IPP, Emile Duclaux, in his "Preface," *BIP* 1 (1903): 1–3. The journal was designed to reflect the whole of the Pastorian mission, embracing veterinary medicine, agriculture, and chemistry—any scientific development relating to microbiology.

171. On Mesnil, see the *IPP Archives* Web site.

172. The Nicolle–Mesnil correspondence is among the typed transcriptions that Pierre Nicolle prepared: AIP FR IP NCP.11. Despite Mesnil's valiant efforts to make his overseas colleagues' work known in Paris, he met with only partial success.

173. The society's journal was originally called the *Bulletin de la Société des Sciences Médicales de Tunis*. It added an "*et Travaux*" in 1911, then shifted to the *Revue Tunisienne des Sciences Médicales* in 1914. In 1929, the society finally settled on *La Tunisie Médicale*. Zitouna, *Médecine en Tunisie*, 169.

174. With the exception of the journal's collaborative publication with the Institut Pasteur d'Alger, the *Archives de l'Institut Pasteur de Tunis* was under Nicolle's editorial control until his death.

175. See the introductory quotation in Chapter 5.

176. The *AIPT*'s growing prestige helped solve another problem created by colonial distance: journal availability. In his early years in Tunis, Nicolle had to rely on Mesnil for access to articles published by other researchers. As his own journal grew in popularity, his institute received increasing numbers of journals in a reciprocal subscription exchange.

Chapter 2

1. August Hirsch, *Handbook of Geographical and Historical Pathology*, 3 vols., trans. Charles Creighton (London: New Sydenham Society, 1883–86), 1: 545. Emphasis in original. Creighton translated the second German edition, which was published in three volumes from 1881. Hirsch's first edition appeared in two volumes between 1860 and 1864.

2. Bertholon, "Étude Statistique" (1894), 365. See also Bertholon and Ernest Chantre, *Recherches Anthropologiques dans la Berberie Orientale, Tripolitaine, Tunisie, Algérie* (Lyon: A. Rey, 1912–13). Bertholon did, however, have an agenda in promoting Tunisia's salubrity: he hoped to attract more French *colons* to his adopted country ["Etude Statistique" (1894), 377–78]. He developed the argument later in his "Mentalité Française" (1901).

3. Loir, "Démographie: Statistique de la Population de Tunis," *Revue Tunisienne* 5 (1898): 348–453, 353. Leaving aside the category of *"maladies non classés,"* Loir included smallpox, diphtheria, typhoid, and measles; he included statistics from 1886–97 for Arabs, Israelites, and Europeans. As we will see, there was some trouble with typhus *outside* the city. Such outbreaks tended to be seen as circumscribed and *imported*.

4. Like "germ theory" (see the Introduction), "Romanticism," "center/periphery," and most other broad descriptive categories applied to complex movements and patterns, "scientific revolution" is a contested term. Was there one? Many? None at all? (see, for example, Trevor H. Levere, "Romanticism, Natural Philosophy and the Sciences: A Review and Bibliographic Essay," *Perspectives on Science* 4 [1996]: 463–88; Latour, *We Have Never Been Modern*, trans. Catherine Porter [New York: Harvester Wheatsheaf, 1993]). For the purposes of this book, debates about revolutionary dynamics are less important than is the observation that Enlightenment rationalism deeply influenced Nicolle's early ideals of scientific process.

5. Francis Bacon, *The New Organon*, ed. Fulton H. Anderson (Indianapolis: Bobbs-Merrill, 1960), I.3. This book was first published in 1620.

6. On specificity, see the Introduction; and Mendelsohn, " 'Like All That Lives' "; Amsterdamska, "Medical and Biological Constraints"; Mazumdar, *Species and Specificity*.

7. Moulin, "Pasteur Institute's International Network," 135, 139–40.

8. This debate, as one would expect, extended well beyond medical circles. For an example of the laissez-faire capitalist approach to medicine in the colonies, see Bertholon, "Mentalité Française et Colonisation Tunisienne," *Revue Tunisienne* 8 (1901): 379–406. An impressive program for the socialist approach to medicine—which contains a helpful sketch of the extant medical landscape in Tunisia—is M. Malinas and M. Tostivint, "Mutualité Coopérative et Projet Général d'Assistance Médical Indigène," *Revue Tunisienne* 12 (1905): 283–304, 386–422, 480–515. For a West African example, see Conklin, *Mission to Civilize*, Chapter 2, "Public Works and Public Health," on Pastorian influence, bacteriology, and hygiene, 59–65.

9. The first part of Malinas and Tostivint's 1905 article includes numbers of doctors (and, in the same table but separately, pharmacists and *sages-femmes*) in Tunisia. These numbers are broken down, on the one hand, by city and its surrounding area, and, on the other, by categories of "French," "Foreign" ["*Étrangers*"], and "*Toléré*." Tunis and its environs, with a

population of 275,000, included 29 French doctors, 49 foreign, and 7 *toléré*. Around Thala, on the other hand, a population of 73,000 was served by just 1 regular doctor and 11 *toléré*. Sousse, with a population roughly three-quarters that of Tunis (204,495), had only 3 French, 9 foreign, and 7 *toléré*. Totals for the whole of Tunisia were, respectively, 55, 76, and 44. Malinas and Tostivint, "Mutualité Coopérative" (1905), 292–95.

10. On Brunswic's project, see Zitouna, *Médecine en Tunisie*, 212–13. Zitouna includes a list of the initial articles defining the school and its functions.

11. The second licensed Tunisian doctor was Hassen Bouhageb. Bouhageb, like Dinguizli, was trained at Bordeaux; he was licensed in 1902. Ibid., 29.

12. "Séance du 8 Juin 1904," *Bulletin de la Société des Sciences Médicales de Tunis* 2 (1904): 274–76; "Séance Extraordinaire du 11 Juin 1904," *Bulletin de la Société des Sciences Médicales de Tunis* 2 (1904): 289–93. The charge against the school was led by Dr. Cattan.

13. "Séance du 8 Juin 1904" (1904), 290. Specifically, Nicolle argued that they might wait to discuss the subject, at the very least, until Brunswic himself was present, as "the work of the Medical School is the project of one particular medical personality."

14. The article, written in the style of a descriptive short story, was published in the *Presse Médicale* on January 23, 1904. In particular, Nicolle and Brunswic, as medical experts, condemned the local practice of using a thick rope, coiled several times around the condemned's neck, coupled with a short drop, which resulted in slow strangulation. An excerpt of the piece was published as Nicolle and Brunswic-le Bihan, *Une Pendaison à Tunis* (Paris: C. Naud, 1904).

15. "Séance du 8 Juin 1904" (1904), 275. Emphasis added.

16. Later, he would chastise Georges Duhamel about his overtly political actions. See, for example, Nicolle to Duhamel, July 23, 1925, and August 4, 1925, AIP FR IP NCP.8–10.

17. "Séance Extraordinaire du 11 Juin 1904" (1904), 292.

18. The final vote was 19 for, 8 opposed, with 2 abstentions. Ibid., 292.

19. The school, in the end, persevered, and the Tunisian medical profession continued to be a profession. For a concise overview of Brunswic's school, see Zitouna, *Médecine en Tunisie*, 213. Zitouna notes that the school's numbers remained low. Yet, during World War I, when most of the Sadiki's doctors, and all of its interns, were mobilized, three Medical Auxiliaries were assigned the functions of the interns. (This was a general pattern in Tunisia during the war, and it did much to help the economic fortunes of Tunisians—until the Europeans returned. Perkins, *History of Modern Tunisia*, 73–76.) See also Grandsire, "L'Hôpital Sadiki," 243.

20. "Discours du Dr. Nicolle, Président Sortant," *Bulletin de la Société des Sciences Médicales de Tunis* 8 (1909): 8–10.

21. This alignment was evident in the medical "cosmos" Nicolle effectively created in Tunisia. See Chapter 1. I'm using "*hygiene*" as a generic term containing both epidemiology and prophylaxis. This was, functionally, how the term was used by Nicolle.

22. "La 'Tunisie Médicale,'" *Tunisie Médicale* 1 (1911): 1–2, 1. The journal is listed at the Bibliothèque Nationale as existing only until 1914; Zitouna mentions a *Tunis Médicale* with which the Society of Medical Science's journal merged in the early 1920s. (To confuse matters further, the society's journal became *La Tunisie Médicale* in 1929.)

23. Ibid., 2.

24. Ibid., 1.

25. The journal's opening claim was striking to this end: "A country's scientific activity and its economic activity are quite similar [*assez semblable à*]: the same laws direct their production and exchange." Ibid., 1.

26. Nicolle, "Nouvelles Acquisitions . . . Typhus" (1911). J. Plancke, Doctor of the Primary Schools of Tunis, also contributed a lead article. J. Plancke, "Hygiène dans les Écoles Primaires de Tunis," *Tunisie Médicale* 1 (1911): 23–25.

27. Zinsser, *Rats, Lice and History* (1934, 1935), 216–17. Zinsser described typhus in its "classic" form—that is, as known through the symptoms it caused in European bodies. Variations on this description will be seen in Nicolle's work, notably in the way typhus presented itself in Tunisian, particularly Arab-Tunisian, bodies.

28. *Typhus* is from the Greek "*typhos*," referring to any fever-related stupor. Though generally perceived as a frightening stage of the disease, delirium was, according to Paul Weindling, experienced by some as a relief from the horrors of concentration camps in World War II. Paul Julian Weindling, *Epidemics and Genocide in Eastern Europe, 1890–1945* (Oxford: Oxford University Press, 2000), 3–5.

29. I will treat the ongoing debates on the causal organism of typhus only tangentially, as they relate to Nicolle's larger understanding of disease. Nicolle did not directly participate in the "hunt" for the causal microbe of typhus.

30. I qualify the outcome as "somewhat more positive" because Nicolle's bout of typhus, though not fatal in itself, is thought to have caused the heart troubles that eventually led to his death. See Chapter 8.

31. Conseil, "Le Typhus Exanthématique en Tunisie," *AIPT* 2 (1907): 145–54, 146. Bertholon, still *médecin en chef* of Tunisian prisons, contracted typhus during the 1906 outbreak. He recovered.

32. In Hirsch's words, "where the misery is felt more or less uniformly by all classes of the population, the disease has . . . sought out chiefly the crowded and filthy quarters, streets, or houses inhabited by the proletariat, or has even been confined to them." Hirsch, *Handbook* 1: 587–88.

33. Ibid, 1: 581. Emphasis in original. August Hirsch was Professor of Medicine at the University of Berlin.

34. Zinsser, *Rats, Lice, and History*, esp. Chapter 8, "On the Influence of Epidemic Diseases on Political and Military History, and on the Relative Unimportance of Generals."

35. Hirsch, *Handbook of Geographical and Historical Pathology* (1883), 1: 555.

36. Ibid., 1: 574.

37. Hirsch did not specifically call attention to the fact that the countries listed tended also to border Europe and the United States; still, the fact remains that they did. Peru, he noted, also had had outbreaks—"probably imported from Spain at a very early period"—and Persia had more limited problems with typhus. Ibid., 1: 570–71, 568. The quotation is on 571.

38. Ibid., 581. Emphasis in original.

39. Ibid., 1: 583. Hirsch did not believe that famine was the direct *cause* of typhus, but, following Virchow, was a *predisposing* cause: "famine and typhus, then, have no necessary connexion as cause and effect, as Virchow has already pointed out in his history of the typhus epidemic of 1847–48 in Upper Silesia. The typhus poison, it is clear, finds a

particularly suitable soil wherein to develop and acquire potency in a populace reduced by hunger; but that detriment only amounts to a material predisposing factor of disease, and it will make itself felt all the more where other lowering causes have been reducing the power of resistance in the individual at the same time" (1: 580–81).

40. Hirsch's two-volume first edition appeared between 1860 and 1864.

41. Dale C. Smith, "The Rise and Fall of Typhomalarial Fever: I. Origins," *JHM* 37 (1982): 182–220, 191–96. See also Smith, "Gerhard's Distinction between Typhoid and Typhus and Its Reception in America, 1833–1860," *BHM* 54 (1980): 368–85; and, on the larger fever project, Leonard G. Wilson, "Fevers and Science in Early Nineteenth Century Medicine," *JHM* 33 (1978): 386–407.

42. Nathan E. Brill, "A Study of Seventeen Cases of a Disease Clinically Resembling Typhoid Fever, But Without the Widal Reaction," *New York Medical Journal* 67 (1898): 48–54; 77–82.

43. John F. Anderson and Joseph Goldberger, "The Relation of So-Called Brill's Disease to Typhus Fever," *Public Health Reports* 27 (1912): 149–60. Brill never mentioned typhus as the disease's possible identity in 1898, but did raise the possibility in 1910, after examining more than two hundred cases. Brill, "An Acute Infectious Disease of Unknown Origin: A Clinical Study Based on 221 Cases," *American Journal of Medical Sciences* 139 (1910): 484–502, 501. On Goldberger, see Alan M. Kraut, *Goldberger's War: The Life and Work of a Public Health Crusader* (New York: Hill and Wang, 2003). So-called Brill's disease had an important role to play in typhus research in the 1930s. See Chapter 6.

44. Bertholon, "Étude Statistique" (1894), 365.

45. The year 1906 also marked the start of systematic study of the variability of bacterial species in terms of "mutation," particularly following the work of Rudolf Neisser. Amsterdamska, "Medical and Biological Constraints," 659–60, 671–73.

46. Dmitri Ivanovski published his findings in 1892, Martinus Beijerinck in 1898. On early tobacco mosaic disease research, see Ton van Helvoort, "What Is a Virus? The Case of Tobacco Mosaic Disease," *Studies in History and Philosophy of Science* 22 (1991): 557–88, 559; and Angela N. H. Creager, *The Life of a Virus: Tobacco Mosaic Virus as an Experimental Model, 1930–1965* (Chicago: University of Chicago Press, 2002), 23–27. On the history of virus research more generally, A. P. Waterson and Lise Wilkinson, *An Introduction to the History of Virology* (Cambridge: Cambridge University Press, 1978). See Chapter 5.

47. Creager includes a table of early filterable virus discoveries. Creager, *Life of a Virus*, 30. Harvard's S. B. Wolbach listed some thirty known filterable viruses in 1912: S. B. Wolbach, "The Filterable Viruses, a Summary," *Journal of Medical Research* 22 (1912): 1–25.

48. Emile Roux, "Sur les Microbes Dits 'Invisibles,'" *BIP* 1 (1903): 7–12. Roux noted that Pasteur had, in 1881, hypothesized that the causal organism of rabies was "so small that we would never see it" (7). Pastorian Paul Remlinger demonstrated the filterability of rabies in 1903 (Creager, *Life of a Virus*, 30).

49. On defining filterable viruses (by that time, just "viruses") by "negative properties," see the review of Thomas M. Rivers, "The Nature of Viruses," *Physiological Reviews* 12 (1932): 423–52.

50. This does not necessarily mean that researchers did not attempt to inoculate themselves with typhus. On human experimentation, see Susan E. Lederer, *Subjected to Science: Human Experimentation in America before the Second World War* (Baltimore: Johns

Hopkins University Press, 1995). On rickettsial diseases, see Victoria A. Harden, *Rocky Mountain Spotted Fever: History of a Twentieth-Century Disease* (Baltimore: Johns Hopkins University Press, 1990); and Willy Burgdorfer and Robert L. Anacker, eds., *Rickettsiae and Rickettsial Diseases* (New York: Academic Press, 1981). For a perspective a bit closer to Nicolle's own, see Thomas M. Rivers, ed., *Viral and Rickettsial Infections of Man* (Philadelphia: J. B. Lippincott, 1948).

51. Conseil reported the disappointing results of laboratory tests on typhus patients in his "Typhus . . . en Tunisie" (1907). He further noted that he tended to give patients suspected of suffering from typhus quinine, to rule out malaria: with typhoid, it was the disease most often confused with typhus (152).

52. Nicolle, *Introduction*, 114. Nicolle gave the longer version in this book and a shorter one in his Nobel speech. Nicolle, "Conférence du Docteur Charles Nicolle sur les Travaux qui lui ont Valu l'Attribution du Prix Nobel de Médecine," *AIPT* 19 (1930): 113–21.

53. Nicolle, "Prix Nobel" (1930), 114.

54. See Chapter 6.

55. Conseil, "Typhus . . . en Tunisie" (1907), 145.

56. Ibid.

57. Ibid., 146. "*La vie au grand air*" was Conseil's exact phrase.

58. Ibid., 146–47.

59. Ibid., 147.

60. Ibid., 151.

61. Ibid., 153. Conseil explicitly mentioned typhoid and paratyphoid among the diseases they needed to eliminate, to be more certain of their typhus diagnoses.

62. Conseil, "Le Typhus Exanthématique en Tunisie Pendant L'année 1909," *AIPT* 5 (1910): 19–42, 19–20. "Typhus has become a rare disease, little known to doctors; and so typhus is often, outside of epidemics, diagnosed as typhoid" (18).

63. Ibid., 21–22. Conseil suspected that two of the foyers had been started by cases brought in from Algeria.

64. Ibid., 23 ("*cafés maures*").

65. The lazaret was soon made into a permanent hospital for contagious diseases. Upon Conseil's death in 1930, it was renamed in his honor. In 1985, it was renamed the Hôpital la Rabta. Zitouna and S. Haouet, "Du Lazaret à l'Hôpital de la Rabta," *Tunisie Medicale* 76 (1998): 311–13.

66. Conseil, "Typhus . . . 1909" (1910), 39.

67. Ibid., 24.

68. Conseil, "Rapport . . . 1909" (1910), 157.

69. At the end of his longer report on the 1909 epidemic, Conseil thanked all the doctors who had supplied him with information by name. His list included some three dozen practitioners. Conseil, "Typhus . . . 1909" (1910), 42. Later, Nicolle, too, would thank "the Tunisian medical corps, ever devoted to the progress of medicine and hygiene," who "have been the best, most devoted, and most constant collaborators to our Institute." Nicolle, "L'Oeuvre de l'Institut Pasteur de Tunis," *Tunisie Médicale* 1 (1911): 253–63, 262–63.

70. Neither this neat, if thick, descriptive formula for scientific discovery, nor Nicolle's later "epiphany" narrative, is likely to reflect the actual processes by which Nicolle et al.

came to their typhus realizations. Nicolle was, however, masterful at covering up any evidence that was not tidy, whatever the discovery theory motivating the master narrative. As we move through Nicolle's life, we will see moments that smudged some of the neat edges of his accounts.

71. Conseil, "Typhus . . . 1909" (1910), 20.

72. Ibid., 27, 24.

73. Ibid., 35–36, 35.

74. Ibid., 29–30.

75. Ibid., 34.

76. Ibid., 24. Diagnosis of typhus, particularly at the start of an epidemic, remained tricky; patients, Conseil noted, were only gathered together after they had been diagnosed.

77. Ibid., 34. In this article, Conseil gave an explanation not just for the differences between Arab and White patients' expressions of the classic typhus rash, but also for their different expressions of stupor: Europeans, whose "nervous system is more differentiated, present more marked cerebral symptoms" (32). Conseil did not, however, elaborate on this *particular* racist assumption, nor does it seem to have played a lasting part in typhus work at the IPT.

78. Ibid., 35.

79. M. Baltazard, "Le Respect des Conditions de la Nature dans l'Expérimentation," *AIPT* 43 (1966): 35–46, 37.

80. See Chapter 1. Nicolle used monkeys for experiments on other diseases in Tunisia before turning to monkeys for typhus.

81. Alhough Alfred Conor is not listed as a coauthor on any of Nicolle's earliest typhus articles, he did, as Nicolle acknowledged at the conclusion of a 1911 article, assist with the monkey work. Nicolle, "Nouvelles Acquisitions . . . Typhus" (1911), 9.

82. Nicolle, "Reproduction Expérimentale du Typhus Exanthématique chez le Singe," *CRAC* 149 (1909): 157–60, 160. Emphasis in original.

83. Conseil, "Discours du Docteur Conseil," *Revue Tunisien des Sciences Médicales* 22 (1926): 123–31, 127.

84. Roux to Nicolle, May 26, 1909, ASM 146 J 33. The chimp was sent from Marseille and cost the IPP 550 francs. Roux was not wholly comfortable about spending so much money. In the same letter, he commented to Nicolle that M. Rimbaud at Marseille "charged us a bit much for the animal, but this isn't important. What is important is the success of your experiment."

85. With other typhus patients by that date, the man was transferred to La Rabta after being diagnosed.

86. Roux to Nicolle, June 30, 1909, ASM 146 J 33.

87. Nicolle, "Reproduction Expérimentale du Typhus Exanthématique" (1909), 157.

88. Nicolle, "Prix Nobel" (1930). See Chapter 5.

89. Nicolle, "Nouvelles Acquisitions . . . Typhus" (1911), 8.

90. Nicolle, C. Comte, and E. Conseil, "Transmission Expérimentale du Typhus Exanthématique par le Pou du Corps," *CRAS* 149 (1909): 486–89. Though "transmitted" by Roux, this note was in fact presented by Metchnikoff: Roux was on annual holiday at the time. Roux to Nicolle, September 7, 1909, ASM 146 J 33.

91. Nicolle, Comte, and Conseil, "Transmission Expérimentale du Typhus Exanthématique" (1909), 487. The trio noted that they had in fact been trying to transmit typhus between monkeys via the body louse from the "the start of our research," but had failed. Here again, chimpanzee infection proved to be the missing link.

92. F. Percival Mackie, "The Part Played by Pediculus Corporis in the Transmission of Relapsing Fever," *BMJ* 2 (1907): 1706–9.

93. J. Everett Dutton and John L. Todd, "The Nature of Tick Fever in the Eastern Part of the Congo Free State," *BMJ* 2 (1905): 1259–60; Philip H. Ross and A. D. Milne, "Tick Fever," *BMJ* 2 (1904): 1453–54.

94. X. de la Tribonnière, "Edmond Sergent (1876–1969) et l'Institut Pasteur d'Algérie," *BSPE* 93 (2000): 365–71. On Foley, with much on his collaborations with Sergent, Paul Doury, "Henry Foley et la Découverte du Rôle du Pou dans la Transmission de la Fièvre Récurrente et du Typhus Exanthématique," *Histoire des Sciences Médicales* 30 (1996): 363–69.

95. Edmond Sergent and H. Foley, "Fièvre Récurrente du Sud-Oranais et *Pediculus vestimenti*. Note Préliminaire," *BSPE* 1 (1908): 174–76; and idem., "Recherches sur la Fièvre Récurrente et son Mode de Transmission, dans une Epidémie Algérienne," *AIP* 24 (1910): 337–73.

96. According to Nicolle, Sergent launched his campaign to claim priority for the louse as vector in 1914. A striking example of Sergent's efforts may be found in his later contribution to a special edition of the *AIPT* honoring Nicolle: Sergent, "Le Pou, Inoculateur de Maladies Humaines (Aperçu Historique)," *AIPT* 36 (1959): 307–10. The Nicolle–Sergent dispute continues to be discussed to this day, with historians coming across one account or the other and transmitting it as fact. I am examining this debate in a separate article. A preliminary version, "A Louse, Divided," was delivered at the annual meeting of the American Association for the History of Medicine, Birmingham, Alabama, April 2005.

97. In fairness, Sergent and Foley did transmit the disease by using a blanket laden with lice that had fed on an infected patient. Nicolle denied that the experiment was rigorous enough to carry the weight of demonstration. Further discussion of the Nicolle–Sergent dispute over relapsing fever is in my "A Louse, Divided."

98. For an insightful discussion of Nicolle's standards of demonstration and their impact on his collaborators, see Baltazard, "Respect des Conditions de la Nature."

99. Conseil, "Typhus . . . 1909" (1910), 37.

100. Roux to Nicolle, August 18, 1909, ASM 146 J 33.

101. "These experiments show that it is possible to transmit typhus from an infected Chinese monkey to a new one by means of the body louse. The application of this fact to the etiology and prevention of the disease in man is essential. Measures taken against typhus must have as their object the destruction of these parasites; they should principally target the body, the linen, the clothing and the bedding of the sick." Nicolle, Comte and Conseil, "Transmission Expérimentale du Typhus Exanthématique" (1909), 489.

102. Nicolle, "Nouvelles Acquisitions . . . Typhus" (1911), 3.

103. Conseil, "Typhus . . . 1909" (1910), 37.

104. Ibid., 39.

105. Ibid., 40.

106. Ibid., 41.

107. Ibid., 19.

108. Conseil, "Le Typhus Exanthématique en Tunisie pendant l'Année 1910," *AIPT* 6 (1911): 134–49, 148. On surveillance by colonial doctors in the countryside (135).

109. This is the pattern Charles Rosenberg made famous in his classic *The Cholera Years: The United States in 1832, 1849, and 1866* (Chicago: University of Chicago Press, 1962).

110. A. Poirson, "L'Epidémie de Typhus du Goubellat (1912)," *AIPT* 7 (1912): 140–43, 141–42.

111. Poirson, "L'Epidémie de Typhus" (1912), 143. Poirson admitted, "I saw these things with my own eyes, to my pleasant surprise." He further noted, in a footnote that "the women even began cleaning the *gourbis* with boiling water, although we had never told them to do this" (143). In an article from the previous year, Conseil had observed that boiling water could work to disinfect clothing but that, in the Tunisian countryside, both water and the materials to heat it were often scarce. He also added that many of the poor people living in the countryside had only, quite literally, the shirt on their back: further complicating cleansing efforts.

112. I have used the phrase "rational hygiene" several times. The Pastorians themselves used the phrase, and variations on it, frequently, when describing the prophylactic measures that followed from the discovery of the louse transmission of typhus.

113. Conseil, "Typhus … 1910" (1911), 147.

114. Ibid., 149.

115. Nicolle and Conseil, "Nécessité des Mesures à prendre pour Préserver nos Armées en Campagne du Typhus Exanthématique et du Typhus Récurrent," *Tunisie Médicale* 4 (1914): 291.

116. Conseil, "Typhus … 1910" (1911), 144. Emphasis added. It will be remembered that Conseil, in his 1910 *AIPT* article, considered familial contagion to be more common in the country than in the city, but still the exception.

117. Conseil, "Typhus … 1910" (1911), 138.

118. Mary Douglas, *Purity and Danger: An Analysis of Concepts of Pollution and Taboo* (London: Routledge, 1966, 1984); Timothy Burke, "Colonialism, Cleanliness, and Civilization in Colonial Rhodesia," in Alice L. Conklin and Ian Christopher Fletcher, *European Imperialism* (Boston: Houghton Mifflin, 1999), 86–95.

119. Nicolle, "Recherches Expérimentales sur le Typhus Exanthématique," *AIPT* 6 (1911): 1–109, 92.

120. Conseil explained the mildness of typhus among the male nomadic population as a result of having "already been vaccinated by a previous attack"; it seems probable that he assumed the same was the case for the females. Conseil, "Le Typhus Exanthématique … 1909" (1910), 41.

121. Conseil, "Typhus … 1910" (1911), 148–49. "A doctor traveling in these places, who attends to the strict application of the prescribed measures and who has with him the materials necessary to carry out those measures will successfully extinguish persistent foyers" of typhus.

122. Conseil, "Résultats de la Prophylaxie du Typhus Exanthématique à Tunis de 1909 à 1912," *Tunisie Médicale* 2 (1912): 401–2. Nicolle (with Georges Blanc and Conseil) would

claim a few years later that typhus in Tunisia had been so rare that they had to rely on cases imported from other countries to renew their laboratory supplies. Nicolle, Blanc, and Conseil, "Nouvelles Recherches Expérimentales sur le Typhus Exanthématique Pratiquées a l'Institut Pasteur de Tunis Pendant l'Année 1914," *AIPT* 9 (1914–16): 84–121, 84.

123. Nicolle, "Recherches Expérimentales sur le Typhus" (1911), 1. The "bishop of Carthage" here appears to be St. Cyprian, who wrote a treatise on the "plague" that struck the city in the third century C.E.

124. Ibid., 1. Later, Nicolle would return to this rhetoric of "birth" and "death" and would extend it to the very existence of disease species. See Chapters 6 and 7.

125. Nicolle, "Nouvelles Acquisitions . . . Typhus" (1911), 4.

126. Ibid., 6.

127. Ibid., 4.

128. Ibid., 9. One may, of course, read this as a classic example of Foucault's "disciplining" of the body. Yet, it seems more fruitful to view it at one remove from such a punitive vision, as an important part of the shifting identity of Charles Nicolle and medicine in Tunisia.

129. Nicolle, "L'Oeuvre de l'Institut Pasteur de Tunis" (1911), 254. Along these lines, Nicolle observed disapprovingly in a letter to Alfred Conor that Remlinger had decided to study rabies in North Africa—something that could be done in "any European laboratory." Nicolle to A. Conor, January 10, 1909, ASM 146 J 37.

130. Nicolle, "L'Oeuvre de l'Institut Pasteur de Tunis" (1911), 261.

131. Nicolle to Alfred Conor, January 26, 1909, ASM 146 J 37.

132. Marthe Conor to Pierre Nicolle, July 18, 1963, ASM 146 J 39.

133. Ibid.

134. After Nicolle devised the revelatory "Door of the Sadiki" narrative, Comte published a number of articles claiming that the louse hypothesis was his, not Nicolle's, and that Nicolle had essentially stolen the credit for the famous discovery. See Chapter 5.

135. Nicolle, "Fonctionnement . . . 1910" (1911), 159. The article, though technically devoted to the IPT's functions in 1910, listed Blaizot's promotion as dating from January 1, 1911. On Blaizot, see "Ludovic Blaizot," *AIPT* 32 (1955): 11–15.

136. See, for example, Roux to Nicolle, August 18, 1909, and September 7, 1909, ASM 146 J 33.

137. Moreover, Nicolle was having trouble with an apparent decrease in the virulence of typhus after continued monkey passage.

138. Guinea pigs were often favored by bacteriological researchers if they could be inoculated with the disease under investigation. Ilana Lowy discusses guinea pig use in her article "From Guinea Pigs to Man."

139. Nicolle, Conseil, and A. Conor, "Le Typhus Expérimentale du Cobaye," *Comptes Rendus de l'Académie des Sciences* 152 (1911-I), 1632.

140. It was in the course of this work that Nicolle noticed that many of the inoculated guinea pigs remained healthy. Eventually, this observation would lead him to construct the concept of "inapparent infection." See Chapter 3.

141. Mendelsohn, "Cultures of Bacteriology"; Moulin, "Patriarchal Science." For a historical perspective on the use of killed vaccines, see Peter Keating, "Vaccine Therapy and the Problem of Opsonins," *JHM* 43 (1988): 275–96. On typhus vaccine work specifically,

see Paul Weindling, " 'Victory with Vaccines': The Problem of Typhus Vaccines During World War II," in *Vaccinia, Vaccination, Vaccinology: Jenner, Pasteur and Their Successors*, eds. S. Plotkin and B. Fantini, 341–47 (Paris: Elsevier, 1996).

142. See Nicolle and Ludovic Blaizot, "Les Vaccins Fluororés dans les Vaccinations Préventives et la Vaccinothérapie," *AIPT* 9 (1914): 1–29. Alfred Conor was ill at the time they wrote this article.

Chapter 3

1. This story was told quite persuasively by Marcel Baltazard nearly three decades after Nicolle's death. Baltazard, director of the Pasteur Institute of Teheran, was at the IPT in the later years of Nicolle's directorship and had worked under Georges Blanc at the IP in Morocco. Baltazard, "Respect des Conditions de la Nature," 36. Baltazard's article would have been more persuasive still if he had actually listed the sources from which he quoted.

2. See Roux to Nicolle, September 9, 1909, ASM 146 J 33, and the discussion following Nicolle and Conseil, "Nos Connaissances sur l'Etiologie du Typhus Exanthématique et de la Fièvre Récurrente: Leur Application à la Prévention de ces Maladies en Particulier dans nos Armées en Campagne," *Revue d'Hygiène* 37 (1915): 172–208, 205–8. Although Nicolle thought that the body louse was the primary culprit in typhus transmission, he believed that head lice might also pass on the disease.

3. Blanc would be appointed *chef de laboratoire* on July 1, 1914; he arrived in Tunisia that May.

4. Nicolle, Georges Blanc, and Conseil, "Nouvelles Recherches . . . Typhus" (1914), 84. In March 1914, Edmond Sergent claimed to have demonstrated that typhus was hereditary in the louse, which, once infected, passed the disease on to its offspring. Sergent, H. Foley, and C. Vialatte, "Transmission à l'Homme et au Singe du Typhus Exanthématique par les Poux d'un Malade Atteint de Fièvre Récurrente et par les Lentes et Poux issus des Précédents," *CRAS* 158 (1914): 964–65.

5. Baltazard, "Respect des Conditions de la Nature," 40. Again, Baltazard gives no source for Nicolle's statement.

6. Nicolle and Conseil, "Nécessité des Mesures" (1914), 290. In this same paragraph, Nicolle observed that the "excreta" has no virulence; however, he was talking about the patient's excreta, not the louse's.

7. Nicolle, Blanc, and Conseil, "Nouvelles Recherches . . . Typhus" (1914–16), 96. Emphasis in original. Also in 1915, Nicolle used the "fact" of typhus transmission by louse feces to criticize Edmond Sergent's experiments "proving" that typhus transmission was hereditary in lice. Nicolle and Conseil, "Connaissances sur l'Etiologie du Typhus" (1915), 184–85.

8. The Nicolle–Sergent dispute(s) live on to this day through the arguments of their respective descendents. We will have some occasion to visit this competitive relationship in this book; however, I develop it more fully in my manuscript "A Louse, Divided."

9. "The climate here at once calms me and energizes me to work, and it has completely vanquished my fatigue and anemia; and I have also found here an organization very favorable to all research." Ludovic Blaizot to Emile Brumpt, February 6, 1910, AIP FR IP

BPT.B1. Brunswic, Blaizot, and, later, Etienne Burnet, all chose to go to Tunis to improve their health, as well as to work.

10. Blaizot to Brumpt, February 6, 1910, ibid.

11. L. Blaizot and E. Gobert, "Deux Epidémies de Fièvre Récurrente en Tunisie: Leur Origine Tripolitaine," *AIPT* 6 (1911): 278–80. Ernest-Gustave Gobert was a colonial doctor with a deep interest in Tunisian history. Briefly director of the IPT's antimalaria services, he was later appointed Director of Hygiene and Public Health.

12. The term *Borrelia* was one of many possibilities being used by researchers in Nicolle's time: *Spirillum* was another popular choice. As a general rule, Nicolle disapproved of the tendency to name microbes after microbiologists; later, he would be particularly annoyed by the choice of *Rickettsia* for the causal agent of typhus and related diseases. For basic information on relapsing fever, Thomas Butler, "Relapsing Fever," in *Hunter's Tropical Medicine and Emerging Infectious Diseases*, 8th ed., ed. G. Thomas Strickland (Philadelphia: W. B. Saunders, 2000), 448–52. A far more detailed, and Pastorian-oriented, account is in Oscar Felsenfeld, *Borrelia: Strains, Vectors, Human and Animal Borreliosis* (St. Louis: Warren H. Green, 1971). Among those to whom Felsenfeld dedicates the volume are Baltazard and Brumpt, with whom he had worked on the disease. Nicolle's influence on the field is evident in Felsenfeld's account.

13. See Chapter 2. It is now known that a multitude of *Borrelia* species convey tick-borne relapsing fever, which also enjoys a number of reservoirs, from rodents and rabbits to lizards and toads. Butler, "Relapsing Fever," in *Hunter's*, 449. Nicolle worked on the tick-borne form of relapsing fever from the mid-1920s and became quite fascinated with both the nature of reservoirs and the question of the evolutionary relations between the two broad disease species. See also Chapter 6.

14. Frederick G. Novy and R. E. Knapp, "Studies on *Spirillum Obermeieri* and Related Organisms," *Journal of Infectious Diseases* 3 (1906): 291–393, esp. 379–86, for a discussion of their position.

15. This is yet another story of the ambiguities often found when one tries to date discoveries. To this day, sources may credit Mackie, Sergent and Foley, or Nicolle; some mention Mackie for epidemiology and *either* Sergent and Foley or Nicolle for laboratory demonstration.

16. See Chapter 1, and Moulin, "Les Instituts Pasteur de la Méditerranée Arabe."

17. Once again, dates given in various sources do not necessarily correlate. The IP of Algeria's Web site, which gives the December 31, 1909 creation date, has Calmette as director from 1910 to 1912, and Sergent as director from 1912 (www.ands.dz/ipa/sommaire.htm); the IPP's Web site, under Sergent's biography, has Sergent directing the institute from 1910 (www.pasteur.fr/infosci/archives/f-bio.html).

18. See Chapter 2.

19. Sergent and Foley, "Recherches sur la Fièvre Récurrente" (1910): 337–73. Their description of the blanket experiment, which must resonate unfavorably with anyone familiar with the history of smallpox in America, is on pages 367–71.

20. Ibid., 372–73. They further suggested that the virulence of relapsing fever was quite variable, especially in experimental conditions.

21. Many of Nicolle's articles drew attention to the experience of IPT researchers with lice. See, for example, Nicolle, Blaizot, and Conseil, "Études sur la Fièvre Récurrente.

I. L'Epidémie Tunisienne de 1912 et la Démonstration Expérimentale de la Transmission de la Fièvre Récurrente par les Poux," *AIPT* 8 (1913): 1–30, 13; Nicolle and Blanc, "Études sur la Fièvre Récurrente, poursuivi à l'Institut Pasteur de Tunis. Deuxième Mémoire (1914)," *AIPT* 9 (1914–16): 69–83, 70.

22. Nicolle, Blaizot, and Conseil, "Études sur la Fièvre Récurrente. I" (1913) [on 1912 work], 12–13.

23. Ibid., 18.

24. Although full details of these experiments appeared in the 1913 *AIPT* article (ibid.), the initial announcements were published in 1912: Nicolle, Blaizot and Conseil, "Etiologie de la Fièvre Récurrente: Son Mode de Transmission par le Pou," *CRAS* 154 (1912-I): 1636–38; Nicolle, Blaizot, and Conseil, "Conditions de Transmission de la Fièvre Récurrente par le Pou," *CRAS* 155 (1912-II): 481–84. See also Huet, "L'Expérimentation Humaine au Temps de Charles Nicolle," *Histoire des Sciences Médicales* 34 (2000): 409–14.

25. Nicolle, "Mon Camarade Habib," unpublished manuscript, ASM 146 J 14, 27–32.

26. Nicolle and Blanc, "Etudes sur la Fièvre Récurrente, Poursuivi à l'Institut Pasteur de Tunis. Deuxième Mémoire (1914)," *AIPT* 9 (1914–16): 69–83, 80.

27. Nicolle, Blaizot, and Conseil, "Conditions . . . Fièvre Récurrente" (1912), 483.

28. For a review of early "granular" relapsing fever studies, see William B. Leishman, "An Experimental Investigation of *Spirochaeta duttoni*, the Parasite of Tick Fever," *Lancet* 2 (1920): 1237–44. The article includes sketches of "Young Spirochaetes observed . . . by Dark-ground Illumination" (1240). Leishman devoted the final section of this lengthy review to "the recent work of Nicolle and his colleagues in Tunis," "in view of its importance" (1243). Leishman published on this subject from 1907.

29. Nicolle, Blaizot, and Conseil, "Conditions . . . Fièvre Récurrente" (1912), 482. Emphasis added.

30. Nicolle, Blaizot and Conseil, "Études sur la Fièvre Récurrente. I" (1913), 25.

31. Nicolle and Charles Lebailly, "L'évolution des Spirochètes de la Fièvre Récurrente Chez le Pou, Telle Qu'on Peut la Suivre sur les Coupes en Série de ces Insectes," *CRAS* 169 (1919-II): 934–36, 936. A cynic, unimpressed by all the ultramicroscopic pathological studies, might point out that Nicolle simply concluded what Sergent and Foley had shown in 1908: that relapsing fever is transmitted by crushed lice. To be fair to Nicolle's standards of demonstration, however, the early Algerian experiments showed only that this was a *potential* path of transmission.

32. Nicolle and Blanc, "Les Spirilles de la Fièvre Récurrente Sont-ils Virulents aux Phases Successives de leur Evolution Chez le Pou? Démonstration de Leur Virulence à un Stade Invisible," *CRAS* 158 (1914): 1815–17.

33. Nicolle and Blanc, "Études sur la Fièvre Récurrente. II" (1914–16), 78. They noted that Sergent and Foley had conducted similar experiments, and come to similar conclusions, independently and at about the same time.

34. The title of the 1914 Nicolle/Blanc article explicitly drew attention to the possibility of microbe evolution in the louse. Nicolle was already thinking about spirochete evolution in 1912–13. See Nicolle, Blaizot, and Conseil, "Études sur la Fièvre Récurrente. I" (1913), 13. Connections with virulence encouraged him to pursue his suspicions.

35. S. B. Wolbach, "Filterable Viruses" (1912), 3, drew attention to protozoa that had "a filterable stage."

36. Nicolle and Blaizot, "Études sur la Fièvre Récurrente: Nouveau Points de l'Etude Expérimentale de la Fièvre Récurrente du Nord de l'Afrique," *AIPT* 7 (1912): 201–12, 212.

37. Nicolle, Blaizot, and Conseil, "Conditions . . . Fièvre Récurrente" (1912), 483.

38. Biology as a discipline was in a state of fairly constant redefinition at the time. See Kevles and Geison, "Experimental Life Sciences in the Twentieth Century."

39. Nicolle to Marthe Conor, February 21, 1908, ASM 146 J 37.

40. Nicolle to Marthe Conor, March 5, 1909, ibid.

41. After citing a letter written by his father describing the Tunis institute's ceremonial opening, in which Nicolle made disparaging comments about some of the speeches, Pierre Nicolle commented in a footnote: "The partially deaf, or, if you prefer, the hard of hearing, often tend to project the reason for their misunderstandings on the speaker whom they have misunderstood." Pierre Nicolle, "Premières Années," 65 n1.

42. Marthe Conor to Pierre Nicolle, July 18, 1963, ASM 146 J 39. "Heurtebise" refers to the essay, "La Chronique de Maître Heurtebise."

43. Huet, *Pommier*, 190.

44. Nicolle's salary was paid by the Tunisian government. In 1913, it was twelve thousand francs per year (ASM 146 J 57, folder "Traitement"). The novel's publication and promotion cost approximately twenty-five hundred francs (Huet, *Pommier*, 190).

45. Nicolle eventually published seven novels: *Le Pâtissier de Bellone* (Calmann-Lévy, 1913); *Les Feuilles de la Sagittaire* (Calmann-Lévy, 1920); *La Narquoise* (Calmann-Lévy, 1922); *Les Menus Plaisirs de l'Ennui* (Calmann-Lévy, 1924); *Marmouse et ses Hôtes* (Reider, 1927); *Les Deux Larrons* (Calmann-Lévy, 1929); and *Les Contes de Marmouse et de ses Hôtes* (Reider, 1930). Numerous unpublished plays and poems remain unstudied in the Nicolle archives in Rouen.

46. Nicolle to Ludovic Blaizot, October 25, 1918, ASM 146 J 36.

47. In a codicil to her will, written days after her husband's untimely death, Marthe Conor noted that the contract, signed by Nicolle, Blaizot, and husband Alfred, was dated September 11, 1913. Upon her death, she wished to divide her share equally between Nicolle and Blaizot. She sent her will with a letter to Nicolle. Marthe Conor to Nicolle, April 9, 1914, ASM 146 J 25.

48. Blaizot to Nicolle, February 18, 1919, ASM 146 J 23.

49. Blaizot to Nicolle, June 13, 1915, ibid.

50. Blaizot to Nicolle, February 27, 1914, ibid.

51. Liebenau and Robson, "L'Institut Pasteur," 57.

52. See Moulin, "La Métaphore Vaccine," for the Pastorian tendency to group both preventive and curative products under the broad heading "vaccine."

53. If medical research facilities could not profit from the development of new pharmaceutical products, there was little incentive to invest much money in such development. Evidence for the efficacy of the positive profit incentive abounds in the present day, when many drug companies jealously guard their patents and go to great lengths to extend extant ones.

54. Terry Shinn, "The Genesis of French Industrial Research, 1880–1940," *Social Science Information* 19 (1980): 607–40. The Serum Commission reported in the *Bulletin de l'Académie de Médecine* (see, for example, 55 [1906]: 165).

55. Liebenau and Robson, "L'Institut Pasteur," 54.

56. Ibid., 57–59; Moulin and Guénel, "L'Institut Pasteur et la Naissance de l'Industrie." Directed by Ernest Fourneau, Poulenc's laboratory developed a nonaddictive cocaine substitute, Stovaine. Fourneau's success drew Roux's attention, and he hired Fourneau in 1911 to create a chemotherapy department at the Pasteur Institute. Fourneau's move to the Pasteur Institute did not, however, symbolize a new Pastorian commitment to industrial alliance: it was predicated upon Fourneau's resignation from Poulenc. Although he encouraged Fourneau to maintain his contacts with the Poulenc staff, Roux did not, apparently, ever sign a formal contract with Poulenc for vaccine manufacture.

57. Shinn, "Genesis of French Industrial Research," 627. Shinn continues, "albeit a badly organized and incomplete one."

58. Among these, see Gwendolyn Wright, *The Politics of Design in French Colonial Urbanism* (Chicago: University of Chicago Press, 1991); Rabinow, *French Modern*.

59. Nicolle's 1910s correspondence with long-time friend Leredde, who was based in Paris and provided Nicolle with a running commentary on Roux's policies, is particularly illuminating. It is contained in the AIP FR IP NIC.3.

60. Marthe Conor to Pierre Nicolle, July 18, 1963, ASM 146 J 39.

61. Marthe Conor was born in 1883, Conseil in 1879, Blaizot in 1882, Georges Blanc and Georges Duhamel in 1884, Pasteur Vallery-Radot in 1886, and Hélène Sparrow in 1891.

62. We have already witnessed other positive advantages Nicolle enjoyed from his colonial isolation. See Chapters 1 and 2.

63. Avice Nicolle to Marcel Nicolle, August 8, 1911, ASM 146 J 36.

64. Avice Nicolle to Marcel Nicolle, September 10, 1911, ibid.

65. Avice Nicolle to Marcel Nicolle, September 22, 1911; Avice Nicolle to Maurice Nicolle, October 1, 1911, ibid.

66. Avice Nicolle to Marcel Nicolle, March 2, 1912, ibid.

67. See, for example, Avice Nicolle to Marcel Nicolle, September 5, 1912, ibid.

68. Avice Nicolle to Nicolle, May 2–6, 1914, ibid.

69. Maurice Nicolle to Marcelle Nicolle, November 28, 1914, ASM 146 J 37. Marcelle, who did become a doctor and eventually returned to live, work, and tend to her father in Tunis, politely declined her uncle's offer, as it would have upset her father.

70. Avice Nicolle to Marcel Nicolle, April 9, 1921, ASM 146 J 36.

71. Nicolle's children, however, continued to have close ties with their father, particularly later in life.

72. Huet, *Pommier*, 99–103. Shortly before he died, Conor, who, in addition to being assistant director of the IPT, was also director of the military bacteriology laboratory in Tunisia, was awarded the Legion of Honor.

73. Nicolle and Marthe Conor, "La Toxoplasmose du Gondi: Maladie Naturelle; Maladie Expérimental," *BSPE* 6 (1913): 160; "Difficulté de Conservation du Virus de la Leishmaniose Canine par les Passages," *BSPE* 7 (1914): 481.

74. Marthe Conor to Pierre Nicolle, 1961–63, ASM 146 J 39.

75. Nicolle, "Fonctionnement . . . 1913" (1914–16), 189. There seems to be some confusion as to whether Blanc arrived in 1913 or 1914, correspondence places his arrival in Tunis in May 1914.

76. Etienne Burnet was named *sous-directeur* of the IPT on December 31, 1920.

77. Nicolle to Pasteur Vallery-Radot, January 3, 1920, ASM 146 J 39.

78. Blaizot to Nicolle, July 19, 1914, ASM 146 J 23. Blaizot was delighted by Nicolle's "gaiety" and "good humor."

79. Nicolle, "Fonctionnement . . . 1914" (1914–16).

80. Ibid., 189. Conseil was assigned to the Tunis military hospital; Gobert, to the Eighth Regiment in Sousse. The *AIPT* reports on Conseil's assignment to Serbia in the "Fonctionnement . . . 1915" (1914–16), 201.

81. Fussell, *Great War and Modern Memory*, 48–49, 189.

82. Isaac Rosenberg, "The Immortals," in *Poems of the First World War: 'Never Such Innocence,'* ed. Martin Stephen (London: Everyman, 1988; 1993), 110–11. Rosenberg also wrote a poem called "Louse Hunting."

83. Nicolle and Conseil, "Nécessité des Mesures à Prendre pour Préserver nos Armées en Campagne des Typhus Exanthématique et Récurrente," *Presse Médicale* 23 (1915): 18–19. (Typhus fever and relapsing fever are the "two typhuses" to which Nicolle referred in this section's opening quotation—not, as today's readers might well expect, classic and murine typhus: these two diseases had yet to be differentiated from each other. Technically, of course, relapsing fever is not typhus); and, under the same title, in *Tunisie Médicale* 4 (1914): 290–92; also in the *Bulletin de l'Académie de Médecine* (1915), 37. The longer paper is Nicolle and Conseil, "Connaissances sur l'Etiologie du Typhus" (1915), which includes a transcript of the discussion that followed its presentation.

84. Nicolle and Conseil, "Connaissances sur l'Etiologie du Typhus" (1915), 172. It was later in this paper that Nicolle would give chronologies and credits for various discoveries. This point would become central to Nicolle and Sergent's tumultuous relationship. See Chapter 4, and my paper "A Louse, Divided."

85. Nicolle and Conseil, "Connaissances sur l'Etiologie du Typhus" (1915), 172.

86. Ibid., 201–3.

87. Nicolle and Conseil, "Nécessite des Mesures" (1915), 19. Weindling, " 'Victory with Vaccines,' " section "War on the Louse."Tunisia supplied eighty thousand troops to the French Army; twenty thousand died. Perkins, *History of Modern Tunisia*, 74–75.

88. For details on the conditions of Serbia and the force of the epidemic, see Richard P. Strong et al., *Typhus Fever with Particular Reference to the Serbian Epidemic* (Cambridge, MA: The American Red Cross at the Harvard University Press, 1920). For typhus immediately after the war, see Gaines M. Foster, "Typhus Disaster in the Wake of War: The American-Polish Relief Expedition, 1919–1920," *BHM* 55 (1981): 221–32.

89. Strong et al., *Typhus Fever*, 3. Strong argued that typhus was brought in by the Austro-Hungarian Army (19) and that the Serbian Army's official statistics listed typhus deaths in 1915 as numbering 171,725 (93). He noted that 126 of Serbia's 350 doctors contracted typhus.

90. Strong gave details of the project in *Typhus Fever*; documents concerning its foundation may be found at the Rockefeller Archives. On the Rockefeller and hookworm, see John Ettling, *The Germ of Laziness: Rockefeller Philanthropy and Public Health in the New South* (Cambridge, MA: Harvard University Press, 1981).

91. Strong et al., *Typhus Fever*, 88.

92. Blanc to Nicolle, February 27, 1915, ASM 146 J 24.

93. Nicolle, "Fonctionnement . . . 1915" (1914–16), 200. See also Nicolle's wartime correspondence with both Blanc and Conseil: ASM 146 J 24, 25.

94. Conseil to Nicolle, April 7, 1915, ASM 146 J 25. As an indication of the doubts surrounding the louse transmission of typhus, see A. W. Sellards, "Laboratory Examinations in Typhus Fever," in Strong et al., *Typhus Fever* (1920), 243–60. Sellards, then assistant professor of tropical medicine at the Harvard University Medical School, argued in his report of December 1915 that "the evidence regarding the louse transmission is in a somewhat confused condition." Pointing out that even those who agreed about louse transmission—namely, "Nicolle and his associates, Ricketts and Wilder, and Anderson and Goldberger," all having concluded "that typhus is transmissible to the monkey by the body louse," worked on "fundamental premises" that "vary widely and even conflict seriously" (256). Further, Sellards worked on the hypothesis that "the establishment of the louse transmission does not militate against the possibility of the disease being transmitted by other methods also" (258).

95. Conseil to Nicolle, April 22, 1915, ASM 146 J 25. The idea that the effluvia released by cadavers could produce infectious disease is a classic statement of the once-popular "miasmatic theory." Weindling, *Epidemics and Genocide*.

96. Nicolle, "Fonctionnement . . . 1915," *AIPT* 9 (1914–16): 200–208, 200.

97. Blaizot to Nicolle, March 17, 1915, ASM 146 J 23.

98. R. P. Strong papers (GA 82), HML/CLM, box 36b, folder "Letters and Telegrams," which includes Nicolle's note accepting the terms of his contract, was dated April 2, 1915, and the letter from Strong to Nicolle, April 12, 1915.

99. "The Relief of Suffering Non-Combatants in Europe: Destitution and Disease in Serbia," April 28, 1915, 24; folder 590, box 60, series 100, RG 1, Rockefeller Foundation Archives, RAC. This pamphlet was to be released to newspapers for publication on April 29.

100. Conseil to Nicolle, May 14, 1915, ASM 146 J 25.

101. Nicolle mentioned that he had corresponded regularly with Blanc's mother, for example, in Nicolle to Blanc, September 27, 1914, ASM 146 J 37.

102. The replacements were Charles Lebailly, Edward Chatton, and Louis Caillon. Nicolle, "Rôle de l'Institut Pasteur de Tunis Pendant la Guerre 1914–1918," *Notice sur l'Institut Pasteur de Tunis* (Tunis: J. Parlier, 1924).

103. The institute, at the time of mobilization, suspended production only of the antigonnorrhea vaccine; it reestablished this production in April 1915. "Fonctionnement . . . 1914" (1914–16), 196; "Fonctionnement . . . 1915" (1914–16), 206.

104. "*Conseiller technique de l'armée d'Afrique*." Nicolle, "Fonctionnement . . . 1917" (1917–18), 182.

105. "Fonctionnement . . . 1916" (1917–18), 108.

106. Chatton's description of his laboratory appears in the *AIPT*: "Le Laboratoire Militaire de Bactériologie du Sud-Tunisien (à Gabès): Organisation Rendement du 1er Août 1916 au 1er Juillet 1918," *AIPT* 10 (1917–18): 199–242. Chatton's story may be worth uncovering. A *chef de laboratoire* at the Pasteur Institute of Paris, he was a student of Mesnil's and appears to have been sent to Tunisia by Roux; Nicolle wanted his assistance as well. There was some controversy over his proper station during war. See the correspondence between Nicolle and Roux (ASM), Nicolle and Blanc (ASM), and Nicolle and Mesnil (AIP).

107. René Potel, "Observations Cliniques et Etiologiques sur les Cas de Typhus Soignés à l'Hôpital Permanent de la Marine de Sidi-Abdallah: Action du Sérum Exanthématique," *AIPT* 9 (1914–16): 245–85, 245.

108. In the opening of this series of articles on typhus in Tunisia during 1916, Nicolle mentioned that the laboratory samples being used at the IPT, which had been maintained since May 1914, were "designated by the names 'Algerian Virus' or 'Virus I' and 'Moroccan Virus' or 'Virus II'." Nicolle, "Nouvelles Etudes sur le Typhus Exanthématique pratiquées à l'Institut Pasteur de Tunis et dans les Formations Sanitaires de la Régence (1916)," *AIPT* 9 (1914–16): 215–44, 215.

109. I have glossed over a strong challenge that arose to Ricketts's proposed agent during the war, launched by Henry Plotz (a student of Nathan Brill) and his colleagues at Mount Sinai Hospital in New York. Harry Plotz, Peter K. Olitsky, and George Baehr, "The Etiology of Typhus Exanthematicus," *Journal of Infectious Disease* 17 (1915), 1–68.

110. "It does seem that the virus is attenuated by passage in the Chinese monkeys." Roux to Nicolle, September 7, 1909, ASM 146 J 33.

111. Potel, "Observations Cliniques et Etiologiques" (1914–16), 245–46.

112. Nicolle, "Nouvelles Acquisitions . . . Typhus" (1911), 4.

113. Roux enthusiastically—and frequently—encouraged Nicolle to explore these properties. See Roux to Nicolle, May 26, 1909; June 30, 1930; August 18, 1909; September 7, 1909, ASM 146 J 33.

114. Nicolle, with Blaizot, Potel, and Henri Poirson, reviewed the whole of the 1916 Serbian typhus project in the *AIPT* 9 (1914–16): 215–90. On preventive and curative vaccine work, see in particular Nicolle and Blaizot's section, "Sur la Préparation d'un Sérum Antiexanthématique Expérimental et Ses Premiers Applications au Typhus de l'Homme," 225–33. They also tested "anti-exanthematic serotherapy" on several patients. Nicolle was encouraged by the results (232). See also Nicolle's section, "Essai de Vaccination Préventive dans le Typhus Exanthématique," 241–44. Nicolle's most famous convalescent serum work concerned his measles preparation. See Nicolle and Conseil, "Pouvoir Préventif du Sérum d'un Malade Convalescent de Rougeole," *Bulletin et Mémoire de la Société Médicale de Paris* 4 (1917): 336–38.

115. Nicolle, "Identité des Virus Exanthématique Africain et Balkanique," *AIPT* 9 (1914–16): 217–24, 224. This article was part of the larger overview of typhus work at the IPT in 1916. Nicolle would return to these questions of microbial species and their interrelations with extensive work on relapsing fever from the latter half of the 1920s and on typhus from around 1930. See Chapter 6.

116. Potel, "Observations Cliniques et Etiologiques" (1914–16), 246.

117. Nicolle, "Quelques Faits ou Observations d'ordre Expérimental Relatifs au Typhus Exanthématique en Particulier à l'Entretien du Virus par Passage," *AIPT* 9 (1914–16): 235–40, 235.

118. Ibid., 235. Nicolle to Blanc, undated note (between April 11 and May 15, 1916), ASM 146 J 36.

119. J. Henry Dible, *Recent Advances in Bacteriology* (1932), 256–83, 268.

120. Nicolle and C. Lebailly, "L'Evolution des Spirochètes" (1919); Nicolle and Lebailly, "Quelques Notions Expérimentales sur le Virus de la Grippe," *CRAS* 167 (1918-II): 607–10; Nicolle and Lebailly, "Recherches Expérimentales sur la Grippe," *AIP* 33 (1919): 395; Nicolle and Lebailly, "Les Infections Expérimentales Inapparentes: Exemples Tirés de l'Etude du Typhus Exanthématique," *CRAS* 168 (1919-I): 800–1. On Nicolle's

influenza research, J. Vieuchange, "Les Recherches de Charles Nicolle sur l'Etiologie de la Grippe," *AIPT* 43 (1966): 481–90.

121. Delattre, a priest in Cardinal Lavigerie's Tunisian mission, dedicated himself to recovering evidence of Tunisia's glorious Carthaginian past as part of his order's broader mission to convert Muslims in North Africa to Christianity (and, presumably, to reclaim the country's ancient glory in the process). J. Dean O'Donnell, Jr., *Lavigerie in Tunisia: The Interplay of Imperialist and Missionary* (Athens: University of Georgia Press, 1979). Delattre even contributed a medical history paper to Nicolle's journal, following a plague threat in Tunisia: A. L. Delattre, "Documents pour Servir à l'Histoire de la Pathologie Infectieuse de l'Afrique Mineure: La Peste à Carthage en 253," *AIPT* 3 (1908): 133–38. Other contributions to regional medical history were to follow other epidemics and infestations, including the history of grasshopper infestations by Marthe Conor.

122. Elie Metchnikoff, *The Nature of Man: Studies in Optimistic Philosophy*, ed. and trans. P. Chalmers Mitchell (New York: Putnam, 1903), 302. Mitchell's translation appeared the same year as the French original, *Etudes sur la Nature Humaine: Essai de Philosophie Optimiste*.

123. Olga Metchnikoff, *Life of Elie Metchnikoff, 1845–1916* (Boston: Houghton Mifflin, 1921), 245.

124. There was, in fact, a reaction against such naïve faith in science that had taken root before the war; however, it was not a view commonly seen among the Pastorians.

125. Prof. Berdnikoff, of Petrograd, was sent to the IPT in 1916 by the Russian military, on a mission to learn about Nicolle's methods of treatment and control. Nicolle, "Fonctionnement . . . 1916" (1917–18). Others would follow later. Further exchanges of material and personnel were particularly active with Poland.

126. This story was part of a collection published only after the war, as *Les Feuilles de la Sagittaire*. There is some speculation that an earlier version appeared in 1914, but Huet could find no confirmation of this (Huet, *Pommier*, 192–93). My claim that this particular story was finished in 1915, and not in 1914, as it is dated in the 1920 publication, comes from the original manuscript. Held in Rouen, the manuscript of the short story, as well as the introductory piece used to open his book and the first chapter of my own, are clearly dated "1915"—in Nicolle's hand.

127. Indeed, Nicolle would later become fond of presenting Duhamel's interpretation as evidence of the interrelations of science and imagination. Though reviews of Nicolle's literary skills tend toward the critical, his language is often quite beautiful and his images, particularly in this story, are haunting and evocative.

128. Moulin cites Fabiani's interpretation (G. Fabiani, "Genèse et Signification du Concept d'Infection Inapparente dans L'œuvre de Charles Nicolle," *La Semaine des Hôpitaux* 48 [1946]: 2879–88, 2884) in her "Charles Nicolle, Savant Tunisien," 360, n36.

129. The dedication appears on a separate title page immediately preceding the story; the title appears again, with the fictional author's name, with the story itself. Nicolle, "Comme un Souvenir Qui ne Vieillit Point," in *Feuilles de la Sagittaire*, 199–236, 199, 201.

130. "Souvenir," 201–2.

131. Ibid., 209. Here, Nicolle used the French verb *vieillir*.

132. Ibid., 203. Soon, he would even extend his scientific observations through study of an optics textbook, to rule out all logical explanations.

133. Ibid., 203–5.

134. Ibid., 214.

135. Ibid., 216.
136. Ibid., 217.
137. Ibid., 219–20.
138. Ibid., 220.
139. Ibid., 223.
140. Ibid., 225.
141. Ibid.
142. Ibid., 226.
143. Ibid., 228.
144. Ibid., 229.
145. Ibid., 230.
146. Ibid., 231.
147. Ibid., 232.
148. Ibid., 233. He indeed repeats the phrase "perpetual present."
149. Ibid. Nicolle even included a darkly humorous aside here. When Lucie left, she asked him to watch her cats and her parrot. He already had dogs. In his shadowy rapture, he neglected the pets: "it seems that my dogs did not get along with Lucie's cats, and that they would have devoured each other if they had not banded together against the parrot, eating it instead. What will its mistress say?" (233). More seriously, the shadow tells him of the lives of other shadows and our narrator notes that some, "like Sisyphus, push their ridiculous rock, which ceaselessly falls again" (233). Camus had only just been born, but he and Nicolle shared more than their multilayered love of the sea.
150. Ibid., 234.
151. Ibid.
152. Ibid., 235.
153. Ibid.
154. Ibid., 235–36.
155. Huet points out that each short story in the *Feuilles* collection is dedicated to a woman, and suggest that all those women were, in fact, some aspect of Marthe Conor. Huet, *Pommier*, 193–94.
156. Marthe Conor to Pierre Nicolle, June 1, 1962, ASM 146 J 39. Marthe Conor was one of the most vibrant and fascinating of all Nicolle's interesting friends and collaborators. Several years ago, I attempted to track down more of her history. A third marriage later in the 1920s left little trace—except for the bittersweet letters she wrote to Pierre much later.
157. Many historians have argued that all evidence is merely "text," to be "read" like any other piece of literature. The challenge of integrating a scientist's literary efforts into a "scientific" biography reveals just how difficult it is to apply such historiography to the doing of history.
158. Fyodor Dostoevsky, "Dream of a Ridiculous Man," trans. Constance Garnett. The text may be found online at a number of Web sites. See, for instance, on "The European Prospect," www.ellopos.net/politics/eu_dostoyiefsky.html. On the original publication, see Joseph Frank, *Dostoevsky: The Mantle of the Prophet, 1871–1881* (Princeton: Princeton University Press, 2002), 318, 351–58. I would like to thank Catherine LeGouis, who kindly supplied me with information about the French translation of Dostoevsky's "Dream." Catherine LeGouis, e-mail message to the author, July 26, 2004.
159. Marthe Conor to Pierre Nicolle, July 18, 1963, ASM 146 J 39.

160. See Chapter 8.

161. In Doestoevsky's "Dream," the suicide is apparent rather than real, and is "committed" by the writer himself. Still, it is this act that brings him into the mysterious other world. Frank comments on the relations between Dostoevsky's utopia and the French socialist utopias of the 1840s. Frank, *Dostoevsky*, 356–57.

162. Dostoevsky, "Dream," IV. I am using section headings for the quotation references.

163. Ibid., V.

164. Ibid.

165. There is another element of inapparent infections that seems prefigured in "Souvenir." Later, when Nicolle began to apply the concept of inapparent infection to his explanation of the rise and fall, not just of epidemics, but of disease species as well, he described a process of gradual adaptation of disease and host that, over time, became less violent and more harmonious until, eventually, pathogen became saprophyte.

166. As with his other significant typhus discoveries (animal inoculation and louse transmission), Nicolle reported first to the Académie des Sciences, then expanded the concept in the *AIPT* (Nicolle and Lebailly, "Infections Expérimentales Inapparentes," also in *AIPT* 11 [1919–20]: 1–5). I will be quoting from the *AIPT* article, unless otherwise noted.

167. Nicolle and Lebailly, "Infections Expérimentales Inapparentes" (1919–20), 2–3.

168. Ibid., 3–4. On "inapparent infection," Fabiani, "Genèse et Signification du Concept d'Infection Inapparente"; idem., "L'Intérêt Toujours Actuel des Infections Inapparentes," *Annales d'Hygiène de Langue Française* 3 (1967): 58–67; idem., "Un Problème de Pathologie Générale: La Définition de l'Infection Inapparente," *Revue de Pathologie Comparée et de Médecine Expérimentale* 68 (1968): 217–22; P. Giroud and J. B. Jadin, "Les Maladies Inapparentes de Charles Nicolle, les Affections Superposées sont à la Base des Faillites de l'Immunité," *AIPT* 63 (1986): 97–99; P. C. C. Garnham, "Charles Nicolle and Inapparent Infections," *American Journal of Tropical Medicine and Hygiene* 26 (1977): 1101–1104.

169. On latent infections, see Judith Walzer Leavitt, *Typhoid Mary: Captive to the Public's Health* (Boston: Beacon Press, 1996), and Andrew Mendelsohn, " 'Typhoid Mary' Strikes Again: The Social and the Scientific in the Making of Modern Public Health," *Isis* 86 (1995): 268–77. See Chapter 5.

170. Nicolle and Lebailly, "Infections Expérimentales Inapparentes" (1919–20), 5. Emphasis added.

171. Nicolle, "L'Etat de Nos Connaissances Expérimentales sur le Typhus Exanthématique," *BIP* 18 (1920): 1–12, 49–60, 57.

172. Ibid., 1. Nicolle used *oeuvre*, but, I think, meant it in its broader sense of "achievement" rather than its narrower one, "work."

173. Nicolle, "Fonctionnement . . . 1918" (1919–20), 58. See also "Fonctionnement . . . 1917" (1917–18), 182, where Nicolle describes the two months following Blaizot and Bance's departure, when he was left to direct the institute alone.

174. Moulin, "Pasteur Institute and the Logic of Non-Profit," 10.

175. Nicolle to Blanc, July 6, 1919, ASM 146 J 36. A reverent sketch of Roux dressed in swaddling clothes and sporting a halo (included in Lagrange's biography) takes on a different meaning in the light of Nicolle's descriptions.

176. Timothy Lenoir, "A Magic Bullet: Research for Profit and the Growth of Knowledge in Germany around 1900," *Minerva* 26 (1988): 66–88.

177. For Calmette's public response to the occupation, see Albert Calmette et al., "Protestation des Savants de Lille contre les Actes de Barbarie des Allemands," *Presse Médicale* 26 (1918): 557–58.

178. Blaizot to Nicolle, November 20, 1918, ASM 146 J 23.

Chapter 4

1. René Vallery-Radot, "Pourquoi le Monde Entier Glorifie Pasteur," *Dépêche Tunisienne,* December 24, 1922. René Vallery-Radot was well prepared for the task, having written his famous biography of Pasteur earlier.

2. Ibid. On the exhibit, see "Le Centenaire de Pasteur: Une Exposition Pastorienne au Palais des Sociétés Françaises," *Dépêche Tunisienne,* December 26, 1922.

3. Pierre Nicolle both outlined the friendship and summarized the concerns of his father and Vallery-Radot on the occasion of Nicolle's manuscripts being given to the Rouen Library in 1970. (Nicolle's personal papers were presented to the Rouen archives some years later.) The text of his speech, "Charles Nicolle et Louis Pasteur Vallery-Radot, d'après leur Correspondance," was printed in the *Académie des Sciences, Belles-Lettres et Arts de Rouen* 47 (1971): 9–14 and was reprinted as an independent text by the *Bulletin de Liaison*. All references to "Vallery-Radot" are to son Louis Pasteur. All references to the father will add "René."

4. Nicolle, "Le Sillon de Pasteur," *Dépêche Tunisienne,* December 27, 1922.

5. On festivals and other rituals, see Catherine Bell, *Ritual: Perspectives and Dimensions* (New York: Oxford University Press, 1997), esp. 104–8; 120–28.

6. Nicolle and Conseil, "Nécessité des Mesures à Prendre" (1915), 18. See Chapter 3.

7. To an extent, I am taking Nicolle's word for this, as I have not been able to find the "circular" that Sergent apparently distributed to French doctors in North Africa (Nicolle to Vallery-Radot, July 2, 1923, AIP FR IP NCP.12). Subsequent developments suggest that Nicolle's account was accurate.

8. George H. F. Nuttall, "The Part Played by *Pediculus humanus* in the Causation of Disease," *Parasitology* 10 (1917): 43–79: 44 ("the investigation of this disease [relapsing fever] by Sergent preceded and stimulated similar researches into the etiology of typhus by Nicolle and his collaborators"). Nuttall, at the Quick Laboratory at Cambridge, was editor of the journal *Parasitology*. He also included an extensive bibliography, published separately in the same volume: idem., "Bibliography of Pediculus and Phthirus, Including Zoological and Medical Publications Dealing with Human Lice, Their Anatomy, Biology, Relation to Disease, etc., and Prophylactic Measures Directed Against Them," *Parasitology* 10 (1917): 1–42.

9. Louis Pasteur, *Œuvres de Pasteur*, ed. Louis Pasteur Vallery-Radot, 7 vols. (Paris: Masson et Cie, 1922–39). Vallery-Radot was also interested in the arts, and counted among his close friends Claude Debussy and Paul Valéry. On Vallery-Radot, www.pasteur.fr/infosci/archives/f-bio.html

10. This was Laurent Victor Louis Emile Leredde (1866–1926). See the Leredde/Nicolle correspondence: AIP FR IP NIC.3. Leredde and Nicolle were friends from Nicolle's student days and shared an interest in syphilis research and treatment. Leredde

would go on to specialize in the subject. On Leredde's medical reform work, see Weisz, "Reform and Conflict," in Fox and Weisz, *Organization of Science and Technology*, 90.

11. Brumpt himself visited the IPT in 1920. "Fonctionnement . . . 1919" (1920), 247–48.

12. Mesnil authored a detailed obituary of Nicolle. Born two years after Nicolle, he died two years after him. See Chapter 1. Obituaries of Mesnil may be found in *Annales de l'Institut Pasteur* 60 (1938): 221–26; *Bulletin de l'Académie de Médecine* 119 (1938): 241–47; *Presse Médicale* 21 (1938): 401–2. Hints of Mesnil's difficulties with collaborator Laveran appear in correspondence with Nicolle between 1904 and 1910.

13. Mesnil to Nicolle, February 11, 1919; March 19, 1919, AIP FR IP NCP.11. Moulin has argued that it was "logical to associate the institutes of Algiers, Tangiers, Casablanca, and Tunis, with those of Constantinople (1888), Alexandria (1927), Jerusalem (1913), and Athens (1921), even if all but Athens of these latter institutes disappeared after WWII." Moulin, "Instituts Pasteur de la Méditerranée Arabe," 136.

14. Moulin, "The Pasteur Institutes Between the Two World Wars: The Transformation of the International Sanitary Order," in *International Health Organizations and Movements, 1918–1939,* ed. Paul Weindling, 244–65 (Cambridge: Cambridge University Press, 1995). The French doctor in Greece was Arnaud; the wealthy sponsor, Basil Zaharoff. See also Mesnil to Nicolle, December 8, 1918, AIP FR IP NCP.11.

15. Mesnil to Nicolle, February 11, 1919, AIP FR IP NCP.11. Mesnil told Nicolle that Roux had decided that Mathis was better suited for Constantinople than Athens.

16. Mesnil to Nicolle, March 19, 1919, ibid.

17. Mesnil to Nicolle, March 22, 1919, ibid. Mesnil added parenthetically that Roux's reasoning might apply to the first year as director, but was hardly the case thereafter.

18. Calmette to Nicolle, March 24, 1919, AIP FR IP NCP.11. Emphasis in original. Metchnikoff's laboratory, Calmette noted, had gone to Besredka—which is unsurprising, given the delay between Metchnikoff's death (1916) and Calmette's arrival in Paris (1919). On Calmette, Noel Bernard, *La Vie et l'Oeuvre d'Albert Calmette* (Paris: La Colombe, 1961).

19. Calmette to Nicolle, May 31, 1919, AIP FR IP NCP.11.

20. Nicolle to Blanc, November 14, 1918, ASM 146 J 36.

21. Calmette made this prediction to Nicolle: Calmette to Nicolle, December 24, 1919, AIP FR IP NCP.11. See this letter also for Calmette's critique of Abt.

22. Calmette to Nicolle, ibid. It was clear in the October 21, 1919, letter that Blanc would be offered the position.

23. Abt asked to leave Greece in the fall of 1921, and Blanc was given his position (Calmette to Nicolle, October 30, 1921, ibid.).

24. Nicolle to Blanc, December 9, 1921, ASM 146 J 36. Note the possessive tone of Nicolle's rhetoric—a tone that, except for the formal "*vous*," was more appropriate for a father to use with a favored son than for a researcher to use with a colleague.

25. Nicolle to Blanc, April 18, 1926, ASM 146 J 36.

26. Calmette to Nicolle, October 21, 1919, AIP FR IP NCP.11.

27. Nicolle to Vallery-Radot, January 3, 1920, AIP FR IP NCP.12.

28. Calmette to Nicolle, October 21, 1919, AIP FR IP NCP.11.

29. Charles Lebailly to Nicolle, March 18, 1919, ASM 146 J 30.

30. Lebailly to Nicolle, December 20, 1919, ibid. Thereafter, Nicolle frequently visited Lebailly during his summer vacations—returning, in a sense, to his childhood summers on the sea. Nicolle, "Mémoires," 88.

31. Nicolle to Vallery-Radot, January 3, 1920, AIP FR IP NCP.12.

32. "Fontionnenent [sic] . . . 1920," *AIPAN* 1 (1921): 201–13, 202. Nicolle and Sergent agreed to an annual alternation of responsibility for compiling the journal; Sergent was to fill that role first. Whether or not the typographical error in the title was Sergent's final responsibility, Nicolle rarely made any such mistakes while editing his journal.

33. Ibid., 201. See also Nicolle, *Notice* (1924): 3.

34. "Fontionnenent [sic] . . . 1920" (1921).

35. Nicolle to Blanc, January 6, 1921, ASM 146 J 36.

36. Nicolle to Mesnil, January 9, 1921, AIP FR IP NIC.11.

37. Nicolle to Vallery-Radot, February 2, 1925, AIP FR IP NCP.12. In this quotation, Nicolle was referring to Albert Calmette. Additionally, Nicolle had earlier assured Blanc that the merger with hygiene was in no way causing him to neglect original research. Nicolle to Blanc, March 11, 1922, ASM 146 J 36.

38. "Fonctionnement du Laboratoire Régional de Sousse (année 1922)," *AIPT* 12 (1923): 254–59.

39. A. Espie, "Fonctionnement du Laboratoire Régional de Sfax (année 1925)," *AIPT* 15 (1926): 194–96.

40. "Fonctionnement . . . 1927" (1928), 168.

41. A listing of IP d'Algérie staff appeared in *AIPT* 11 (1919–1920), 79.

42. Nicolle announced the project as decided in a letter of December 13, 1920.

43. Burnet to Nicolle, July 20, 1920, AIP FR IP NIC.3. Burnet made this proclamation upon hearing that Nicolle was being consulted about the colonial school of bacteriology in Marseille. The letter implies that Nicolle was being considered to head up the laboratory. Clearly, by 1920, Nicolle had positioned himself so that he was naturally consulted about alterations in any bacteriological institution around the Mediterranean.

44. Nicolle to Mesnil, May 10, 1921, AIP FR IP NCP.11. Emphasis added.

45. Mesnil to Nicolle, December 20, 1921, ibid.

46. Nicolle to Vallery-Radot, February 14, 1921, AIP FR IP NCP.12.

47. Nicolle to Vallery-Radot, January 3, 1920, ibid.

48. Nicolle to Vallery-Radot, January 27, 1920; Vallery-Radot to Nicolle, February 15, 1920, ibid.

49. Nicolle to Vallery-Radot, August 5, 1920, ibid.

50. Nicolle to Vallery-Radot, ibid.

51. "Conseil is well, but his patients have rendered him nearly invisible." Nicolle to Blanc, March 11, 1922, ASM 146 J 36.

52. Blaizot to Nicolle, September 30, 1921, ASM 146 J 23. It is probable that Blaizot's clinical aspirations were being driven by wholly different forces than were Conseil's. Blaizot, who had pressed for profits and gleefully anticipated their arrival with the Poulenc scheme, was eager to find new sources of revenue. Conseil, on the other hand, frequently treated poor Tunisian patients. Moreover, Conseil was not specifically a researcher at the IPT, but the city's Director of Hygiene. Blaizot, as a researcher, was

expected to devote himself to the laboratory. Despite Blaizot's departure, however, he and Nicolle did later visit with each other. Correspondence to Nicolle from other Pastorians *suggests* that he and Blaizot quickly set aside their personal animosity and simply decided it was best to work separately.

53. Nicolle to Vallery-Radot, September 18, 1918, attached manuscript, "The Peril of Microbiological Studies in France," AIP FR IP NCP.12. In the copy of his book *Responsabilités, I,* that Nicolle inscribed to Emile Brumpt, there was only one added mark, presumably Brumpt's. Next to Nicolle's statement, "my conscience obliges me to conclude, once more, that the soul [*esprit*] of the educator is in opposition to the soul of the researcher" (28), was a large "?."

54. Nicolle to Vallery-Radot, September 6, 1920, AIP FR IP NCP.12. Despite his admitted fascination with the plan for industrial alliance, Nicolle confessed that he himself had "no skills for setting this plan in motion. No taste for it, either."

55. Moulin, "Bacteriological Research and Medical Practice."

56. Nicolle, text of "Peril," in Nicolle to Vallery-Radot September 18, 1920, AIP FR IP NCP.12; also in *Le Temps*, October 8, 1920, 1.

57. Roux to Nicolle, October 18, 1920, ASM 146 J 33.

58. Ibid. Nicolle was himself to adopt a position similar to Roux's in the 1930s; Nicolle, however, substituted the corrupting influence of money with the distracting influence of women.

59. Calmette even warned Nicolle that his campaign in the press "highly displeased the Patron." Calmette to Nicolle, March 14, 1921, AIP FR IP NCP.11.

60. Calmette's involvement with the Association was substantive enough that Mesnil later attributed its existence to him. See Mesnil to Nicolle, September 29, 1923, AIP FR IP NCP.11.

61. Association pour l'Extension des études Pastoriennes (Paris: R. Tancrède, 1921).

62. Ibid., 22.

63. Ibid., "Extraits des Statuts," 25. The rhetoric suggests that Nicolle had a hand in writing this.

64. Vallery-Radot to Nicolle, February 7, 1921, AIP FR IP NCP.12.

65. Nicolle to Vallery-Radot, February 14, 1921, ibid. Nicolle referred to the organization sometimes as "the Society," sometimes as "the Association."

66. Vallery-Radot to Nicolle, March 17, 1921, ibid.

67. There has been much interest in the Rockefeller Foundation's influence on the development of medicine and public health, nationally and internationally, during the twentieth century. A recent volume of *Studies in History and Philosophy of Biological and Biomedical Sciences* (31 [2000]) was devoted to the subject. See, in particular, Lion Murard and Patrick Zylberman, "Seeds for French Health Care: Did the Rockefeller Foundation Plant the Seeds between the Two World Wars?," 463–75; Marta Aleksandra Balinska, "The Rockefeller Foundation and the National Institute of Hygiene, Poland, 1918–45," 419–32; Anne-Emanuelle Birn, "Wa(i)ves of Influence: Rockefeller Public Health in Mexico, 1920–50," 381–95; and Ilana Löwy and Patrick Zylberman, "Introduction: Medicine as a Social Instrument: Rockefeller Foundation, 1913–45," 365–79. See also Moulin, "Pasteur Institutes between the Two World Wars," 244–65, and A. Opinel and G. Gachelin, "The Rockefeller Foundation and the Prevention of Malaria in Corsica, 1923–1951: Support

Given to the French Parasitologist Emile Brumpt," *Parassitologia* 46 (204): 287–302. Etienne Burnet played a far larger role in this story than did Nicolle.

68. "Executive Committee Meeting of March 22, 1921," *Minutes of the Rockefeller Foundation*, 21046–7, folder 16, box 2, RG 1.1, Rockefeller Foundation Archives, RAC. Moulin also discusses the Rockefeller–Pasteur Institute connection, and the AEEP, in "Pasteur Institute and Non-Profit," 8–11.

69. Nicolle to Mesnil, May 21, 1921, AIP FR IP NCP.11.

70. Nicolle, "Sillon de Pasteur" (1922), and "Inauguration d'un Buste de Pasteur" (1923).

71. Nicolle did welcome a female *boursier* at the IPT: Mlle Thielle. Nicolle, "Fonctionnement . . . 1923" (1924), 138.

72. Nicolle, "Sillon de Pasteur" (1922).

73. Ibid. (1922).

74. I am not arguing that Nicolle had never before commented on Pasteur's "genius" or that he was in any way unique in focusing on it (the *Résident Général* focused his bust inauguration speech on Pasteur's genius). Instead, by the early 1920s, Nicolle was more focused on genius, and was more actively integrating his own interpretations of Pasteur's methods and missions into his self-image and actions. Like so many things in history, it is a matter of a shift in cumulative focus rather than the creation of some new element.

75. "Inauguration d'un Buste de Pasteur" (1923), 264–65.

76. Ibid., 266. Pasteur's words were literally, "one must work." For one of the many references to this story in secondary sources, Lot, *Charles Nicolle*, 21.

77. Sergent, Foley, and Ch. Vialatte, "Transmission de Laboratoire du Typhus Exanthématique par le Pou," *AIPAN* 1 (1921): 218–30. The 1921 version elaborated on the clinical dimensions of the experiments.

78. Nicolle to Vallery-Radot, July 2, 1923, in Huet, *Pommier,* 119–21, 120. The letter is also in the Nicolle correspondence at the AIP.

79. Nicolle, "L'Infection par le Virus du Typhus Exanthématique Est-Elle Héréditaire Chez le Pou," *AIPAN* 1 (1921): 433–36. In his response, Nicolle revealed a bit more of what was at stake in Sergent's claims: "it would suggest that our desinsectation procedures, which are only partially effective against nits, would be incapable of stopping an epidemic of typhus, when it is a common observation that these procedures do stop the epidemics" (436).

80. The warning is recounted in Nicolle to Vallery-Radot, July 2, 1923, in Huet, *Pommier,* 120; the published response was Nicolle, "L'Infection par le Virus du Typhus" (1921).

81. "Experimental Transmission of Typhus to Man," *Lancet,* 1 (1922): 445. Nicolle told Vallery-Radot (in the July 2 letter) that Nuttall himself was behind the review.

82. Nicolle to Vallery-Radot, July 2, 1923, Huet, *Pommier*, 121.

83. Marthe Conor to Pierre Nicolle, July 18, 1963, and August 30, 1963, ASM 146 J 39.

84. These "later events" refer to the succession dispute of 1933–34 (Chapter 7) and various of Sergent's arguments and actions. On the latter, see my "A Louse, Divided."

85. Correspondence indicates that the surgery took place in the spring of 1918 and was for a stomach problem.

86. Marthe Conor to Pierre Nicolle, June 1, 1962, ASM 146 J 39. Conor, almost eighty when she wrote these letters to Pierre, remained vital and insightful.

87. Marthe Conor to Nicolle, undated letter from the personal collection of Dr. Huet. Huet suspects that Marthe wrote this to Nicolle around 1928, when she remarried. Huet, *Pommier,* 114.

88. Georges Duhamel, *Light on My Days,* trans. Basil Collier (London: J. M. Dent & Sons, 1948), 199. This book combines translations of the first two volumes of Duhamel's autobiography: *Inventaire de l'Abîme* and *Biographie de mes Fantômes.*

89. His collaborators on this project were R. Arcos, Charles Vildrac, G. Chennevière, and Luc Durtain. Patrick Edward Charvet, *A Literary History of France: The Nineteenth and Twentieth Centuries* (New York: Barnes and Noble, 1967), 106.

90. Ibid., 106.

91. The Abbaye published, for example, Duhamel's first book of poetry, *Des Légendes, des Batailles,* in 1907.

92. Pierre-Henri Simon, *Georges Duhamel, où le Bourgeois Sauvé* (Paris: Editions du Temps Présent, 1946), 9–10.

93. Duhamel, *Civilization, 1914–17* (1919), 283. Duhamel's secular humanism did not simply condemn technology but, instead, warned of the dangers of a technology that outstripped human capacity to employ it wisely.

94. Bettina L. Knapp, *Georges Duhamel* (New York: Twayne Publishers, 1972), 52. Duhamel had originally published the book under the pseudonym "Denis Thévenin" and only came forward after the book won the prestigious prize.

95. L. Clark Keating, *Critic of Civilization: Georges Duhamel and His Writings* (Lexington: University of Kentucky Press, 1965), 44.

96. His book about the United States, *Scènes de la Vie Future* (Paris: Mercure de France, 1930), was scathing. Translated into English as *America the Menace,* it found acclaim in France (particularly from Nicolle) and condemnation in the States. After World War II, Duhamel made another visit to the United States; this time, his assessment was much more favorable.

97. Reino Virtanen, "Claude Bernard's Prophesies and the Historical Relation of Science to Literature," *Journal of the History of Ideas* 47 (1986): 275–86, 279. Duhamel's two great novel-cycles focused on two characters: Salavan (five volumes, 1920–32) and Pasquier (ten volumes, 1933–44). This was, of course, the format explored earlier by novelists such as Balzac and Zola.

98. Ibid., 279. Today, however, Duhamel's name is rarely recognized in the United States.

99. Duhamel served as *secrétaire perpétuel* of the Académie Française from 1942 to 1946, was president of the Alliance Française in 1937, and even was president of the Académie de Médecine in 1960.

100. The voluminous correspondence between Duhamel and Nicolle has been collected together, edited, and annotated in J.-J. Hueber, *Entretiens d'Humanistes: Correspondance de Charles Nicolle et Georges Duhamel, 1922–1936* (Rouen: Académie des Sciences, Belles-Lettres et Arts de Rouen, 1996). See also Pierre Nicolle, "Débuts," 6.

101. Founded in 1905 by Alexandre Fichet, *l'Essor* started as a society of amateur actors who performed for profit and for charity in the theaters of Tunis and Carthage. Gradually, it extended its interests to other arts and to politics, sponsoring readings and lectures. Chatelain, *Vie Littéraire,* 36–7.

102. Nicolle to Duhamel, January 17, 1923, AIP FR IP NCP.8–10.

103. After Duhamel had agreed to stay with Nicolle, Nicolle wrote to warn his prospective visitor of his deafness. Nicolle to Duhamel, January 17, 1923, ibid.

104. See, for example, Nicolle to Duhamel, November 29, 1923, ibid.

105. Duhamel, *Le Prince Jaffar* (Paris: Mercure de France, 1924, 1946), 46. In these lines, Nicolle emerges again as the passionate man revealed a decade earlier by Marthe Conor.

106. Ibid., 39. It should be noted that Delattre also remained "Delattre."

107. Hueber, *Entretiens d'Humanistes,* provides a number of examples of Nicolle's post-*Jaffar* enthusiasm for discussing "Habibisms." Also, Marthe Conor spoke of the profound affection evident between Nicolle and Habib in her letter to Pierre of June 1, 1962 (ASM 146 J 39). She urged the younger Nicolle, then preparing his father's biography, to do justice to "this incomparable servant and collaborator, without whose absolute devotion your Father would have had great trouble successfully completing his early typhus research and experiments." She also mentioned that the trio had tea together in Sidi Bou Saïd almost every afternoon. It should be noted that Conor did not escape from employing paternalistic tones when describing the relationship of Nicolle and Habib.

108. Nicolle to Duhamel, May 30, 1926, AIP FR IP NCP.8–10. Returning to a favored theme, Nicolle continued: "No one can know what I owe him. With him dies my second childhood, which was my only childhood."

109. Nicolle, "Mon Camarade Habib," manuscript, ASM 146 J 14. The typed manuscript is nearly forty pages long.

110. See the Nicolle–Duhamel correspondence dated May 30, 1926, AIP FR IP NCP.8–10. The Nicolle–Habib dynamic is a striking example of the kind of colonial paternalism that infantilizes the recipient of that affection. The stock nature of the dynamic does not negate the authenticity of the affection; it does, however, color it—in too-familiar hues.

111. Pierre Nicolle, "Débuts," 34, n. 35. The Fichets became friends with Habib Bourguiba, future president of Tunisia and champion of cultural integration, including women's liberty. At the time, Tunisia, like many other colonial possessions, was witnessing the rising frustration—and effective organization—of its own people against colonial control. (See, for example, Conklin, *A Mission to Civilize;* Perkins, *History of Modern Tunisia.*) Despite his new social connections, however, Nicolle remained publicly silent about the developments in Tunisia. See Chapter 8 for more on Nicolle's "Tunisian" identity.

112. Nicolle not only associated with members of *Tunis-socialiste,* but also with high-ranking members of France's far-right Action Française—including Leon Daudet. Nicolle's aversion to outward political ties is evident in his critique of Duhamel's public protest against the war in Morocco. Other letters, however, make it clear that Nicolle did discuss politics *privately.*

113. Chatelain, *Vie Littéraire,* 44.

114. Objectives quoted in ibid., 40.

115. Ibid., 6, 38. Pellegrin argued that French should be used for practical reasons: literary Arabic was unknown to most Europeans *and* to most Arabs (40).

116. Relations between SEAN branches, despite harmonious intentions, were not always cordial. Tension with Algerian writers caused a schism that resulted in the formation of the Association des Ecrivains Algériens. Eventually, however, the two groups became conciliatory, and several members of the Algerian group also joined SEAN. Ibid., 40.

117. Ibid., 41. Jules Romains, for example, gave a SEAN-sponsored lecture. On the Institut de Carthage, see Chapter 1.

118. Chatelain, *Vie Littéraire,* 69. The works considered had to be written in French.

119. The journal's name was suggested by Pierre Hubec, after a Berber woman who, "like an African Joan of Arc," fought against the Islamic invasions (ibid., 41). The choice needs no commentary.

120. Nicolle to Duhamel, July 25, 1924, AIP FR IP NCP.8–10.

121. Nicolle to Blanche Duhamel, September 18, 1924, ibid. Blanche, an actress, was greatly admired by Nicolle, who continued to write to her frequently after this trip. Nicolle also seemed genuinely to admire the Duhamels' strong relationship.

122. Duhamel, "Voies de Communication," *Mercure de France* 280 (1937): 5–8, 6.

123. Nicolle to Blanc, May 4, 1925; see also March 11, 1922, ASM 146 J 36.

124. Nicolle to Blanc, June 28, 1923 (ASM 146 J 36); to Mesnil (AIP FR IP NCP.11).

125. In his general article on typhus of 1920, he mentioned inapparent infection in passing, in relation to its potential use to explain interepidemic reservoirs of disease. Nicolle, "L'Etat de nos Connaissances . . . Typhus" (1920), 56.

126. Nicolle to Blanc, June 3, 1924, ASM 146 J 36.

127. Nicolle, "Contribution à la Connaissance des Infections Inapparentes," *CRAS* 179 (1924): 375–77.

128. Duhamel to Nicolle, October 25, 1924, AIP FR IP NCP.8–10. Duhamel's image is, literally, more fluid—rationing something out in dribs and drabs rather than breaking it into pieces. Hueber read the date of this letter as October 21.

129. Nicolle to Duhamel, October 29, 1924, ibid.: "it will only be after careful research that I will be able to extract from my experiments the book that you wish me to publish." Despite his tendency to reshape history, Nicolle did have a sense of evidence that would warm the hearts of many historians.

130. This work and its philosophic expression will be dealt with in the remainder of this book.

131. Duhamel, "Voies de Communication," 6–7.

132. Nicolle to Duhamel, November 16, 1924, AIP FR IP NCP.8–10. Emphasis added.

133. Nicolle to Duhamel, March 2, 1923, ibid.

134. Nicolle to Vallery-Radot, August 22, 1928, AIP FR IP NCP.8–10.

135. "The pen is thoughtful; its action lasts longer than the spoken word." Nicolle, *Introduction,* 31.

136. From the time Duhamel and Arcos told Nicolle of their initial intervention with Bloch on his behalf (Arcos to Nicolle, February 25, 1923 [in the Duhamel file]; Duhamel to Nicolle, March 1, 1923, AIP FR IP NCP.8–10), their correspondence is flooded with publishing inquiries through 1929.

137. Nicolle to Duhamel, August 6, 1926, ibid.

138. If Duhamel declined further travels in a manner reflective of his literary-explorer inclinations, he always remained fiercely loyal to Nicolle. His publicity campaigns on Nicolle's behalf, both before and after Nicolle's death, are moving and remarkable.

139. Duhamel to Nicolle, June 29, 1925, AIP FR IP NCP.8–10.

140. Duhamel to Nicolle, August 31, 1925, ibid. One wonders what Blanche Duhamel, who had recently given birth, thought of Nicolle's relentless plea that her

husband leave her for a few months to travel with him. Ever polite to his friend, however, Duhamel never mentioned to Nicolle any discomfort his persistence may have caused.

141. Nicolle to Vallery-Radot, July 2, 1925, AIP FR IP NCP.12.

142. Carlos Chagas to Nicolle, April 9, 1917, ASM 146 J 25.

143. Nicolle, "Rapport sur une Mission Scientifique en Argentine," *AIPT* 15 (1926): 166–72, 167.

144. Ibid., 169.

145. Ibid., 167.

146. Nicolle, "Rapport Présenté par le Docteur Charles Nicolle à S. E. Monsieur Clinchant, Ambassadeur de France auprès de la République Argentine," *AIPT* 20 (1931): 94–97, 95.

147. Nicolle, corrected galley of the article "Allocution Prononcée à l'Occasion de sa Visite au Centre Médical Argentine, Centre des Etudiants en Médicine le 23 Octobre 1925": 1473–76, 1473, ASM 146 J 57. Though the page numbers are crossed out in the proof, I am using them for sake of simple reference.

148. Ibid., 1474. Emphasis added.

149. As will become clear in later chapters, Nicolle believed that only men could be true "geniuses." The French were particularly inclined toward genius.

150. Nicolle, "Allocution" (1925), 1475.

151. Presumably because of the European influence in Argentina, Nicolle checked his paternalism to an extent, conceding that the country—again, if it followed a kind of European mind-set—could itself achieve works of genius. Ibid., 1475–76.

152. Nicolle, "Rapport Présenté par le Docteur Charles Nicolle à S. E. Monsieur Clinchant"(1931), 95.

153. Nicolle to Vallery-Radot, December 10, 1925, AIP FR IP NCP.12. Nicolle arrived in France on December 26 and returned to Tunis in early January.

154. See, for example, Nicolle to Vallery-Radot, November 11, 1930, ibid. Nicolle also presided over the inauguration of Flaubert's centennial bust in Carthage. Flaubert was often claimed by the literary French inhabitants of Tunisia (such as Nicolle) on the basis of his visit to Carthage and subsequent novel, *Salammbo*.

155. Nicolle to Blanc, August 8, 1922, ASM 146 J 36.

156. Nicolle to Blanc, May 4, 1925, ibid.

157. Nicolle to Blanc, February 5, 1928, ibid.

158. It will be remembered that the IPT, in its new location, began functioning in 1904, though it was not inaugurated until 1905.

159. "Employing only minimal services until its 1903 reorganization, the early institute merely succeeded in identifying several animal diseases previously unknown or debated in Tunisia." Nicolle, *Notice* (1924), 3–4.

160. Ibid., 9. The section is "Vaccinothérapie." Indeed, most sections began with a variation on "With X and Y, Nicolle. . . ."

161. Nicolle listed his visiting guests in each year's "Fonctionnement." Some of these visitors, as we shall see later in this and in subsequent chapters, would be of great consequence to Nicolle.

162. Lucien Saint, Tunisia's *Résident Général*, was honorary president. Nicolle acted as vice president, and committee members included Pastorians Burnet, Conseil, and

Gobert (Nicolle's hand-selected Director of Hygiene), along with numerous hospital doctors and veterinarians. *Revue Tunisienne des Sciences Médicales* 20 (1926): 27.

163. Nicolle, "Discours du Dr. Charles Nicolle," in "Les Journées Médicales Tunisiennes, 2–5 Avril 1926," *Revue Tunisienne des Sciences Médicales* 20 (1926): 6–11. (When citing Nicolle's presentation, I will use his title; otherwise, I will simply refer to the "Journées Médicales" article as a whole.) The conference is included as a special, repaginated section in this volume of the journal. An official dignitary opened the conference, but Nicolle gave the first talk. Participants attended meetings on gastro-duodenal surgery, Mediterranean fever, the prophylaxis and treatment of measles, and trachoma. Of these, Nicolle had done significant work on all but the first.

164. Nicolle, "Discours" (1926), 11.

165. "Journées Médicales Tunisiennes" (1926). Bernard's quotation is on page 14. The other two are, in order, from Professor Sanarelli, director of the Microbiological Institute of the University of Rome (21); and Lucien Saint (25).

166. Ibid., 22.

Chapter 5

1. This was Brumpt's lab. According to the IPT annual reports, Brumpt himself, with his *chef de laboratoire* Dr. Langeron, were at the institute in 1919. Langeron returned in 1920. The IPT's first AEEP *boursier*, Charles Anderson, had been a *préparateur* at the parasitology lab. (In 1922, Anderson was officially appointed *chef de laboratoire* at the IPT.) Prof. Charles Joyeaux spent the summer of 1922 in Tunis.

2. "Fonctionnement . . . 1924" (1925). The Rouen file on Nicolle's 1925 Mission contains an ornate, hand-decorated menu for a dinner organized by Mazza in Nicolle's honor: ASM 146 J.

3. Nicolle to Vallery-Radot, October 23, 1923, AIP FR IP NCP.12.

4. Latour underscores the importance of such networks in his *Science in Action*.

5. Nicolle, "Contribution à l'Etude des Infections Inapparentes: Le Typhus Exanthématique Inapparent," *AIPT* 14 (1925): 149–212; Nicolle, "Les Infections Inapparentes à propos du Typhus Exanthématique Inapparent," *Presse Médicale* 33 (1925): 1169–70. In the *AIPT* volume appeared other articles relating to specific applications of inapparent infections.

6. On the Mallon case and its context, see Leavitt, *Typhoid Mary*. Mary Mallon was reintroduced to the general public in the PBS special "The Most Dangerous Woman in America" (associated Web site at www.pbs.org/wgbh/nova/typhoid/). Leavitt was a consultant for the show.

7. Charles-Edward Amory Winslow, *The Conquest of Epidemic Disease: A Chapter in the History of Ideas* (Princeton: Princeton University Press, 1943), esp. Chapter 16, "The Concept of the Carrier" (336–46). Winslow notes that the concept was systematically outlined by Reed, Vaughan, and Shakespeare in 1900 (340). For a thorough and perceptive review of the challenges the concept presented to the germ theory of disease, see Mendelsohn, "Cultures of Bacteriology," and idem., "Medicine and the Making of Bodily

Inequality in Twentieth-Century Europe," in *Heredity and Infection: The History of Disease Transmission,* eds. Jean-Paul Gaudillière and Ilana Löwy (London: Routledge, 2001), 21–79.

8. Frederick G. Novy, "Disease Carriers," *Science* 36 (1912): 1–10. Paying particular attention to the healthy carrier, Novy also considered insect vectors. He divided carriers into "chronic," "convalescent," and "healthy," and provided several examples of each.

9. Nicolle, "Contribution à l'Etude des Infections Inapparentes" (1925), 159. Emphasis in original. Not everyone accepted Nicolle's contention that inapparent infection was different from latent infection: Edmond Sergent was particularly virulent in his attacks on the concept. For a more recent assessment of the concept's continued relevance (admittedly by a Nicolle supporter), see Giroud and Jadin, "Maladies Inapparentes de Ch. Nicolle."

10. Nicolle, "Contribution à l'Étude des Infections Inapparentes" (1925), 164.

11. In the process, he also substantially rewrote the history of his inapparent infection work, pressing the "discovery" date back to 1911.

12. Ibid., 150.

13. Ibid., 150–52. As he elaborated later in the article, "When facing a doubtful [inoculation] result, or even a negative one, after the first set of inoculations of a virus, it might be necessary to conduct a passage from the animal that displayed no symptoms to a new animal" before determining with finality that no disease existed (158). The Poulenc reference is on page 172.

14. Ibid., 166–67.

15. Ibid., 210.

16. Ibid., 164. Emphasis in original. Concerning individual resistance, Nicolle only drew attention to the tendency of typhus to be benign in children, particularly in infants (163).

17. Nicolle, "Les Infections Inapparentes" (1925), 1169.

18. Ibid., 1170.

19. Nicolle, "Contribution à l'Étude des Infections Inapparentes" (1925), 166.

20. An excellent review of experimental epidemiology in the 1920s may be found in Dible's *Recent Advances in Bacteriology,* 113–28. On epidemiology in the interwar years, Mendelsohn, "From Eradication to Equilibrium: How Epidemics Became Complex after World War I," in *Greater Than the Parts: Holism in Biomedicine, 1920–1950,* eds. Christopher Lawrence and George Weisz (New York: Oxford University Press, 1998), 303–31. Also, on experimental epidemiology in 1920s Britain and America, Amsterdamska, "Standardizing Epidemics: Infection, Inheritance, and Environment in Prewar Experimental Epidemiology," in Gaudillière and Löwy, eds., *Heredity and Infection,* 135–79.

21. Nicolle, "Contribution à l'Étude des Infections Inapparentes" (1925), 209. Emphasis in original.

22. Nicolle, "Les Infections Inapparentes" (1925), 1170.

23. Ibid., 1169. Emphasis in original. The concept of *inapparent* would eventually lead Nicolle to his formulation of the "birth, life, and death of epidemic diseases." It would also be at the center of an international debate about the nature of typhus. See Chapters 6 and 8.

24. The search for a typhus vaccine became an international quest in the 1930s, with Georges Blanc following one of Nicolle's lines of thought and Hans Zinsser following another. The complexity of the story is far outside the scope of this book; however, for a review, see Weindling, *Epidemics and Genocide,* esp. 212–18.

25. Nicolle, "Essai de Vaccination Préventive dans le Typhus Exanthématique," *CRAS* 163 (1916-II): 38. See Chapter 3. Nicolle claimed to have first discovered the value of convalescent serum for typhus in 1910; subsequently, he applied it to measles. Dible, *Recent Advances in Bacteriology*, 290–93, on Nicolle and convalescent serum for measles. Nicolle and Conseil, "Sur la Production d'un Sérum Expérimental Préventive du Typhus Exanthématique: Étapes et Solution du Problème," *AIPT* 14 (1925): 355–83, 356.

26. Nicolle and Conseil, "Production d'un Sérum . . . Préventive du Typhus" (1925), 358–60.

27. On Polish typhus research (including information on Weigl), Balinska, "Rockefeller Foundation and the National Institute of Hygiene, Poland"; and Weindling, *Epidemics and Genocide,* Chapter 7: "The Sanitary Iron Curtain: The Relief of Polish and Russian Typhus."

28. Nicolle to Calmette, October 22, 1926, AIP FR IP NCP.11.

29. Huet, *Pommier,* 156–58.

30. Nicolle, Sparrow, and Conseil, "Vaccination Préventive de l'Homme contre le Typhus Exanthématique par Inoculations Répétées de Petites Doses de Virus: Étapes et Solution du Problème," *AIPT* 16 (1927): 1–32.

31. Sparrow later indicated to Blanc that the "happy" collaboration with Nicolle was not always so happy—nor so equitable: "It is not my intention to lay claim to any corner of our Master's glory, but I owe it to the truth to tell you that all the preliminary experiments concerning the proportioning of the virus . . . were made by me only." Sparrow to Blanc, January 17, 1938, AIP FR IP BLA.4.

32. Blanc, J. Caminopetros, and E. Manoussakis, "Mémoires: Quelques Recherches Expérimentales sur la Dengue," *BSPE* (1928): 525–37. Nicolle's elaboration on Blanc's work, and his fatherly claim on Blanc, came in Nicolle, "Un Nouvel Exemple d'Infections Inapparentes, à propos de la Découverte, faite par G. Blanc, J. Caminoptros et E. Manoussakis de la Dengue Inapparente de l'Homme et de celle du Cobaye" *AIPT* 17 (1928): 356–62, 362.

33. Nicolle, "Nouvel Exemple d'Infections Inapparentes" (1928), 362.

34. S. Ramsine, "Sur l'Existence de la Forme Inapparente du Typhus Exanthématique Chez l'Homme," *AIPT* 18 (1929): 247–57.

35. Ibid., 248.

36. Ibid., 249.

37. Dible notes that "Wilson, of Belfast," devised a similar test in 1910. Though careful to emphasize that Weil and Felix made their discovery independent of Wilson's work, he did offer comment when noting that "the reaction, although not quite fairly to other and earlier observers, is generally known by" Weil and Felix's names. Dible, *Recent Advances in Bacteriology,* 324.

38. John C. Snyder, "Typhus Fevers," in *Viral and Rickettsial Infections of Man,* ed. Thomas M. Rivers (Philadelphia: J. B. Lippincott, 1948), 462–92, 476.

39. Victoria Harden, "Koch's Postulates and the Etiology of Rickettsial Diseases," *JHM* 42 (1987): 277–95, 291; 286–7.

40. Ramsine, "Sur l'Existence de la Forme Inapparente" (1929), 250.

41. Ibid.

42. Ibid., 254. Emphasis added.

43. Nicolle, "À Propos du Mémoire de S. Ramsine sur l'Existence du Typhus Inapparent Chez l'Homme," *AIPT* 18 (1929): 255–57, 255. Nicolle dated the piece (May 15, 1929), something he did not do with articles.

44. Ibid., 256. Though Nicolle's prescription might sound at once ominous and racist to today's readers, two points should be considered. First, much advice relating to latent infections at the time was similarly ominous in tone, warning of unseen dangers harbored by carriers (Novy, "Disease Carriers" [1912], 2, 3). There was, however, awareness of the importance of finding a balanced approach to dealing with the threat (J. C. G. Ledingham and J. A. Arkwright, *The Carrier Problem in Infectious Diseases* [London: Edward Arnold, 1912], 1–2). Second, Nicolle applied his formulation to all individuals living in places where typhus was active. It applied in North Africa, but also in Belgrade or Russia— and would presumably apply to French populations so stricken, whether they were in France or Tunisia. In this way, it seems to be more revealing of Nicolle's thinking about typhus (or disease more generally) than about typhus-ridden populations. That said, the concept did have elements that would certainly have invited abuse.

45. W. Barykine, S. Minervine, and A. Kompaneez, "Le Typhus Exanthématique Inapparente et Son Importance Epidemiologique," *AIPT* 19 (1930): 422–32.

46. Ibid., 422, 432.

47. See Weil, Singer, and Breinl, Institute of Hygiene of the German University in Prague [E. Weil and F. Breinl, "Über die Erzeugung von Inapparenten, zu Aktiven Immunität Fuhrended Fleckfieberinfektionen bei Passiv Immunisierten Meerschweinchen," *Wiener Klinische Wochenschrift* 35 (1922): 458]; Otto and Munter, the Robert Koch Institute [R. Otto and H. Munter, "Beiträge zur Immunität beim Experimentellen Fleckfieber des Meerschweinchens," *Zeitschrift für Hygiene und Infektions-Krankheiten* 104 (1925): 408–35]; Wilhelm Kolle, director, Staatsinstitut für Experimentelle Therapie and Georg-Speyer-Haus, Frankfurt. [W. Kolle, "Aktive Immunisierung und Schutzimpfung," *Zentralblatt für Bakteriologie, Parasitenkunde und Infektionskrankheiten* 104 (1927): 90–115]. See also K. F. Meyer, "Latent Infections," *Journal of Bacteriology* 31 (1936): 109–35.

48. The Americans tended to be far more skeptical about Nicolle's reliance on inapparent infections to explain disease conservation. On the international discussion of typhus reservoirs (and varieties), see Chapters 6 and 8.

49. Nicolle, "Sur la Nature des Virus Invisibles: Origine Microbienne des Inframicrobes," *AIPT* 14 (1925): 105–20, 108. Nicolle credited his work with Blanc in 1914, rather than his earlier ultramicroscopic investigations with Blaizot, with starting his interest in filterable viruses.

50. See Chapter 3. Nicolle's observation of an invisible stage for what is now called *Borrelia recurrentis* was supported by a number of other researchers and was not finally disproved until Oscar Felsenfeld brought an electron microscope to the subject in 1965. Felsenfeld, *Borrelia,* 17–18.

51. Dible qualifies Nicolle's contribution to influenza studies. Dible, *Recent Advances in Bacteriology* (1932), 268. See the surrounding chapter for a concise review of the science surrounding influenza research during and after World War I. The influenza pandemic has been the subject of much historical study, moving well beyond the status of "forgotten pandemic," as it had been dubbed in one such early study. Alfred W. Crosby, *America's Forgotten Pandemic: The Influenza of 1918* (Cambridge: Cambridge University Press, 1989). (Crosby

entitled the first edition, published by Greenwood Press in 1976, *Epidemic and Peace.*) More recently, see Gina Kolata, *Flu: The Story of the Great Influenza Pandemic of 1918 and the Search for the Virus That Caused It* (New York: Farrar, Straus and Giroux, 1999).

52. On d'Herelle, see Summers, *Félix d'Herelle*. Summers notes that d'Herelle was at the IPT from April until August 1915. Nicolle had recommended to the Tunisian government that d'Herelle be brought in to deal with the locust infestation that had been decimating Tunisia for three years (43–44). The discovery of the bacteriophage has long been attached to a priority dispute over whether the substance of d'Herelle's famous 1917 paper had already been laid out by Britain's Frederick Twort in 1915. Summers deals with the controversy (59, 70–72). See also the work of Ton van Helvoort, "Félix d'Hérelle en de Controverse rond het Twort-d'Hérelle Fenomeen in de Jaren 1920: Ultrafiltreerbarr Virus of Lytisch Ferment," *Tildschrift voor de Geschiedenis der Geneeskunde, Natuurwetenschappen, Wiskunde en Techniek* 8 (1985): 58–72.

53. On Wendell Stanley and his work, see Creager, *Life of a Virus*.

54. For an immensely helpful overview of the conceptual development of virus studies, see Ton van Helvoort, "History of Virus Research in the Twentieth Century: The Problem of Conceptual Continuity," *History of Science*, 32 (1994): 185–235. Also see Waterson and Wilkinson, *Introduction to the History of Virology*.

55. Nicolle, "Sur la Nature des Virus Invisibles" (1925), 107. Emphasis in original. As with inapparent infections, I have chosen to retain Nicolle's exact term, in an effort to underscore the historical disconnect between his interpretations and later, more familiar—but often modified—concepts (such as subclinical infections and viruses).

56. See Chapter 2.

57. Nicolle, "Sur la Nature des Virus Invisibles" (1925), 105–6.

58. Ibid., 106.

59. Ibid., 110.

60. "Fonctionnement . . . 1924" (1925), 243.

61. Nicolle, "Sur la Nature des Virus Invisibles" (1925), 111. See also Frederic Breinl, "Sur les Relations du Virus Exanthématique et des Bacilles Proteus X," *AIPT* 13 (1924): 208–11.

62. On the d'Herelle-Bordet debate, Summers, *Félix d'Herelle*, 64–66, and Ton von Helvoort, "Bacteriological and Physiological Research Styles in the Early Controversy on the Nature of the Bacteriophage Phenomenon," *Medical History* 36 (1992): 243–70.

63. Nicolle, "Sur la Nature des Virus Invisibles" (1925), 112–13.

64. Philip Hadley, "Microbial Dissociation," *Journal of Infectious Disease* 40 (1927): 1–312. On Hadley and cyclogenic theory, see Summers, "From Culture as Organism," 178–81; and Amsterdamska, "Stabilizing Instability," 204–20. Amsterdamska in particular elucidates Hadley's interpretation of cyclogeny.

65. Nicolle, "Sur la Nature des Virus Invisibles" (1925), 115. Nicolle, like most bacteriologists, believed bacteria reproduced through transverse division—except that, eventually, he came to believe that inframicrobes divided into granules—a means of reproduction that would be far faster.

66. On Robert Green, Patrick Laidlaw, and their hypothesis of retrograde evolution in viruses, see van Helvoort, "History of Virus Research," 196–99. Nicolle himself was to offer an explanation that was quite close to Green and Laidlaw's.

67. On Leishman and the granular theory, see Chapter 3. It was Leishman who used Nicolle's relapsing fever work to support his interpretation of granules. Also, Amsterdamska, "Stabilizing Instability," 196.

68. Nicolle, "Sur la Nature des Virus Invisibles" (1925), 116.

69. Ibid., 119. The second ellipsis is in Nicolle's text.

70. Ibid., 120. This is the quotation with which I opened this chapter.

71. Nicolle to Blanc, November 21, 1928, ASM 146 J 36.

72. I am thinking of his appeals to Blanc to take over the IPT. It is plausible that, had Blanc accepted and returned to Tunis, Nicolle might have formally retired. Plausible, but not likely: along with his missionary commitments, he was still actively involved in research whose results were important to him. See Chapter 6.

73. Nicolle repeated these views often, in letters and publications, throughout his career. The quotation is from his article of October 8, 1920, in *Le Temps*, "Le Péril des Études Microbiologique en France," in Nicolle to Vallery-Radot, September 18, 1920 (AIP FR IP NCP.12). The charge of *"fausse monnaie"* can be found, among other places, in his Introduction (80). For more information on the prize system of nineteenth- and early-twentieth-century French scientific funding, see Elisabeth Crawford, "The Prize System of the Academy of Sciences, 1850–1914," in Fox and Weisz, *Organization of Science and Technology*, 283–307; and Paul, *From Knowledge to Power*, Chapter 8, "Science Funding in the Twentieth Century: Laying the Foundations of the Science Empire."

74. Dinguizli was dropped from the IPT story almost immediately after Nicolle became director. Private correspondence suggests that Nicolle was not as impressed by the Tunisian doctor's abilities as his predecessor had been.

75. One such invitation was sent to longtime typhus researcher S. Burt Wolbach, head of pathology at Harvard University. Wolbach graciously accepted the invitation and sent in his 250-franc "subscription." S. Burt Wolbach to F. Gerard, December 30, 1927, and Gerard to Wolbach, January 20, 1928. Harvard Medical School, Department of Pathology, Office Files (AA 168), HML/CLM, box 11, folder G., 1927–28.

76. "La Célébration du 25me Anniversaire du Docteur Charles Nicolle à la Direction de l'Institut Pasteur de Tunis, 28 Avril 1928," *Revue Tunisienne des Sciences Médicale* 22 (1928): 119–48, 123. Conseil's speech is on pages 123–31. The event is described on pages 119–20, with texts of speeches following.

77. "Célébration du 25me Anniversaire du Docteur Charles Nicolle" (1928), 124.

78. Ibid., 125.

79. Ibid., 142–47, 145–46.

80. Ibid., 143. Nicolle even mentioned the contributions of the absent director of the IP of Algeria, Edmond Sergent. As one might suspect, Sergent's acknowledged contributions concerned malaria prophylaxis rather than typhus.

81. Ibid., 146.

82. Ibid., 144.

83. Moulin has reflected on Nicolle's "Tunisian" identity in "Charles Nicolle, Savant Tunisien." See also Chapter 8.

84. Ibid., 145.

85. Nicolle to Duhamel, November 2, 1926; Duhamel to Nicolle, November 8, 1926, AIP FR IP NCP.8–10.

86. Nicolle to Duhamel, December 1, 1927, ibid.

87. Huet, *Pommier*, 123–26. Burnet was not alone in having such an experience with Nicolle. Nicolle had virtually no relations with his brother Marcel; ties with his brother Maurice went from strained to severed. He and Sergent broke off cordial communications on more than one occasion.

88. Nicolle to Duhamel, August 24, 1928, AIP FR IP NCP.8–10. Nicolle used the same image when describing his plight to Vallery-Radot; August 28, 1928, AIP FR IP NCP.12.

89. Nicolle to Blanche Duhamel, November 6 or 8, 1928, AIP FR IP NCP.8–10.

90. Nicolle to Blanc, November 19 and 21, 1928, ASM 146 J 36. The quotation is from November 21; the tone is, again, familial.

91. Blanc to Nicolle, November 11, 1928, ibid.

92. Nicolle to Vallery-Radot, May 16, 1934, AIP FR IP NCP.12.

93. Nicolle to Mesnil, October 8, 1935, AIP FR IP NCP.11. "I am most concerned about the question of my successor. . . . Blanc is my first choice; but I have asked him, and he has rejected my request."

94. Nicolle to Vallery-Radot, June 22, 1930, AIP FR IP NCP.12.

95. Nicolle, "Fonctionnement . . . 1928" (1929), 222. Whereas Nicolle had most commonly referred to female doctors as "*la doctresse*," he referred to Marcelle, then to most women doctors after her, simply as "doctor." Nicolle followed the same practice with BCG that he had with his own vaccines: free initial production and distribution.

96. Jean Friéderich, "Un Grand Savant Français: Une Heure avec le Docteur Charles Nicolle," *Journal de Rouen*, February 1, 1932. In ASM 146 J, folder "Charles Nicolle."

97. Nicolle had few women on his scientific staff and only began to report the number of Tunisians he employed after his longtime friend and companion, Habib, died in 1926. The presence of any women in his lab at all is striking when one reads the misogynistic comments Nicolle makes in his philosophical texts of the early 1930s. His friendship with Habib, as well as with "israélites tunisiens," and even with Jewish Pastorians, stands in marked contrast to the xenophobic stance of brother Maurice, who was involved with the Action Française—and to the occasional comment by Charles. See Huet, *Pommier*, 108–9.

98. Friéderich, "Grand Savant Français" (1932).

99. On the Society of Biology, see the exchange between Blanc and Nicolle, autumn 1924; on the Prix Montyon and the Academy of Medicine, Nicolle to Blanc, October 27, 1927, ASM 146 J 36.

100. Calmette to Nicolle, January 2, 1927, AIP FR IP NCP.11.

101. The five Academies are l'Académie Française, l'Académie des Inscriptions et Belles-Lettres, l'Académie des Sciences, l'Académie des Beaux-Arts, and l'Académie des Sciences Morales et Politiques.

102. "The Osiris Prize, worth 100,000 francs, awarded every three years by the Institut de France, is intended to reward the most remarkable discovery or work in the sciences, letters, arts, industry, and generally all things that affect the public interest." "Compte Rendu de la Réception Faite le 22 Octobre 1927, à l'Hôtel de Ville, par M. le Maire et le Conseil Municipal, en l'Honneur du Dr. Charles Nicolle, Lauréat du Prix Osiris," pamphlet, 3, n. 1, in ASM 146 J.

103. Roux, "Rapport sur les Titres Scientifiques de M. le Docteur Charles Nicolle," in M. E. Roux, *Rapport sur le Prix Osiris* (1927): 6–11, 10, ASM 146 J 66.

104. Ibid., 7. Also in his report, Roux presented one of the earliest published formulations of Nicolle's "Door of the Sadiki" narrative—another essential component, from that time forth, of any sanctioned "telling" of the Nicolle story.

105. Huet, *Pommier*, 36. Nicolle asserted at the end of his own speech, "for now, let me return to Africa, where my work is not yet finished." "Charles Nicolle, Lauréat du Prix Osiris," 14.

106. See the correspondence between Nicolle and Mesnil for 1927 (AIP FR IP NCP.11) and also Huet, *Pommier*, 139–40.

107. Mesnil to Nicolle, October 15, 1929, AIP FR IP NCP.11.

108. These were Camille Sauvageau (1861–1931) and Lucien Cuénot (1866–1951). On Cuénot's early work, see Camille Limoges, "Natural Selection, Phagocytosis, and Preadaptation: Lucien Cuénot, 1886–1901," *JHM* 31 (1976): 176–214.

109. Mesnil to Nicolle, November 19, 1929, AIP FR IP NCP.11.

110. Mesnil to Nicolle, December 3, 1929, ibid. Nicolle faced a similar anti-Pastorian campaign in his 1931–32 efforts to become chair of experimental medicine at the Collège de France; Vincent, who also was to play a role in this struggle, played an ambiguous role here (Mesnil to Nicolle, December 17, 1929, AIP FR IP NCP.11). In the final vote, Nicolle defeated Sauvageau 26–14; Mesnil revealed how he had, at the last moment, persuaded a pro-Sauvageau member to vote for Nicolle. Pastorians who voted included Mesnil, Calmette, Roux, and Gabriel Bertrand.

111. For more on Nobel networks, see Elisabeth Crawford, *The Beginnings of the Nobel Institution: The Science Prizes, 1901–1915* (Cambridge: Cambridge University Press, 1984).

112. Nicolle to Vallery-Radot, January 3, 1927, AIP FR IP NCP.12. The Faculties included those in Paris, Bordeaux, Dijon, Brussels, Florence, and Crakow.

113. Nicolle to Vallery-Radot, January 3, 1927, ibid. Note his use of "*poids*" ("weight") when speaking about authority through prestige.

114. Vallery-Radot to Nicolle, January 22, 1928, ibid.

115. Nicolle to Vallery-Radot, January 27, 1928, ibid.

116. Reenstierna to Nicolle, November 25, 1927, ASM 146 J 29. Willem Einthoven received the prize in 1924 for inventing the electrocardiograph; Julius Wagner von Jauregg won in 1927. The Swedish position to which Nicolle was elected was Einthoven's.

117. Ibid.

118. Vallery-Radot and Nicolle remained relatively silent about the prize until Nicolle had received it.

119. Reenstierna to Nicolle, December 28, 1927, ASM 146 J 29. Perhaps it was the lack of specificity in Nicolle's previous nominations that had lessened his chances for success.

120. Vallery-Radot to Nicolle, October 31, 1928, AIP FR IP NCP.12.

121. Nicolle to Vallery-Radot, January 3, 1929, ibid. Roux had written to Nicolle: "I would have been happy to talk with you about the present and the future. This present and future depend on your health." Roux to Nicolle, December 7, 1928, ASM 146 J 33.

122. Nicolle to Vallery-Radot, January 3, 1929, AIP FR IP NCP.12.

123. Bergson was proposed for the Nobel Prize in 1927, but questions were raised about awarding the prize in literature to a philosopher. Upon further study, Bergson was officially announced as the winner in 1928. He is sometimes listed as having won in 1927, sometimes as the winner for 1928. Pierre Nicolle, "Un Evénement Capital dans la Vie

Passionnée de Charles Nicolle: Le Prix Nobel de Physiologie ou Médecine," *BSPE* 74 (1981): 101–18, 102 n. 1.

124. There was some question as to whether Nicolle would have attended regardless. He was scheduled to preside over an important medical conference in Egypt at that same time and, in letters to friends, expressed reservations about canceling.

125. The assorted texts relating to Nicolle's award are gathered together in "Le Prix Nobel de Médecine de 1928," *AIPT* 19 (1930): 105–21. Here, see "Lettre du Docteur Charles Nicolle Lue par M. le Ministre de France à Stockholm," 112–13.

126. Nicolle to Vallery-Radot, August 22, 1928, AIP FR IP NCP.12.

127. Nicolle, "Contribution à l'Étude des Infections Inapparentes" (1925), 149–50.

128. This was in fact the first main heading of the *AIPT* article: "The Knowledge of Inapparent Infection Was Born Out of the Experimental Study of the Guinea Pig." Nicolle, "Contribution à l'Étude des Infections Inapparentes" (1925), 149. The evidence-oriented Nicolle made sure to include instances demonstrating his claim that he knew about inapparent infections in 1911. He cited unpublished laboratory experiments of the inoculation of asymptomatic blood into monkeys, and then into guinea pigs; he even found a reference to these infrequent experiments in a 1912 paper on typhus (153–55). His case observations were most probably accurate. However, as late as his 1918 paper on guinea pig susceptibility to typhus, he showed no evidence of having made the crucial break between "symptoms" and "virulence."

129. "Conférence du Docteur Charles Nicolle sur les Travaux qui Lui Ont Valu l'Attribution du Prix Nobel de Médecine," 113–21, 114; in "Prix Nobel" (1930).

130. Ibid., 117. Emphasis in original.

131. Ibid., 120.

132. I have used my own translations of Nicolle's Nobel lecture. The full text, in English translation, is at the Nobel Foundation's "Nobel Prize" Web site: http://nobelprize.org/medicine/laureates/1928/nicolle-lecture.html

133. Indeed, a kind of "rough" form of the story appears in Nicolle's "Notice sur l'Institut Pasteur de Tunis," AIPT 15 (1926): 8. However, there is nothing similar in his Notice (1924).

134. It is distinctly odd that Nicolle, who dated everything, never dated this narrative, particularly in light of his priority disputes with Sergent. See my paper "A Louse, Divided." On the dating of scientific discoveries more generally, see Steve Woolgar, "Discovery: Logic and Sequence in a Scientific Text," in *The Social Process of Scientific Investigation. Sociology of the Sciences*, Volume IV, eds. Karin D. Knorr, Roger Krohn, and Richard Whitely, 239–68 (Dordrecht, Holland: D. Reidel, 1980).

135. "Charles Nicolle . . . Prix Nobel" (1930), 114–15.

136. Comte's charges may be found in his articles, "Contribution à l'Histoire du Typhus Exanthématique," 83–85; "Contribution à l'Historie du Rôle du Pou dans la Transmission du Typhus Exanthématique," 303–6, 331–34, both in *Revue Moderne de Médecine et de Chirurgie* 30 (1932). For an assessment of the legitimacy of Comte's claims (and there is at least plausibility there), see Huet, *Pommier*, 90–94. To underscore: Nicolle laid sole claim to the *discovery* aspects of the research.

137. "Charles Nicolle . . . Prix Nobel" (1930), 121. Emphasis added.

138. Nicolle frequently disavowed any interest in what he called "purely morphological" studies. Pasteur himself had expressed a similar position.

139. "Charles Nicolle . . . Prix Nobel" (1930), 121.

Chapter 6

1. Geison notes that Davaine and his collaborators had shown that "virulence could be modified by passage through living animals. But the meaning of this isolated fact was obscure." Geison, "Pasteur," 390.

2. Mazumdar, *Species and Specificity,* 73. (See my Introduction.) Duclaux's attribution of "specificity" to Pasteur concerned work on the fermentation of alcohol, rather than directly about causal microbes of disease (Duclaux, *Traité* [1898], 1: 18–19). As I mention in the notes to Chapter 1, and again underscore, Duclaux took a broadly biological approach to microbes, and was greatly interested in their variable qualities of function and structure. It is likely that the perceived connections between Pasteur and specificity grew stronger in the years after his death, so that, by 1930, when Nicolle wished to question strict specificity, it was natural that he would attribute the doctrine to Pasteur. In a sense, then, Nicolle returned to the beginnings of Pastorism near the end of his life to reformulate Pastorian disease concepts.

3. Geison, "Pasteur," 390, 399. Andrew Mendelsohn has pressed Pasteur's interest in variable virulence still further—and has also shown that Koch, at least briefly, entertained the possibility of its broader significance. Mendelsohn, " 'Like All That Lives.' " I think the extent to which ideas on variable virulence implied an openness to something beyond strict specificity among early microbiological investigators requires further exploration.

4. Geison, "Pasteur," 400; Mendelsohn, " 'Like All That Lives,' " 11.

5. Historians of medicine have recently (again) taken an interest in the history of "the ecology—or 'natural history'—of disease" (Warwick Anderson, "Natural Histories," 41). As is the case with much of the history of microbiology, however, there tends to be a divide between French sources on the one hand, and English-speaking sources (extending sometimes to German) on the other. Anderson, for example, examines the work of Theobald Smith, F. Macfarlane Burnet, and René Dubos (Dubos, though born in France, spent his professional career in the United States). Though he mentions Zinsser, he does not mention Nicolle, whose ideas certainly influenced Zinsser and seem also to have influenced Macfarlane Burnet (see, for example, Anderson's discussion of Burnet's 1935 work on "latent, inapparent infection," and its influence on his ideas about disease ecology [48]). On the other hand, Nicolle's French advocates tend to credit him with the very idea that infectious disease had an evolutionary history (Harant, "Charles Nicolle, 'Inventeur' de l'Ecologie Médicale"). Anderson is quite right in his assertion that "each of the major pioneers of a broader biological conception of disease processes tended to represent himself as singular, as the sole author of the idea" (41). An influential source for medical ecology was Theobald Smith, *Parasitism and Disease* (Princeton: Princeton University Press, 1934).

6. Nicolle revised *NVM* for his Collège de France lectures, publishing it under the title *Destin des Maladies Infectieuses* in 1933.

7. The book was in part a response to Duhamel's 1924 challenge that Nicolle think more generally about the significance of inapparent infections.

8. Nicolle, Blaizot, and Conseil, "Études sur la Fièvre Récurrente. I" (1913).

9. In his initial experiments on the hereditary nature of relapsing fever in lice, Nicolle had rather unconvincing evidence that such transmission might be possible. He was not convinced that the phenomenon was extensive enough to explain the disease's continued

existence between epidemic outbreaks. Ibid., 27. Later, however, he would become more confident that hereditary transmission in lice was a central component in such preservation. In this, history did not bear him out: however, in his excellent review of relapsing fever research, Felsenfeld, in noting that hereditary transmission in the louse had been disproved, incorrectly attributed that proof to Nicolle: Felsenfeld, *Borrelia*, 31.

10. Nicolle, Blaizot, and Conseil, "Études sur la Fièvre Récurrente. I" (1913), 27–29. Mesnil provided the IPT with a sample of the tick-borne virus (28).

11. Nicolle and Charles Anderson, "Fièvre Récurrente Transmise à la Fois par Ornithodores et par Poux," *CRAS* 182 (1926-I): 1450–51, 1451. Relapsing fever is transmitted by soft ticks of the *Ornithodorus* genus. For the purposes of this basic description of Nicolle's work, I have chosen to translate "*Ornithodores*" simply as "ticks."

12. Ibid., 1451. An overview and analysis of Nicolle's relapsing fever work can be found in F. Rodhain, "Les Fièvres Récurrentes dans l'Oeuvre de Charles Nicolle," in Pierre Nicolle's files for his father's biography, AIP FR IP NCP.6–7.

13. Nicolle and Anderson, "Étude Comparative de Quelques Virus Récurrents, Pathogènes pour l'Homme," *AIPT* 16 (1927): 123–206, 203.

14. Ibid., 205.

15. Though he had worked out most of these details for his earlier 1927 *AIPT* article (ibid.), Nicolle wrote a summary of his findings for the larger audience of the *Bulletin de l'Institut Pasteur* [*BIP*] that August. Nicolle and Anderson, "Sur l'Origine des Fièvres Récurrentes Humaines," *BIP* 25 (1927): 657–65.

16. Nicolle and Anderson, "Origine des Fièvres Récurrentes" (1927), 662–63.

17. Ibid., 660.

18. Nicolle and Anderson, "Étude . . . Quelques Virus Récurrents" (1927), 203.

19. Nicolle and Anderson, "Origine des Fièvres Récurrentes" (1927), 661.

20. Ibid., 664.

21. Ultimately, Nicolle concluded that one could not speak of "species" of tick-borne relapsing fever in any meaningful sense. There were only "groups" of very similar individuals. Nicolle, C. Mathis, and Ch. Anderson, "Sur l'Unicité des Spirochètes Récurrents du Groupe Dutton," *CRAS* 187 (1928-II): 631–32.

22. Constantin Mathis was working on relapsing fever in Dakar. For a sense of the nature of spirochete exchange, see Nicolle, Anderson, and Colas-Belcour, "Recherches Expérimentales, Poursuivies à l'Institut Pasteur de Tunis, sur les Conditions de la Transmission des Spirochètes Récurrents par les Ornithodores," *AIPT* 19 (1930): 133–227, 135.

23. Nicolle and Anderson, "Note au Sujet des Deux Précédents Mémoires," *AIPT* 18 (1929): 188–98, 191.

24. Nicolle, "L'évolution des Spirochètes et le Mécanisme de la Crise dans les Spirochètes," *AIPT* 16 (1927): 207–17, 207. (This article was included within the larger study by Nicolle and Anderson, "Fievre Recurrente . . . Ornithodores et Poux" [1927]. I am using a separate citation when referring to this particular section.) I was tempted to open the book with this quotation.

25. Nicolle, "L'Évolution des Spirochètes" (1927), 207.

26. Nicolle, "À Propos de la Posologie des Vaccins Microbiens," *AIPT* 17 (1927): 400–11.

27. Ibid., 408.

28. Ibid., 401–3, on preventive vaccines; 403–10, on curative.

29. Maurice Nicolle, *Les Antigènes et les Anticorps: Caractères Généraux—Applications Diagnostiques—Applications Thérapeutiques* (Paris: Masson et Cie, 1920).

30. An excellent statement of the difference between the two notions of virulence is in W. W. C. Topley and G. S. Wilson, *The Principles of Bacteriology and Immunity*, 2 vols. (London: Edward Arnold, 1929): "It is convenient to have some term to denote this power of rapid spread within the tissues, and the term 'virulence' has, by common usage, come to be accepted in this sense. Unfortunately, it is also employed in a much wider and looser sense, to denote the power of bringing about the rapid death of a particular host, irrespective of the kind of process which leads up to the fatal issue. Thus, all bacteriologists refer freely to virulent and avirulent strains of diphtheria bacilli, although this organism is a typical exotoxin producer, with no tendency to tissue invasion. The student, in his reading, must accustom himself to the use of the term with two different connotations: the implication of poisonousness, irrespective of the way in which the poisonous effect which is brought about, which is clearly warranted by the deviation of the word: and the more restricted implication of power to overrun the tissues, for which 'invasiveness' would probably be an adequately descriptive term. As will be seen, it is usually the power to produce death which we measure, when we attempt to apply quantitative methods in the determination of virulence," 2: 617.

31. Nicolle, "Posologie des Vaccins Microbiens" (1927), 403–5.

32. Silverstein, *History of Immunology*, esp. Chapters 2–6; Moulin, *Dernier Langage*.

33. Nicolle, "Posologie des Vaccins Microbiens" (1927), 406.

34. "Except for virulence, which is not at issue here and which would be difficult to define materially, that which is specific in microbes is the property of certain of its constituent parts. In the case before us, it is the curative antigen that is specific." Ibid., 409.

35. Maurice appealed to a "mosaic" metaphor to define the specificity of pathogenic microbes themselves. Nicolle, as we shall see, adopted this explanation directly by 1930, then altered it shortly thereafter.

36. Nicolle, "Posologie des Vaccins Microbiens" (1927), 409.

37. Ibid., 406. Nicolle believed that the curative vaccine should be injected, in very small quantities, just as the patient's temperature was beginning to lower. It served in this way to reinforce the body's natural responses (and resonates with nineteenth-century ideas on medical interventions following "reaction").

38. Nicolle, *NVM*, 37, 41.

39. Nicolle, "Mémoires," ASM 146 J 13. See Chapter 1.

40. I have taken the chronology of Nicolle's illness and publications from letters exchanged with Georges Duhamel.

41. Nicolle, *NVM*, 1–3.

42. Ibid., 35.

43. Ibid., 37.

44. Ibid., 40.

45. Ibid., 41.

46. For Nicolle's early investigations, see Chapter 1. For a good period overview of work on variations in microbial colonies, see Dible, *Recent Advances* (1932), 42–74. Though Nicolle remained interested in microbial variability—alternately called "mutation" and

"dissociation"—he did not work on the kinds of diseases that could be artificially cultured. His perspective was greatly shaped by the diseases he studied.

47. Nicolle, *NVM*, 41–46.

48. Ibid., 48. Emphasis in original.

49. I use the term "element" intentionally. See Chapter 7.

50. "Among microbes, as among other living beings, there are only individuals more or less similar to each other, groups and not species." Nicolle, *NVM*, 50.

51. Ibid., 48–49.

52. Ibid., 49. "Virulence, toxic power are not more essential to a germ than are other of their characters that are less interesting to us, such as their power of fermenting sugars."

53. Ibid., 62. Nicolle used the word *pénètre* to describe the invasive process; however, he used the two interchangeably when describing the infection of a human host.

54. Nicolle would clearly label the many microbial species living happily in the host's intestines as "saprophytes." The connection between virulence and toxicity appears to have rested on the purpose of microbial adaptation to host: its *function*, once adapted, which was to release its toxins or somehow have a pathogenic effect. See also Chapter 5, on virulence in inapparent infection.

55. In his relative use and judgment of experimental and observational evidence, Nicolle was mirroring the extant tensions not only between "experimental" and clinical medicine, but also in various biological disciplines, including evolutionary theory. In the latter field, tensions were diminished with the formulation of the "evolutionary synthesis" in the 1930s. Peter J. Bowler, *Evolution: The History of an Idea*, 3rd ed., rev. (Berkeley: University of California Press, 2003), Chapter 9, "The Evolutionary Synthesis."

56. Nicolle, *NVM*, 77.

57. Ibid., 79. It was in this context that Nicolle used the ecstatic description of intuition. As we shall see in Chapter 7, his enthusiasm for genius continued to escalate over time.

58. In a book of nearly 220 pages, "individual" disease merits roughly 25 pages. The relapsing fever example alone takes up nearly a third of the 12 pages devoted to individual disease "birth."

59. Nicolle, *NVM*, 59–60. Nicolle's description of the "life" of individual disease, which follows this section, fills less than four pages.

60. Ibid., 68.

61. Ibid., 74. Nicolle made far more explicit appeal to military metaphors in this popular formulation of disease than he ever did when discussing disease in other contexts. In this tendency, he was far from alone.

62. See Chapter 5 for a review of Nicolle's 1925 article on "inframicrobes."

63. Nicolle, *NVM*, 72.

64. Ibid.

65. Ibid., 73–74. Nicolle concluded his treatment of the death of individual disease with a two-page section on the varieties of immunity that might follow a disease.

66. Ibid., 74.

67. On the epidemiological debates, Mendelsohn, "From Eradication to Equilibrium"; Amsterdamska, "Standardizing Epidemics."

68. Nicolle, *NVM*, 82–83.
69. Ibid., 83–87, 84.
70. Ibid., 87.
71. Ibid., 89–90.
72. Ibid., 91–92.
73. Ibid., 149.
74. Ibid., 152–60.
75. Ibid., 94–95. On historical evidence for disease birth and death, ibid., 93–106; 164–70.
76. Among the diseases Nicolle listed were plague, syphilis, and Mediterranean fever.
77. Nicolle, *NVM*, 108–10.
78. Ibid., 110–13, 111–12.
79. These were the typhus vaccine experiments that Nicolle and his colleagues conducted on donkeys. Ibid., 117.
80. Ibid., 114–16, 115.
81. Ibid., 121.
82. Ibid., 122.
83. Ibid., 124–25. Nicolle was beginning to think about the structural basis and functional nature of virulence, even suggesting here that it was one of the "vital functions" and was similar to "an act of memory." As he developed his thinking on the subject only after publishing *NVM*, I will wait until Chapter 7 to treat it in more detail.
84. Ibid., 125.
85. After becoming an advocate for inapparent infection, Nicolle regularly used the noun *costume* ("costume") and the verb *revêtir* ("to dress") when describing the relationship between "symptoms" and disease or virulence: "How will we even suspect their existence," he asked of "new" disease species, "before they have donned their costume of symptoms [*revêtu leur costume de symptômes*]?" Ibid., 130.
86. Ibid., 126.
87. Ibid., 129. In *Destin,* Nicolle used the Greek gods instead, replacing Minerva with Athena and Jupiter with Zeus.
88. Ibid., 131–32.
89. Though Nicolle had published on such questions after Hugo de Vries published his theories on evolution by mutation in 1901 (in French), there is no indication that Nicolle was in fact exploring their implications in this work. Sharon Kingsland provides a nice summary of de Vries's mutation theory in her "The Battling Botanist: Daniel Trembly MacDougal, Mutation Theory, and the Rise of Experimental Evolutionary Biology in America, 1900–1912," *Isis* 82 (1991): 479–509, esp. 484–85. On connecting de Vries to the French scene, see Limoges, "Natural Selection," 210–13. This was the same Cuénot who was Nicolle's rival for the Académie des Sciences position in 1929 (Chapter 5). On de Vries and the reception of genetics in France, see Burian, Gayon, and Zallen, "Singular Fate of Genetics."
90. Nicolle, *NVM,* 133–35. Nicolle extended the example with reference to studies of Chaumier and Netter. On rabies, see Chapter 7.
91. Nicolle, *NVM,* 139.
92. Ibid., 146.

93. Ibid., 148.
94. Ibid., 174.
95. Ibid.
96. Ibid., 176–83.
97. Ibid., 184–85.
98. Ibid., 206.
99. Nicolle frequently qualified his use of "path" and "method" when he applied it to nature: nature followed no logic and, therefore, "followed" paths and "employed" methods only figuratively.
100. Nicolle, *NVM*, 206–7. Nicolle was thinking of this phenomenon when he argued that preventive vaccines appeared to act in a manner that approximated nature.
101. Ibid., 210–11.
102. Ibid., 205. In this passage, Nicolle, who constantly emphasized the randomness of nature's seeming methods, actually used the adjective *aveugle* ("blind") to describe nature.
103. For one of Nicolle's many rhetorical battle presentations, see ibid., 184.
104. In showing how humanity might bring about disease death, Nicolle laid out four diseases that might, with extant knowledge and technologies, be vanquished: syphilis, typhoid, malaria, and typhus.
105. This exclusivity was in the process of being upended by work on typhus in Mexico, as discussed later.
106. Nicolle did emphasize that human reservoirs acted to preserve the virus: if typhus rickettsia were to be wholly banished by global cleanliness, there would be nothing (at least no typhus) to feed upon our uncivilized tendencies when they erupted.
107. Nicolle, *NVM*, 195–96.
108. Ibid., 16.
109. Ibid., 216.
110. Ibid., 218.
111. Nicolle, "Discours Prononcé aux Obsèques du Docteur Ernest Conseil le 6 Juin 1930," *AIPT* 19 (1930): 387–89, 387. Nicolle also wrote a review of Conseil's work, which was published with a photograph and prefaced Conseil's bibliography. Appearing in the *AIPT* (19 [1930]), it was also published as a separate pamphlet by Joseph Aloccio, Tunis.
112. Zinsser to Nicolle, November 8, 1928, Hans Zinsser papers (H MS c73), HML/CLM, box 2, folder 90.
113. For Nicolle's fears about the stability of Blanc's vaccine, see Nicolle to Zinsser, December 23, 1933, ibid.
114. In light of its impact on Nicolle's thinking about disease, I will concentrate on his work on typhus varieties: in itself a complex story. On typhus vaccines, see Weindling, *Epidemics and Genocide*, esp. 212–18 for the 1930s work.
115. Presenting these anomalies in a narrative frame that leads directly to Brill-Zinsser disease implies a straight-line, progressive historical path that does not at all reflect the actual development of the work. However, as they are important to the later story, I offer them with cautions against Whiggish interpretations.
116. On Brill's early work, see also Chapter 2.
117. In fact, M. H. Neill, the second of these researchers, was familiar with Brill's work when he wrote up his interpretation of his apparently erratic laboratory findings in

1917. M. H. Neill, "Experimental Typhus Fever in Guinea Pigs: A Description of a Scrotal Lesion in Guinea Pigs Infected with Mexican Typhus," *Public Health Reports* 32 (1917): 1105–8, 1106.

118. Brill, "Acute Infectious Disease" (1910).

119. Brill, "Pathological and Experimental Data Derived from a Further Study of an Acute Infectious Disease of Unknown Origin," *American Journal of Medical Sciences* 142 (1911): 196–218. Ottenberg is known for his work on blood transfusion and blood typing.

120. Ibid., 217. Brill did qualify, "We still have before us the work to prove that the disease differs from typhus fever of the Old World."

121. Ibid., 217–18.

122. Anderson and Goldberger, "Relation of So-Called Brill's Disease" (1912), 151. See also Kraut, *Goldberger's War.*

123. Nicolle, "Nouvelles Études sur le Typhus" (1914–16), 217–24; and "État de nos Connaissances Expérimentale sur le Typhus Exanthématique (Suite et Fin)," *BIP* 18 (1920): 49–60, 50.

124. Brill, "On the Identity of Typhus Fever and Brill's Disease," *Medical Record* 81 (1912): 1037–38, 1038. Brill also reminded readers that the mild vaccinia vaccinated against variola, but no one would confuse the two as identical diseases. It appears that similar reasoning encouraged Maurice Nicolle to posit his "mosaic" of antigens.

125. Brill, "The Form of Typhus Fever That Is Now Endemic in New York City," *Medical Record* 88 (1915): 914–17, 915. Plotz was proved wrong in his etiological assertions, but he would continue to work on typhus—and on Brill's disease—for many years to follow, conducting some of that work at the IPP in the 1930s. Harry Plotz, "The Etiology of Typhus Fever (and of Brill's Disease): Preliminary Communication," *JAMA* 62 (1914): 1556; Plotz, Olitsky, and Baehr, "Etiology of Typhus" (1915).

126. Brill, "Typhus . . . Endemic in New York City" (1915). Nicolle was familiar with Brill's work. Brill's image of typhus "masquerading in strange garments," coming four years before Nicolle published on inapparent infection, is intriguing. On the other hand, metaphors abounded in bacteriological discourse. The theater was not nearly as popular as the battlefield, but had its place, nonetheless.

127. Ibid., 916.

128. The name persisted, despite Dr. Brill's "funeral oration." Reports of "Brill's disease, or endemic typhus," came from the Rio Grande Valley, Atlanta, Boston, Georgia, Chicago, Maryland, Milwaukee, New Orleans, and California. See, for example, Solomon Strouse, "Brill's Disease, Mild Typhus Fever, in the Michael Reese Hospital," *Illinois Medical Journal* 23 (1913): 37–41; E. F. Smith, "Endemic Typhus Fever (Brill's disease): A Case in Sussex County," *Delaware State Medical Journal* 2 (1930): 139–40; A. E. Roussel, "Brill's Disease, a Comparison of Four Cases with Four Cases of Typhus Fever Treated by the Author," *Maryland Medical Journal* 57 (1914): 729–35; W. C. Rucker, "Mild Typhus Exanthematicus (Brill's Disease), with Report of a Case," *New Orleans Medical and Surgical Journal* 82 (1929): 177–79.

129. Neill, "Experimental Typhus in Guinea Pigs" (1917).

130. S. Burt Wolbach, John L. Todd, and Francis W. Palfrey, *The Etiology and Pathology of Typhus: Being the Main Report of the Typhus Research Commission of the League of Red Cross Societies to Poland* (Cambridge, MA: League of Red Cross Societies at the Harvard University Press, 1922).

131. Mooser would later argue that Neill's neglect was the fault of Harvard's S. Burt Wolbach: "to ascribe to Wolbach and Todd the discovery of the agent of murine typhus sounds amusing to those who know that it was due to Wolbach's great authority on typhus that in the U.S.A. Neill's paper of 1917 was—except Wolbach's critical comments—completely disregarded in the United States." Herman Mooser, "*Rickettsia typhi* (Wolbach and Todd 1920) Philip 1943, a synonym of *Rickettsia prowazeki* Rocha Lima 1916," *AIPT* 36 (1959): 301–6, 302.

132. Kenneth F. Maxcy, "Clinical Observations on the Endemic Typhus (Brill's Disease) in Southern United States," *Public Health Reports* 41 (1926): 1213–20.

133. Maxcy, "An Epidemiological Study of Endemic Typhus (Brill's disease) in the Southeastern United States, with Special Reference to its Mode of Transmission," *Public Health Reports* 41 (1926): 2967–95. This article (December) followed up the questions he had raised in his first article (June).

134. Ibid., 2973. Emphasis in original.

135. Ibid., 2967.

136. Ibid., 2987. Maxcy was, quite impressively, up on the latest laboratory literature, citing in his bibliography both Nicolle's 1925 article on inapparent infection and his 1926 follow-up article on typhus.

137. Ibid.

138. Ibid., 2968.

139. Ibid., 2990.

140. Zinsser, "Recent Advances in the Study of Typhus Fever," *Transactions of the College of Physicians of Philadelphia,* 3rd ser. 1 (1934): 1–15, 7.

141. Herman Mooser, "Contribución al Estudio de la Etiología Tifo Mexicano," *Gaceta Medica de Mexico* 59 (1928): 219; "Experiments Relating to the Pathology and the Etiology of Mexican Typhus (Tabardillo)," *Journal of Infectious Diseases* 43 (1928): 214–60; 261–72; "Contribution to the Etiology of Mexican Typhus," *JAMA* 91 (1928): 19–20; "An American Variety of Typhus," *Transactions of the Royal Society of Tropical Medicine and Hygiene* 22 (1928): 175–76; "Ein Beitrag zur Ätiologie des Mexikanischen Fleckfiebers," *Archiv für Schiffs-und-Tropenhygiene* 32 (1928): 261.

142. Zinsser, *As I Remember Him: The Biography of R. S.* (Boston: Little, Brown, 1940), 344. ("R. S." was indeed Zinsser—this was his autobiography.) Zinsser further noted that Mooser "is a little, sturdy bombshell of energy whose brutal honesty has made him many enemies among all but equally honest people." Mooser left Mexico in the mid-1930s to become a professor at the University of Zurich.

143. Mooser, "Reaction of Guinea-Pigs to Mexican Typhus (Tabardillo): Preliminary Note on Bacteriologic Observations," *JAMA* 91 (1928): 19–20, 19.

144. Mooser, "Experiments Relating to . . . Mexican Typhus," (1928), 259. Mooser found that "over 90% of the male guinea-pigs inoculated with the virus of Mexican typhus (tabardillo) presented more or less pronounced swelling and reddening of the scrotum which is due to extensive specific lesions in the tunica cremasterica, tunica vaginalis and testicles" (260). He also mentioned a debate on the question of the identity of Mexican and European typhus that took place in Mexico in 1922 (259).

145. Mooser, "American Variety of Typhus" (1928), 175. Mooser presented a paper on his findings at "the annual meeting of the American Pathologists and Bacteriologists in

Washington, D.C.": Mooser, "Tabardillo, An American Variety of Typhus," *Journal of Infectious Diseases* 44 (1929): 186–93, 187.

146. Mooser, "An American Variety of Typhus" (1929), 176.

147. Ibid.

148. Mooser, "Tabardillo, An American Variety of Typhus" (1929), 190–91. Mooser submitted the paper in November 1928.

149. R. E. Dyer, "A Virus of the Typhus Type Derived from Fleas Collected from Wild Rats," *Public Health Reports* 46 (1931): 334–38.

150. Zinsser, *As I Remember Him,* Chapter 20.

151. For information on Harvard's departments of pathology and bacteriology and immunology I am grateful to the late Dr. Morris F. Schaffer, who was a student in Zinsser's lab from 1934 to 1938. Maxcy had been in contact with Wolbach about his typhus work as early as 1925. See assorted correspondence between Maxcy and Wolbach, Department of Pathology, Office Files (AA 168), HML/CLM, box 10. On Mooser, Zinsser, and Castaneda, see Zinsser Papers (H MS c73), HML/CLM, box 2, folder 88 (Mooser/Zinsser letters) and box 2, folder 70 (M. Ruiz Castaneda/Zinsser letters). Mooser appears to have sent Castaneda to Zinsser around 1929–30.

152. This was the *Journal of Experimental Medicine.* Pinkerton started the tacit debate, however, in the *Journal of Infectious Diseases:* Henry Pinkerton, "Rickettsia-like Organisms in the Scrotal Sac of Guinea-Pigs with European Typhus," *Journal of Infectious Diseases* 44 (1929): 337–46.

153. Sadashivarao R. Savoor and Roberto Velasco, "The Survival of Varieties of Typhus Virus in Mouse Passage, with Particular Reference to the Virus of Brill's Disease," *Journal of Experimental Medicine* 60 (1934): 317–22, 317.

154. Wolbach to S. I Kornhauser, June 15, 1928, Department of Pathology, Office Files (AA 168), HML/CLM, box 10, folder K, 1926–27.

155. Pinkerton, "Rickettsia-Like Organisms" (1929), 338. The European typhus strain that Pinkerton used had been brought to the Harvard lab by Wolbach in 1920 and had been maintained in guinea pigs since then.

156. Pinkerton and Maxcy, "Pathological Study of a Case of Endemic Typhus in Virginia with Demonstration of Rickettsia," *American Journal of Pathology* 7 (1931): 95–104. It is interesting that Maxcy, who had been critical of Nicolle's overreliance on the laboratory, turned to a strongly laboratory-oriented researcher to examine typhus varieties.

157. Zinsser, M. Ruiz Castaneda, and Mooser, "Notes on the Epidemiology of Typhus Fever and the Possible Evolution of the Rickettsia Disease Group," *Transactions of the Association of American Physicians* 47 (1932): 129–42, 138.

158. Zinsser, *As I Remember Him,* 313. See Chapter 19, "Tunis."

159. Ibid., 312. Zinsser's musing takes on added significance when one realizes he wrote it when he was dying: Zinsser died the very year his autobiography was published.

160. Zinsser, *Rats, Lice and History* (1934, 1935), dedication.

161. Zinsser and Castaneda, "Studies on Typhus Fever, II: Studies on the Etiology of Mexican Typhus Fever," *Journal of Experimental Medicine* 52 (1930): 649–58, 658. "Summarizing all these facts, . . . it seems reasonable to assume that we are dealing with two closely related varieties of a single disease group into which, also, Rocky Mountain Spotted Fever may be placed" (650).

162. Zinsser, *As I Remember Him,* 327–29. Small infected animals appear to have been regular companions to bacteriologists traveling aboard passenger ships of the day. (Nicolle was in Paris at this time.)

163. In an effort to minimize terminological confusion, I will initially refer to the typhus of Mexico either as "tabardillo" or "New World," and the European/North African expression as "Old World," until the time when the two were sorted into the "murine" and "classic/epidemic" forms.

164. Less than a year earlier, Nicolle had returned to South America, to lecture at the University of Santiago in Chile and, while he was there, to revisit friends and institutions in Buenos Aires. His daughter, Marcelle, accompanied him. Nicolle to Duhamel, October 5, 1930, AIP FR IP NCP.8–10.

165. Jean Marx [of the Service des Oeuvres Françaises à l'Étranger] to Nicolle, February 18, 1931, ASM 146 J 56.

166. Marx to Nicolle, February 18, 1931, ASM 146 J 31.

167. Nicolle and Sparrow, "Le Typhus Exanthématique Mexicain," *BIP* 29 (1931): 945–59, 947.

168. Ibid., 954.

169. Ibid., 949.

170. Ibid., 955.

171. Ibid., 957.

172. Nicolle and Sparrow, "Le Typhus Exanthématique Mexicain: Rôle du Rat et des Puces dans l'Etiologie du Typhus," *Presse Médicale* 40 (1932): 137–39, 139.

173. See Chapter 7 for more on *Biologie de l'Invention* and the convergence of Nicolle's thinking about genius, virulence, and civilization.

174. "Fonctionnement . . . 1931" (1932), 154. Nicolle's lamentations about the veterinary void in Tunis may be found as another recurrent theme in much of his correspondence. When he was advising the IPP about the proposed new institute in Morocco, he made particular mention of the need for veterinary services, arguing that the only reason the IPT had not been badly harmed by its absence (denied him for assorted political reasons) was, essentially, because of the force of his personal successes.

175. Constantin Mathis, *L'Oeuvre des Pastoriens en Afrique Noire* (Paris: PUF, 1946), 365. According to the IP Dakar Web site, Mathis's father, a colonial doctor, died during a fierce yellow fever epidemic at Saint Louis de Senegal in 1878. "L'Institut Pasteur de Dakar," www.pasteur.sn/pasteur/histo.htm

176. Max Theiler was in the Department of Tropical Medicine of the Harvard Medical School. See his "Studies on the Action of Yellow Fever Virus in Mice," *Annals of Tropical Medicine and Parasitology* 24 (1930): 249–72.

177. Jean Laigret, *Titres et Travaux Scientifiques du Dr. J. Laigret, Chef de Laboratoire à l'Institut Pasteur de Tunis* (Tunis: J. Aloccio, 1936), 5–6. The monkeys were macaques.

178. "The third monkey was injected with material from the forty-second passage in mice 273 days after the establishment of the mouse strain. There was no rise of temperature and the monkey remained well until the forty-seventh day, when he appeared to be ill." The monkey died, but the autopsy revealed that pathological evidence "were consistent with, though not typical of experimental yellow fever in monkeys. . . . All the evidence therefore, pathological and experimental, tends to indicate that this monkey did not die of

yellow fever, but of some intercurrent infection." Theiler, "Studies on the Action of Yellow Fever" (1930), 262–63. Theiler referred to this as "a loss of *virulence* of the virus for monkeys," 271. Emphasis added. I have yet to discern who first referred to this phenomenon as "inapparent infection," but it was most probably Laigret.

179. Mathis, *L'Oeuvre des Pastoriens en Afrique Noire*, 366.

180. Mooser, "Essai sur l'Histoire Naturelle du Typhus Exanthématique," *AIPT* 21 (1932): 1–17. The article is followed by two "addenda" (17–19).

181. Ibid., 4–5.

182. Ibid., 14.

183. Ibid., 15.

184. "Discussion, Nicolle, 'Unité ou Pluralité des Typhus,'" *BSPE* 26 (1933): 331–40, 338. Brumpt insisted that New World typhus be called "Brill's disease." Mesnil, who was present at the paper's discussion, attempted to convince him that "murine" was a more fitting name (339). Nicolle was too sick to attend the meeting, and so sent in his responses for subsequent publication: "I have nothing to add to the terminological questions raised by M. Brumpt. M. Mesnil responded perfectly." Nicolle. "Unité ou Pluralité des Typhus Exanthématiques, à Propos de la Discussion de Mon Rapport à la Séance du 9 Février," *BSPE* 26 (1933): 375–76.

185. Mooser, Gerardo Varela, and Hans Pilz, "Experiments on the Conversion of Typhus Strains," *Journal of Experimental Medicine* 59 (1934): 137–57, 153–54. Emphasis added. They continued: "It is concluded from our experiments that there does not exist any real difference between the virus of historic Old World typhus and the murine New World typhus. Both are considered to be of murine origin. The murine strains represent the original form of the virus of typhus, whereas the epidemic strains are the result of a prolonged propagation in the cycle man-louse-man" (156–57).

186. Mooser would return to his shift from the two- to the one-typhus camp in 1959, explaining how he may have been led to make what he came, by then, to consider an erroneous conclusion. Mooser, "Rickettsia typhi" (1959).

187. Nicolle, "Origine Commune des Typhus et des Autres Fièvres Exanthématique: Leur Individualité Présente," *AIPT* 21 (1932): 32–42, 38. Nicolle wrote a lovely paper on the subject of interpreting laboratory possibility as natural proof: Nicolle and Anderson, "D'une Erreur Commune dans la Conduite des Expériences Portant sur la Détermination des Spirochètes et de la Même Erreur dans Toutes les Investigations Analogues," *AIPT* 16 (1927): 228–32.

188. Nicolle, "Origine Commune des Typhus" (1932), 38–40.

189. Ibid., 41. As murine typhus was found in different seaports around the world, Nicolle not only became increasingly apt to use the term "murine typhus" but also to believe that there were many subspecies of murine typhus itself.

190. Nicolle, "Unité ou Pluralité des Typhus," *BSPE* 26 (1933): 316–31, 328–29.

191. Zinsser, "Varieties of Typhus Virus and the Epidemiology of the American Form of European Typhus Fever (Brill's Disease)," *American Journal of Hygiene* 20 (1934): 513–32, 516. Here, I think Zinsser and Nicolle may have differed. Zinsser implied that he would have taken the laboratory conversion experiments, if positive for producing fixed varieties, as evidence that such transformations occurred in nature. Nicolle would have insisted that the laboratory evidence required field confirmation before it could be accepted as demonstrative.

192. Zinsser, "Varieties of Typhus Virus" (1934), 518.

Chapter 7

1. The Collège de France, which was founded by François I in the sixteenth century (and was given its current name in 1870), is structured around its chairs, who are elected to the position on the basis of the importance and originality of their work. Chairs are expected to conduct research as well as to teach in lectures that are open to the public. The Collège de France neither gives exams nor awards diplomas. On Collège chairs, see Christophe Charle and Eva Telkès, *Les Professeurs du Collège de France: Dictionnaire Biographique, 1901–1939* (Paris: Institut National de Recherche Pédagogique, 1988).

2. Moulin, "Bacteriological Research and Medical Practice."

3. Weinberg to Nicolle, December 1, 1930, ASM 146 J 30.

4. Nicolle to Duhamel, August 19, 1931, AIP FR IP NCP.8–10.

5. Duhamel to Nicolle, August 20, 1931, ibid.

6. Blanche Duhamel to Nicolle, December 10, 1931, ibid. Mme. Duhamel encouraged Nicolle: "The literary scholars" (many of whom were good friends with her husband) "often discuss how much they would like to see the laboratory brought back to life."

7. Nicolle to Delabarre, November 12, 1931, ASM 146 J 34.

8. Joseph Bédier to Nicolle, October 15, 1931, ASM 146 J 61, file "Collège de France." Nicolle expounded upon his doubts about the position: Nicolle to Mesnil, October 21, 1931, AIP FR IP NCP.11; and Nicolle to Vallery-Radot, October 25, 1931, AIP FR IP NCP.12.

9. Netter to Nicolle, October 30, 1933: "You will have heard about Calmette's death and are doubtlessly aware of Roux's fragile state. Thus comes to pass that which I foresaw when I pressed you to come to the Collège." ASM 146 J 28.

10. Nicolle to Mesnil, October 21, 1931, AIP FR IP NCP.11.

11. Nicolle to Blanc, November 12, 1931, ASM 146 J 36.

12. Nicolle to Vallery-Radot, November 6, 1931, AIP FR IP NCP.12. In this letter and in letters to other friends, he used the description "*lutte chaude*" in describing the election before him.

13. Nicolle to Delabarre, November 12, 1931, ASM 146 J 34. The physiologists, with Claude Bernard as their standard, had held the Collège de France's chair of experimental medicine for a century, since Magendie claimed it in 1831. Yet, Pasteur's success with bacteriology and the subsequent rise of Pasteur Institutes in Paris and around the world offered a new model of experimental medicine that could effectively challenge physiology's hegemony. Despite the amicable relations and mutual appreciation of the two men after whom the physiological and bacteriological camps took their names, "Bernardians" and "Pastorians" perceived their medical models to be in competition.

14. Nicolle received a letter from Paris dated January 4, 1932, from a well-connected friend with an illegible signature. Vincent, chair of epidemiology at the Collège, had told him, " 'four or five members of the Collège. . . are not friends of the institute.' " In this case, he is probably referring to the Pasteur Institute. ?? to Nicolle, January 4, 1932, ASM 146 J, file "Collège de France." The quote is also from this letter.

15. Nicolle to Duhamel, October 16, 1931; December 31, 1931, AIP FR IP NCP.8–10; Nicolle to Mesnil, October 21, 1931, AIP FR IP NCP.11; Nicolle to Vallery-Radot, October 25, 1931, AIP FR IP NCP.12.

16. Nicolle sent these letters in early November. Several members replied. Gsell, for example, encouraged Nicolle: "I would very much like our chair of medicine to be filled by a Pastorian." Gsell to Nicolle, November 25, 1931, ASM 146 J 61.

17. Nicolle told Duhamel that his typhus research was at too delicate a point to leave: he would have to bring all his lab animals with him to Paris. Naturally, he didn't. Nicolle to Duhamel, December 2, 1931, AIP FR IP NCP.8–10.

18. Nicolle to Duhamel, December 7, 1931, ibid.

19. Nageotte to Nicolle, January 4, 1932, ASM 146 J 61. Nageotte sent this text to Nicolle before he read it at the election.

20. Lefranc to Nicolle, January 10, 1932, ASM 146 J 61.

21. The reference was of course to Bernard's classic 1865 treatise, *An Introduction to the Study of Experimental Medicine*. Nicolle's *Introduction*—the text of the five lectures—was published in 1932 by Felix Alcan, in Paris. I am using a reissued edition, published in Tunis by the *Maison Tunisienne de l'Edition* in 1981.

22. Nicolle, *Introduction*, 32–36.

23. Ibid., 39–40.

24. In his discussions of invention and the scientific inventor in his third lecture, Nicolle directed his audience to *Biologie* for further details. Ibid., 67.

25. Ibid., 40–41.

26. Ibid. Nicolle provided a poetic description of Metchnikoff and his influence. Roux, though still mentioned, was truncated to two sentences.

27. Ibid., 52–53.

28. Ibid., 94–105.

29. See, for example, Nicolle to Duhamel, September 1, 1931, AIP FR IP NCP.8–10. "I am unknown to all but a few," Nicolle complained. If he didn't introduce his works to his audience, "they would say, 'Who is this obscure individual who presumes to speak of genius?' "

30. He discussed it frequently in letters to Duhamel, Delabarre, and Vallery-Radot.

31. Nicolle to Vallery-Radot, December 31, 1931; March 29, 1932, AIP FR IP NCP.12. Illness delayed his trip until May.

32. Nicolle to Blanche Duhamel, May 20, 1932, AIP FR IP NCP.8–10.

33. Giroud had been one of his *"boursiers"* at the IPT in the 1920s.

34. Nicolle to Delabarre, March 17, 1933, ASM 146 J 22.

35. Nicolle to Vallery-Radot, October 30, 1932, AIP FR IP NCP.12. See also Nicolle to Vallery-Radot, December 1, 1932, ibid.

36. Nicolle to Delabarre, March 17, 1933, ASM 146 J 22. Nicolle wrote to Vallery-Radot about his intention to ask Roux for more lab space in a letter dated December 1, 1932, AIP FR IP NCP.12.

37. See, for example, P. Giroud and H. Plotz, "Étude Expérimentale des Infections, déterminées par les Cultures des Virus Typhiques Historique ou Murin, et des Immunités qu'Elles Déterminent vis-à-vis de Ces Virus ou de Leurs Cultures," *AIPT* 24 (1935): 420–34; and Nicolle and P. Giroud, "Faits Expérimentaux Contraires à l'Hypothèse de la Transformation Naturelle Actuelle du Virus Typhique en Virus Historique, donc à l'Unité Actuelle de ces Virus," *AIPT* 24 (1935): 47–55.

38. Nicolle, *Destin,* 1, 4. Nicolle described similar motives and means in a letter to Duhamel, December 31, 1931, AIP FR IP NCP.8–10.

39. Duhamel to Nicolle, August 29, 1931, AIP NCP.8–10. Duhamel continued: "It is always difficult for the French to deviate from these classical genres." Hueber notes that Nicolle appears to have made the corrections Duhamel suggested. Hueber, *Entretiens d'Humanistes,* 290 n. 1.

40. Duhamel's detailed list of critiques was not preserved with the correspondence.

41. René Vallery-Radot to Nicolle, January 15, 1932, AIP FR IP C.NIC. Readers today would still find a tremendous amount of objectionable material in the text.

42. "The characteristic of life is its tendency toward equilibrium." Nicolle, *Biologie,* 8.

43. Frederic L. Holmes, "Claude Bernard, the 'Milieu Intérieur,' and Regulatory Physiology," *History and Philosophy of the Life Sciences* 8 (1986): 3–25.

44. Ernest Starling, "The Chemical Correlation of the Functions of the Body," *Lancet* 2 (1905): 339–41, 423–25, 501–3, 579–83. Walter B. Cannon, *The Wisdom of the Body* (London: Kegan Paul, 1932). See Stephen J. Cross and William R. Albury, "Walter B. Cannon, L. J. Henderson, and the Organic Analogy," *Osiris* 3 (1987): 165–92. On homeostasis—and for metaphors of adaptation that would have pleased Nicolle—see D. M. Walsh, "Chasing Shadows: Natural Selection and Adaptation," *Studies in History and Philosophy of Science Part C: Studies in History and Philosophy of Biological and Biomedical Sciences* 31 (2000): 135–53: "Homeostasis involves responding to internal and external perturbations by means of compensatory changes. If a system is too robust it cannot implement compensatory changes; if it is too labile any internal change or external perturbation will cause the complete collapse into disorder. . . . among self-organising systems, living things seem to be distinguished by the possession of an extremely fine-honed capacity for maintaining homeostasis, of withstanding and adapting to internal and external perturbations" (147).

45. Andrew Mendelsohn, "From Eradication to Equilibrium." Once again, things were different in France. Mendelsohn, who discusses the rise of the concept of equilibrium among English-speaking epidemiologists in the interwar period, notes that "The Pastorians . . . had conceived of epidemic infectious disease along similar lines and had used the term *equilibrium* as far back as the 1880s" (319).

46. George Weisz, "A Moment of Synthesis: Medical Holism between the Wars," in Lawrence and Weisz, eds., *Greater than the Parts,* 68–93.

47. We will see, in *Destin,* how Nicolle further pressed his concept of the genius, who became not just savior, but also, like a pathogenic microbe, the locus of virulent, adaptive power. Within a Catholic formulation, it is arguable that equilibrium acted more as Holy Spirit than God.

48. Nicolle, *Biologie,* 3–6, 6. The conquest rhetoric, appropriate to both individual (male/female) and social (colonizer/colonized) realms, hardly demands further comment.

49. Ibid., 7.

50. Ibid., 26–27. On French reservations toward Mendelian genetics (even into the 1930s), see Burian, Gayon, and Zallen, "The Singular Fate of Genetics."

51. Nicolle, *Biologie,* 56. Emphasis in original.

52. On Bergson, see Gilles Deleuze, *Bergsonism,* trans. Hugh Tomlinson and Barbara Habberjam (New York: Zone Books, 1988); Mark Antliff, *Inventing Bergson: Cultural Politics and the Parisian Avant-Garde* (Princeton: Princeton University Press, 1993); H. Stuart Hughes, *Consciousness and Society: The Reorientation of European Social Thought, 1890–1930* (New York: Vintage, 1961, 1977).

53. Bergson wrote Nicolle: "It is an honor for me to be awarded a Nobel Prize at the same time as a scientist whose discoveries have done so much to serve science and humanity." Henri Bergson to Nicolle, November 18, 1928, ASM 146 J 19.

54. He commented, for example, on Nicolle's treatment of invention in *Biologie:* "It is a penetrating analysis of the spirit of invention; moreover, it is a thorough study of the conditions in which the inventor works." Bergson to Nicolle, June 12, 1932, ASM 146 J 19.

55. Nicolle, *Biologie,* xv.

56. For a mention of Nicolle's "mutation/genius" concept of creativity in broader context, see Mirko D. Grmek, "A Plea for Freeing the History of Scientific Discoveries from Myth," in *On Scientific Discovery,* eds. M. D. Grmek, R. S. Cohen, and Guido Cimino (Dordrecht, Holland: R. Reidel, 1980), 9–42, 36–37.

57. Nicolle, *Biologie,* 79, 122.

58. Ibid., 27.

59. Ibid., 72–86, for one of Nicolle's many "statements" about women and genius. He would, in fact, develop the argument more fully in subsequent publications. Nicolle's ideas on women were far from original—and, unlike his arguments about equilibrium, reveal little that was unique about him. However, no biographical account of Nicolle could be complete without mentioning their existence, and their continued importance to the way he constructed his world.

60. Nicolle to Vallery-Radot, April 17, 1934, AIP FR IP NCP.12.

61. Nicolle, *Biologie,* 44; 69–72.

62. Ibid., 35–36, 46, 124.

63. Ibid., 93.

64. Ibid., 32 on inapparent infection; 57 on typhus.

65. On Comte, Chapter 5, note 136.

66. Nicolle, *Biologie,* 17.

67. Ibid., 17–24, 139. Joseph-Arthur de Gobineau, Nicolle argued, was wrong: "pure" blood was sterile, and sterility led to death, not life. Nicolle's arguments against mechanism followed Duhamel, whose recent critique of American culture, *Scènes de la Vie Futur* (Paris: 1930), was translated into English in 1931 as *America: The Menace.* By the 1930s, it was quite common to couch racial arguments in biological terms. For a review of French racism, which includes discussions of Gobineau, Ernest Renan, and other nineteenth-century writers Nicolle was influenced by (or reacting against), Tzvetan Todorov, *On Human Diversity: Nationalism, Racism, and Exoticism in French Thought,* trans. Catherine Porter (Cambridge, MA: Harvard University Press, 1993). On the rise of "biological" racism (and the persistence of cultural justifications) in the French military, Osborne and Fogarty, "Views from the Periphery."

68. Nicolle, *Biologie,* 24–25, 25.

69. For more of Nicolle's views on women, see ibid., 36; 74; 141. On French ideas about gender, see Sian Reynolds, *France between the Wars: Gender and Politics* (London: Routledge, 1996), esp. Chapters 4 and 5.

70. Nicolle, *Biologie,* 68.

71. Ibid., 148–52.

72. Ibid., 151–52.

73. Nicolle to the French Minister of Foreign Affairs, August 12, 1931, ASM 146 J, "Vie Professionnel," 3. Unfortunately, I have not seen the text of this speech, which he delivered to the Mexican Alliance Française.

74. Ibid., 8.

75. Ibid., 8–9.

76. Ibid., 11.

77. Ibid.

78. Nicolle and Burnet, "Sur la Restauration du Virus Fixe," *CRSB* 91 (1924): 366–68.

79. In *Destin,* Nicolle commented that Pasteur certainly would never have dared try that first inoculation had he been a physician (see my Introduction). Nicolle, *Destin,* 189.

80. For a larger discussion of this rabies research, see Dible, *Recent Advances* (1932), chapter titled "Rabies," 192–201, esp. 197–201. Dible's book was published in 1932 and so did not include Nicolle's latest findings. Dible did review the work of Remlinger and Levaditi in some detail and mentioned the 1927 International Congress on Rabies, convened by the League of Nations and held at the IPP (196).

81. Nicolle and L. Balozet, "Essai de Restauration du Virus Rabique Fixe par Passages Intra-cerebraux sur le Chien," *CRAS* 194 (1932-I): 1706–8, 1708.

82. Nicolle, *Destin,* 189. Emphasis added.

83. Nicolle, "Lettre aux Sourds" (1929), 4.

84. Nicolle noted on more than one occasion that if the budget of the world war had been placed in the hands of scientists, it would have produced astounding benefits for humanity.

85. Nicolle, *Destin,* 85.

86. Ibid. Emphasis in original.

87. Ibid., 87–88. Here again, Nicolle demonstrated his Bernardian inclinations toward explanations of biological phenomena. He underscored what was not yet known, but held out hope that, one day, it would be known: through science.

88. Nicolle recounted the limitations of specific laboratory tests in *Destin,* 63–71.

89. Allen, "Naturalists and Experimentalists." Mendelsohn argues for the importance of bacteriology for establishing a laboratory tradition in biology (Mendelsohn, " 'Like All that Lives' ").

90. Nicolle was born four days before Morgan in 1866. On Morgan and his work, Robert Kohler, *Lords of the Fly: Drosophila Genetics and the Experimental Life* (Chicago: University of Chicago Press, 1994).

91. T. H. Morgan, "The Relation of Genetics to Physiology and Medicine," PDF file attached to the official Web site of the Nobel Foundation: www.nobel.se/medicine/laureates/1933/morgan-lecture.pdf. On the meanings of "gene," see Raphael Falk, "What Is a Gene?" *Studies in History and Philosophy of Science* 17 (1986): 133–73.

92. Nicolle, *Destin,* 87.

93. Ibid., 224.

94. Ibid., 178. Nicolle mentioned chromosomes in connection with the elements of the mosaic also on page 92.

95. Ibid., 81. Emphasis in original.

96. Ibid., 82.

97. Ibid., 89. Emphasis added.

98. Ibid., 195.

99. I would like to stress again that, despite his separation of virulence from toxicity, Nicolle *did* still think of virulence as having some violent power: "Had it not been acquired, the agents that cause our diseases would remain in the realm of saprophytes." Ibid., 89. As he noted in passing, microbes that could live and reproduce in a host but displayed no toxic functions could be thought of as "*pathogènes d'emblée*": *latent* pathogenic microbes (193). Perhaps, then, Nicolle's "virulence" had only the power to create enough violence to effect a new equilibrium. In this formulation, if that power created too great a disequilibrium, destruction of both host and microbe would result. Thus, successful virulence, like successful genius, disturbed the balance only to an extent that preserved viability.

100. See my Introduction and that of Conklin in her *Mission to Civilize*.

101. There is an enormous literature on metaphor and its significance. For classic studies, George Lakoff and Mark Johnson, *Metaphors We Live By* (Chicago: University of Chicago Press, 1980); Max Black, "Metaphor," in *Models and Metaphors: Studies in Language and Philosophy* (Ithaca, NY: Cornell University Press, 1962); Andrew Ortony, ed., *Metaphor and Thought* (Cambridge: Cambridge University Press, 1979); Peter Galison, "History, Philosophy, and the Central Metaphor," *Science in Context* 2 (1988): 197–212. For applications of metaphor in specific historical cases, see Robert M. Young, *Darwin's Metaphor: Nature's Place in Victorian Culture* (Cambridge: Cambridge University Press, 1985); Daniel P. Todes, *Pavlov's Physiology Factory: Experiment, Interpretation, Laboratory Enterprise* (Baltimore: Johns Hopkins University Press, 2002); and L. J. Rather, *Addison and the White Corpuscles: An Aspect of Nineteenth Century Biology* (London: The Wellcome Institute, 1972). F. L. Holmes structured his final scholarly contribution around the metaphor of the scientific career "path": Frederic Lawrence Holmes, *Investigative Pathways: Patterns and Stages in the Careers of Experimental Scientists* (New Haven: Yale University Press, 2004).

102. Nicolle, *Nature*. See Chapter 8.

103. Nicolle, "Paroles Biologiques sur la Crise Actuelle," *Mercure de France*, January 1, 1934: 5–30, 29.

104. Nicolle to Delabarre, March 28, 1933, ASM 146 J 38.

105. See Chapter 4.

106. This scathing critique is found in Nicolle to Delabarre, March 28, 1933, ASM 146 J 38. Nicolle expressed similar sentiments about Roux and the Pasteur Institute to other friends (Duhamel, Vallery-Radot, Leredde), but this letter is the most complete and emotive.

107. Ibid. In a letter to Duhamel later that year, he called Roux the "most disagreeable character in the world." Nicolle to Duhamel, August 2, 1933, AIP FR IP NCP.8–10.

108. Nicolle to Delabarre, March 28, 1933, ASM 146 J 38.

109. Lagrange, "Monsieur Roux," facing the "Table des Matières."

110. Nicolle to Delabarre, March 28, 1933, ASM 146 J 48. Emphasis added.

111. Nicolle to Vallery-Radot, April 19, 1933, AIP FR IP NCP.12.

112. Ibid. Nicolle was constantly aware that he needed to persuade the public of his abilities if he hoped to succeed. It is conceivable that Vallery-Radot wrote this article specifically to help Nicolle win over Paris.

113. No copy of the letter existed in the Nicolle collections of the ASM or the AIP when I consulted them.

114. Nicolle to Vallery-Radot, April 19, 1933, AIP FR IP NCP.12. Nicolle opened the second section of *Nature* with this quotation.

115. Nicolle to Vallery-Radot, April 27, 1933, ibid.

116. Calmette recounted the outline of the story to Nicolle in his letter of June 3, 1930, AIP FR IP NCP.11. See Marina Gheorghiu, "Le BCG, Vaccin Contre la Tuberculose: Leçons du Passe pour Aujourd'hui," in *L'Aventure de la Vaccination,* ed. Anne Marie Moulin, 219–28 ([France]: Fayard, 1996), 224–25.

117. Calmette to Nicolle, June 3, 1930, AIP FR IP NCP.11.

118. Nicolle to Calmette, March 11, 1931, ibid.

119. Nicolle to Calmette, December 30, 1930, ibid.

120. Calmette to Nicolle, November 3, 1931, ibid.

121. Calmette died October 29, 1933.

122. Lagrange, *Monsieur Roux,* 231.

123. Netter to Nicolle, October 30, 1933, ASM 146 J 32. Vallery-Radot was now on the council.

124. Giroud to Nicolle, November 26, 1933, ASM 146 J 29.

125. Nicolle to Duhamel, November 10, 1933, AIP FR IP NCP.8–10. Nicolle told Duhamel, "If I am to play a role in the *maison,* I would rather be called to it than ask for it."

126. Nicolle, "Paroles" (1934), 29.

127. "Minutes, Conseil d'Administration," Vol. III, October 30 and November 23, 1933; January 28 and May 16, 1934, AIP CA REG 3, show how Vallery-Radot attempted to negotiate a diplomatic path between Nicolle's reform efforts and his colleagues' more conservative tendencies.

128. In a letter from November 23, 1933, Netter informed Nicolle of Vaillard's assertion. The "Pasteur Institute" in general, he explained, thought Nicolle to be the best candidate; Vaillard, however, claimed that Roux had wholly opposed him. ASM 146 J 32.

129. "Minutes, Conseil d'Administration," November 22, 1933, Vol. III, 442, AIP CA REG 2.

130. Vallery-Radot added that, were his grandfather present at the meeting, "he himself would certainly have proposed to modify the institute's statutes, as these were no longer appropriate for an establishment that had grown extensively." "Minutes, Conseil d'Administration," ibid., 445.

131. Vallery-Radot to Nicolle, November 25, 1933, AIP FR IP NCP.12.

132. Nicolle to Delabarre, December 13, 1933, ASM 146 J 38.

133. Nicolle to Vallery-Radot, January 27, 1934, AIP FR IP NCP.12.

134. Frédéric Lefèvre [Charles Nicolle], "Une Heure avec le Docteur Charles Nicolle, Professeur au Collège de France—Prix Nobel 1928. La Grande Misère de l'Institut Pasteur: Un Cri d'Alarme," *Nouvelles Littéraires,* February 3, 1934.

135. Nicolle to Geniaux, February 9, 1934, ASM 146 J 38.

136. Nicolle was unaware that the *Nouvelles Littéraires* would thus present his article. He was annoyed, thinking it needlessly provocative. Nicolle to Vallery-Radot, February 9, 1934, AIP FR IP NCP.12.

137. [Nicolle], "Grande Misère de l'Institut Pasteur" (1934).

138. This was perhaps Nicolle's least sage assertion, alienating, as it must have done, any potential allies at the IPP.

139. I would like to thank Vivian Nutton for locating this passage for me.

140. The whole of the *NL* article was on one page. I have therefore only added notes of commentary.

141. Nicolle, "Paroles" (1934).

142. Ibid., 25.

143. Ibid., 21. Emphasis added. Nicolle continued, eerily outlining a future European Union: "This entente would require the unification of moneys, the suppression of tariffs, and a freedom of exchange."

144. Ibid., 25. It should be noted that Nicolle also laid an enormous share of the blame for international economic woes on women. After the war, they had not returned to their biologically determined roles (the conservers of life, rather than the genius producers of disequilibrium). Obviously, Nicolle, champion of individualism, opposed communism.

145. Ibid., 29.

146. Lagrange, *Monsieur Roux*, 241. For a spectrum of reactions, see Remlinger to Nicolle, February 6, 1934, ASM 146 J 33; Sorel to Nicolle, February 14, 1934, ASM 146 J 34; Delabarre to Nicolle, February 13, 1934, ASM 146 J 26. Indeed, not even the Parisian riots of February 6 could deflect the Pastorians' attentions from their colleague's presumed transgression.

147. Duhamel, Zinsser, and Vallery-Radot were convinced that Nicolle's aspirations for the directorship motivated him to write.

148. Nicolle to Delebarre, February 19, 1934, ASM 146 J 38.

149. Nicolle to Vallery-Radot, April 17, 1934, AIP FR IP NCP.12. Nicolle had just received his first letter from Mesnil since before the article appeared when he wrote this letter. I can only imagine that Mesnil was not charmed by his friend's characterization of Parisian Pastorians as "lazy functionaries."

150. Morax to Nicolle, February 20, 1934, ASM 146 J 32, is the most explicit of these statements. Morax emphasized the need to preserve the public face of the institute, therefore leaving private problems private. Other correspondence on this subject includes Nicolle to Duhamel, March 13, 1934, AIP FR IP NCP.8–10; Nicolle to Delabarre, April 11, 1934, ASM 146 J 38; Nicolle to Marcelle Nicolle, April 19, 1934, ASM 146 J 35.

151. Nicolle to Vallery-Radot, February 9, 1934, AIP FR IP NCP.12. Vallery-Radot's actual response is missing from the collection; all that remains is Nicolle's side of the discussion. Why Vallery-Radot reacted so vehemently against an article that he had had an opportunity to revise before its publication remains a mystery.

152. Nicolle to Duhamel, February 25, 1934, AIP FR IP NCP.8–10.

153. Duhamel to Nicolle, March 3, 1934, AIP FR IP NCP.8–10. In a subsequent letter (March 17, 1934, AIP FR IP NCP.8–10), Duhamel described a medical conference he had attended, at which Nicolle's article was a central topic of conversations. Of the one hundred or so doctors Duhamel spoke with, he told Nicolle, only one disagreed with the article—and within two minutes, Duhamel had persuaded him that Nicolle was right. Earlier, Lasneret had suggested that support for Nicolle existed among the doctors: Lasneret to Nicolle, November 17, 1934, ASM 146 J 30.

154. Remlinger to Nicolle, March 3, 1934, ASM 146 J 33. Nicolle repeated his belief that Martin and Ramon would be appointed in a letter to daughter Marcelle (April 17, 1934, ASM 146 J 35).

155. Nicolle to Vallery-Radot, May 16, 1934, AIP FR IP NCP.12.
156. On the Administrative Council, Vallery-Radot alone pressed for Nicolle's appointment. His success in this delicate task is a testimony to his authority and diplomacy.
157. Nicolle to Vallery-Radot, May 20, 1934, AIP FR IP NCP.12.
158. Nicolle to Delabarre, June 4, 1934, ASM 146 J 38.
159. Nicolle to Duhamel, June 11, 1934, AIP FR IP NCP.8–10.
160. Ibid. The document Nicolle sent was approximately sixty pages long.
161. Nicolle to Duhamel, October 4, 1934, AIP FR IP NCP.8–10.
162. Nicolle to Vallery-Radot, February 17, 1935, AIP NCP.12.

Chapter 8

1. Nicolle addresses the reader using the familiar *"tu"* form of "you," rather than *"vous."* The only people with whom he himself used *"tu"* were childhood friends, children (including his own, fully grown), close family members, and, conceivably, mistresses. The reader is thus meant to be intimately included in Nicolle's observations and interpretations.
2. Nicolle, *Nature*, 1–2.
3. Ibid., 3.
4. Unfortunately, there is no room, within the limits of this book, to review Nicolle's explanations of these phenomena.
5. See my Introduction; on the French civilizing mission and "mastery," see Conklin, *Mission to Civilize,* particularly her introduction. Of course, one could argue the extent to which the Pastorian and French civilizing missions were particularly "Baconian." Here, I refer to the broadest possible sense of the word: the sense that fits with Book I, Aphorism III. See Chapter 2.
6. Nicolle outlined this chronology in his final book, *La Destinée Humaine,* 113. He completed his revisions in September 1934.
7. This was a recurrent theme for Duhamel (and his fellow French interwar holists); see Duhamel, *L'Humaniste et L'Automate* (Paris: Hartmann, 1933). For a broader perspective on the historical persistence of these themes, see Charles E. Rosenberg, "Pathologies of Progress: The Idea of Civilization as Risk," *BHM* 72 (1998): 714–30. On growing despair in Britain over humanity's ability to control disease (and nature more generally), see Tilley, "Ecologies of Complexity," esp. 32–38. The turn toward despair over human power—within a frame of disease ecology, and extending outward toward civilization more generally—characterizes the careers of Warwick Anderson's central figures in his "Natural Histories of Infectious Disease": "Certainly Dubos became a famous critic of the dangers of industrial capitalism and environmentally insensitive modernity. By the end of his career, condemnation of a destructive civilization, and its associated alienated rationalism, dominated his writing, and his arguments came to assume a more traditionally holistic, humanistic, and even mystical cast. Burnet, too, displayed ambivalence toward modernity, pointing to the dangers of overpopulation, biological warfare, antibiotic resistance, and environmental degradation—all, in his opinion, the fruits of a narrowly reductionist—even obscurantist—worldview" (43). Nicolle is obviously a kindred spirit. Further connections remain to be discovered.

8. *Nature,* 37–38.

9. Ibid., 38–40.

10. Ibid., 33–34.

11. *Nature,* 34. Nicolle also observed that typhus, where it continued naturally, gradually lessened in its severity, with each generation less devastated by it. Westerners, long kept from the disease, were destroyed when placed in contact with it (35). Weak vaccines, he further warned, allowed bacteria to proliferate, leading to chronic lesions or even to subsequent disease attacks "of a severity equal to, or even greater than, the attack it initially helped diminish."

12. Ibid., 41.

13. Ibid., 40–41.

14. Ibid., 43: "The brain of the professor, the erudite, is incapable of creating anything. Its functional discipline has killed its initiative capacity."

15. Ibid. Emphasis added.

16. "Comme un Souvenir Qui ne Vieillit Point." See Chapter 3.

17. Again, Nicolle did not cite Dostoevsky directly. One cannot read into this omission any diminution of intellectual debt: even where he was obviously being influenced by men such as Duhamel and Zinsser, Nicolle rarely credited "contemporaries"; by "contemporaries," here, I mean anyone who lived after "antiquity."

18. *Nature,* 45.

19. Ibid., 46–47.

20. Ibid., 47–48. Jean-Jacques Rousseau quite evidently informed Nicolle's choice of metaphor.

21. Dostoevsky, "Dream," V. For the context of this quotation, see Chapter 3.

22. *Nature,* 49.

23. Ibid., 71. "The revolutionary, the destroyer of societies, belongs more to this society than to the one whose arrival he prepares. . . . Let us add that this enterprise is not only a spiritual need; it is also a kind of obligation" (71–72).

24. Ibid., 52.

25. Ibid., 69. Nicolle also cited Epictetus later: " 'Ask not that things happen as you desire, but that you desire what happens. Remember that you are actors in a play' " (125). He concluded his final paragraph, "Places, everyone, in the play that we did not write, to play our role" (131–32).

26. Mooser, Varela, and Pilz, "Conversion of Typhus Strains" (1934), 153. Closer to home, Edmond Sergent, too, began to question the significance of inapparent infection. In the same spirit with which he approached their separate work on louse transmission of typhus and relapsing fever, Sergent eventually laid claim to the concept publicly, arguing that he had himself defined the phenomenon almost a decade before Nicolle, while working on malaria in birds. Moreover, he asserted firmly that Nicolle was wrong in his belief that such infections were diseases. Rather, they were *latent infections.* He emphasized this difference in the name he chose for the process: "*infections latentes d'emblée,*" or "immediate latent infections." Sergent, "Réflexions sur les Modalités de l'Infection," *AIP d'Algérie,* 26 (1948): 91–104, 101–2.

27. Zinsser, *Rats, Lice and History* (1934, 1935), 229. Though he gave a brief description of the recent debate about typhus varieties and the nature of evidence that had been

gathered to resolve it, he left little room for anything but a dualist interpretation of that evidence: "It was necessary . . . to determine whether the two types were permanently fixed . . . or . . . 'dissociations' of one and the same virus, dependent upon or induced by the different hosts through which they passed. This question has, in our opinion, been answered—though in the interests of accuracy . . . we must add that there is still an element of speculation in the explanation" (230–31). Zinsser even gave a description of the laboratory efforts to convert the two varieties into each other.

28. The connections between Nicolle's thinking on disease evolution and Zinsser's is evident. The two did discuss their ideas on this subject in their correspondence—but not in sufficient detail to add much to what can be gleaned from their publications. The correspondence itself is split between Harvard's Countway Library and the ASM in Rouen.

29. Zinsser, *Rats, Lice and History* (1934, 1935), 228. Zinsser did note that inapparent infection had some practical importance for typhus; yet, this was limited to infection in rats.

30. Ibid., 233.

31. Zinsser and Castenada, "On the Isolation from a Case of Brill's Disease of a Typhus Strain Resembling the European Type," *New England Journal of Medicine* 209 (1933): 815–19, 816.

32. Zinsser, "Sur la Maladie de Brill et le Réservoir Interépidémique du Typhus Classique," *AIPT* 23 (1934): 149–54, 152. Correspondence surrounding Zinsser's Brill's study is in the Zinsser papers (H MS c73), HML/CLM, box 2, esp. folder 78, Haven Emerson.

33. A large percentage of these patients were Jewish. Zinsser noted: "typhus, when it is epidemic, spreads equally among Jews and Gentiles, wherever it occurs. The large percentage of Jews in these statistics means merely that the immigration from typhus endemic foci to the United States has largely consisted of the Jewish population of these regions, and the large percentage of Russians means almost entirely Russian Jews." Zinsser, "Varieties of Typhus (Brill's Disease)" (1934), 521. I have worked on the history of Brill's disease and have presented a paper, "Reservoir Docs," on the subject. On Jewish migration to New York and Boston during the time of Brill's work, Gerald Sorin, *A Time for Building: The Third Migration, 1880–1920 (The Jewish People in America)* (Baltimore: The Johns Hopkins University Press, 1992); and Howard Markel, *Quarantine!: East European Jewish Immigrants and the New York City Epidemics of 1892* (Baltimore: Johns Hopkins University Press, 1999).

34. Zinsser, *Rats, Lice and History* (1934, 1935), 234.

35. See, for example, Nicolle to Zinsser, February 22, 1934, in which Nicolle tells Zinsser to send him his results: "Write in French, and I will give it an impeccable style in this language." By April 2, 1934, Nicolle was completing his revisions, commenting to Zinsser that, if he lived nearer, "I would place myself at your disposal to perfect your French. This would not be a difficult task, because you already possess a sense of the *spirit* of our language. The *spirit* is the most important thing." Zinsser papers (H MS c73), HML/CLM, box 2, folder 90. Emphasis in original.

36. Zinsser, "Sur la Maladie de Brill" (1934), 154.

37. Nicolle to Zinsser, March 8, 1935, Zinsser papers (H MS c73), HML/CLM, box 2, folder 90. Zinsser visited Nicolle in mid-April.

38. Nicolle, "A Propos de Six Cas de Typhus Murin Contractés au Cours de Recherches," *AIPT* 24 (1935): 99–113, 111.

39. Ibid., 110. "Doctor P. G., 35 years old, French"—presumably Paul Giroud—also contracted the disease.

40. Nicolle to Vallery-Radot, March 16, 1934, AIP FR IP NCP.12.

41. Nicolle to Vallery-Radot, September 7, 1934, Ibid.

42. See Duhamel to Nicolle, October 25, 1935 (AIP FR IP NCP.8–10) for details on the inner politics of ensuring that his chosen successor (the surgeon Leriche) would be selected. On Leriche, see Weisz, "Moment of Synthesis," 78, 83–85.

43. Huet, Pommier, 182–83. It appears that numerous colleagues believed Nicolle had promised them the position; during his long illness, tensions escalated. Huet has it on apparently excellent but unnamed authority (ultimately confirmed by a letter from Burnet to Ramon, recounting Marcelle's own account of events) that on the final day of Nicolle's life, one of Nicolle's collaborators had a violent altercation with him (apparently over bad research results, of which Nicolle had learned), jumping on the dying Nicolle and grabbing him by the throat. Nicolle died several hours later.

44. It appears that Nicolle and Burnet's wife, Lydia, had met up while Nicolle was in Paris and Burnet was in Brazil. On June 26, 1934, Burnet resumed correspondence with Nicolle, thanking him for his visits to Lydia in his absence. By winter, the ailing Nicolle asked Burnet to take over some of his lecturing responsibilities at the *Collège de France* (Burnet complied). Nicolle, dying, wrote Burnet a farewell letter on December 9, 1935. In his moving final letter to Nicolle, Burnet mentioned their earlier difficulties and suggested neither of them think about past troubles again (January 15, 1936). All in AIP FR IP NIC.3.

45. Nicolle's influence on future research is strikingly evident in relapsing fever studies. See, for example, Felsenfeld's bibliography and narrative in his *Borrellia*.

46. Nicolle, "Signification de la Forme Inapparent dans la Naissance et de le Déclin des Maladies Infectieuses," *AIPT* 24 (1935): 1–7.

47. Nicolle, "Constitution des Cultures Pures et des Virus en Eléments Vivants. Associations de Virus. Variantes chez les Inframicrobes," *AIPT* 24 (1935): 139–78. This is a particularly fascinating article, in which Nicolle returned to his 1902 paper on variability and recounted what he then knew—and what he had yet to suspect—about microbial mutation: "My error, the error of my contemporaries, was to attribute the differences in the appearance of cultures and their variable sensitivity in relation to agglutinins to the action of *exterior* factors on individual microbes that we thought to be the same in a pure culture, instead of thinking that there existed, in the same culture, particular, divergent types. It must also be said that knowledge of the actions of mutation had not yet entered microbiology laboratories. We all followed Roux in attributing the changes that we observed in bacterial properties to a progressive adaptation" (145–46). Emphasis in original.

48. Nicolle, *La Destinée Humaine* (Tunis: Maison Tunisienne de l'Edition, 1981), 113.

49. Ibid., 9.

50. Ibid., 9, 13–14.

51. Ibid., 111.

52. Duhamel, *Light,* 289. Duhamel also discussed this phenomenon on (182). On Cuénot, see Limoges, "Natural Selection." Also see Nicolle's own *Destinée Humaine:* Cuénot is cited on a number of occasions.

53. Nicolle to Duhamel, February 1, 1935, AIP FR IP NCP.8–10.

54. Nicolle, *Destinée,* 114. Nicolle also described his conversion in letters to his closest friends.

55. Marcelle Nicolle to Duhamel, August 30, 1935, AIP FR IP NCP.8–10.

56. Nicolle to Vallery-Radot, October 3, 1935, AIP FR IP NCP.12.

57. Nicolle's life-ordering certainly included editing. As a Nobel Prize winner with strong sense of history, he could not have failed to think of his own historical future. At certain key moments, important letters are missing from otherwise well-preserved stacks.

58. Nicolle, "Testament," February 20, 1936, ASM 146 J 12.

59. Nicolle to Duhamel, February 1, 1936, AIP NCP.8–10. Indeed, Nicolle expressed to Duhamel his wish that "Habib" be published in many of his final letters.

60. "Codicille," February 20, 1936, ASM 146 J 12.

61. Nicolle to Vallery-Radot, January 21, 1936, AIP FR IP NCP.12.

62. Nicolle, "Mémoires," 88.

63. Nicolle, *Responsabilités,* 37–53, 37. This first volume of *Responsabilités* was published in 1935.

64. Ibid., 44–47, 47–48, respectively.

65. Ibid., 53. For Nicolle's list of France's scientific contributions in North Africa, see pages 51–53.

66. Ibid., 8–9. Nicolle's redefinition of the colonial project in no way excluded paternalism; it did, however, temper it a bit.

67. Interview with M. Said ben Chaabane, former vice president of Tunis, December 21, 1990. Current maps show that the street is still named after Nicolle.

68. Moulin, "Charles Nicolle, Savant Tunisien." On Chadli, "Biographie du Professeur Amor Chadli à l'Occasion de Son Election à l'Académie de Médecine de France," *AIPT* 61 (1984): 247–49. For speeches on the occasion of the IPT's centennial, *AIPT* 71 (1994). Subsequently, Moulin reflected on the festivities in her "Une Généalogie Scientifique: l''Isnad' de Tunis (1883–1993)," in *La Mise en Mémoire de la Science: Pour une Ethnographie Historique des Rites Commémoratifs,* ed. P. G. Abir-Am, 207–24 (Paris: Editions des Archives Contemporaines, 1998).

69. Morris F. Shaffer, letter to the author, October 19, 1992. Again, I am grateful to the late Dr. Shaffer, who always provided warm assistance and even moral support. There is a student award in cellular and molecular biology in his name at Tulane University's medical school.

70. Michel Foucault, *Discipline and Punish: The Birth of the Prison,* trans. Alan Sheridan (London: Allen Lane, 1977); and his *Birth of the Clinic: An Archeology of Medical Perception,* trans. A. M. Sheridan Smith (London: Tavistock, 1973); Said, *Orientalism.*

71. Warwick Anderson, "Disease, Race, and Empire," *BHM* 70 (1996): 62–67, and his "Immunities of Empire: Race, Disease, and the New Tropical Medicine, 1900–1920," *BHM* 70 (1996): 94–118. See also Megan Vaughan, *Curing Their Ills: Colonial Power and African Illness* (Oxford: Polity Press, 1991); Shula Marks, "What Is Colonial about Colonial Medicine? and What Has Happened to Imperialism and Health?" *Social History of Medicine* 10 (1997): 205–19.

72. I am deeply grateful to the Countway's Jack Eckert, who was invaluable in helping me uncover the strange history of the Zinsser/Nicolle papers.

73. Soderqvist, "Existential Projects and Existential Choice in Science."

74. One need not spend much time at the IPP today to recognize the persistence of Nicolle's memory. Many of the researchers with whom I spoke knew well the substance of Nicolle's challenge to the Paris administration. Some even argued that he had—though again, only after World War II—been fully vindicated.

75. Lagrange, *Monsieur Roux,* 242. This is one of the few texts that discusses Nicolle's *NL* article in any detail (and quotes from it at length, 238–41).

76. Nicolle, "Paroles" (1934), 20. In this belief, too, Nicolle was quite typical of his times. Without going much further into this field of analysis, I should point out that this was a time of rabid racial and nationalist sentiment, of sweeping eugenic proclamations. Nicolle, as was his tendency in so many things, avoided the extremes. His closest friends included liberal humanitarians such as Duhamel, and also members of the fascist Action Français. In one instance, Nicolle, who stated his belief that the "black" race had contributed nothing of note to civilization (*Biologie*), still condemned Americans for having a culture that could produce so abhorrent a group as the KKK. For Nicolle, all humanity was one in its right to exist, free of disease, of want. Beyond that, other categories applied. See Weber, *The Hollow Years;* Hughes, *The Obstructed Path.*

BIBLIOGRAPHIC NOTE

There are a number of (mostly French) biographical sources on Nicolle. The Pasteur Institute of Tunis's *Archives* (*AIPT*) includes many such articles. These tend to be gathered around anniversaries of Nicolle's birth (1866), death (1936), discovery of the louse transmission of typhus (1909), or one of the many dates connected with the institute's establishment (foundation and direction by Adrien Loir, 1893–94; elevation to the formal rank of "institute," 1900; Nicolle's directorship, 1903; functioning in its new buildings, 1904; official inauguration, 1905). Many are written by former collaborators. Several were written by close friends and supporters, such as Georges Duhamel and Louis Pasteur Vallery-Radot, while Nicolle was still alive—often in an effort to attract Parisian attention to the accomplishments of their colonial compatriot. Nicolle himself had a healthy appreciation for the historical importance of his work and kept up a voluminous correspondence. (Indeed, the letters exchanged between Nicolle and Georges Duhamel have been published in a collection entitled *Entretiens d'Huministes*, by J.-J. Hueber.) Although there is evidence that Nicolle withheld selective pieces of his correspondence from his final collection, he did make arrangements for that collection to be deposited in his hometown, Rouen. Many of these papers were sealed for some fifty years after his death.

Perhaps the greatest contribution to the preservation of Nicolle's papers and memory was made by his son, Pierre. Not only did Pierre Nicolle write numerous articles on his father and his work; he also used his father's private papers and his connections with his father's colleagues to compile information that he had hoped to turn into a complete biography. This was no small task: Nicolle's scientific writings alone range across a broad spectrum of diseases and techniques. There were, in addition, the administrative, literary, philosophical, sociocultural, and personal dimensions of his life and work. Pierre Nicolle sagely chose to ask others with more specialized knowledge to contribute chapters on select aspects of his father's work. He also, just as sagely, had his father's most important correspondence "translated" into typescript. (Nicolle's handwriting was notoriously poor: others commented on it, and he often apologized for it.) The transcriptions, as well as the completed chapters, are in the "Pierre Nicolle" collection at the Archives of the Pasteur Institute of Paris.

Though Pierre Nicolle never completed his project, in 1995, Maurice Huet, who had long worked at the Pasteur Institute of Tunis, published a biography of Nicolle (*Le Pommier et l'Olivier*) that drew upon these sources. I completed my own dissertation on Nicolle in 1994. Dr. Huet and I exchanged information; however, I did not see his manuscript until after my dissertation was complete. Huet's approach, like Germaine Lot's earlier biography (*Charles Nicolle et la Biologie Conquérante*, 1961), reviews the whole of Nicolle's life and work. Huet includes summaries of Nicolle's literary and philosophical works at the end of his book; Lot generally provides extracts. Given the vast amount of material that a biographical overview demanded, both books tend to be more summary in their treatment of the Nicolle's many contributions. Huet also provides thoughtful assessments of a few "sensitive" episodes in Nicolle's life.

I began my archival research on Nicolle in earnest in 1990, with the support of a Fulbright Dissertation Grant. At the time, the Nicolle collection at Rouen's Archives Départementales de la Seine-Maritime had only recently been opened and was not yet catalogued. (Indeed, the only indication of its existence was a reference to the deposit made earlier by Pierre Nicolle.) Additionally, the Pasteur Institute of Paris had no catalogued papers. I therefore started my work in Tunis, where I was able to consult a number of papers that had been stored in folders. There were also laboratory notebooks. Unfortunately, administrative complications in Tunis have prevented me from securing formal permission to cite these archival materials. I would, however, like to thank Prof. Dellagi, who provided me with reprints of a number of Nicolle's published articles as well as copies of commemorative numbers of the *AIPT*. In Paris, the Pasteur Institute, under energetic archivist Denise Ogilvie, was in the process of gathering together documents relating to its own history. Several papers had previously been catalogued at the IP Musée, under the directorship of Mme. Annick Perrot. Now, however, in the process of seeking out new acquisitions, Denise Ogilvie had discovered Pierre Nicolle's papers, including the notes for the biography of his father and the correspondence typescripts. She opened them—and her archives—to me, allowing me to consult them before they were formally catalogued. Several years later, she provided me with a list of contents and classifications. Subsequently, Stephane Kraxner became the IP's archivist. He, too, has been welcoming and enthusiastic. He has also introduced another classificatory system. I have done my best to determine the proper listings for each document I have cited from the IPP collection, and Stephane Kraxner has kindly assisted me in my efforts to attach proper classifications at a distance.

A similar scenario greeted me at the Rouen archives. The archivists had intended to catalogue the Nicolle materials (some one hundred file boxes), but stepped up their schedule to accommodate the limited timing of my research trip. Indeed, they, too, permitted me to consult the materials before they had finished assigning them formal reference numbers. A subsequent, brief research trip to France and access to the Nicolle collection catalogue have enabled me to assign proper numbers to most of the documents I have used. The collection itself is under "146 J." If there was ambiguity about box numbers, I assigned only this general reference. The Rouen archives, too, provided a delightful working atmosphere.

Finally, a note on the way I have cited published sources. The chapters themselves contain full citations for all of Nicolle's published work except for his annual reports on the "Fonctionnement de l'Institut Pasteur de Tunis." As a rule, these appeared in the *AIPT* (or the *AIPAN*) volume for the subsequent year. Consequently, unless I am citing information from a specific page of the report, I have simply referred to each with a basic shorthand: for example, "Fonctionnement . . . 1909" (1910). In the bibliography, I have listed Nicolle's novels and philosophical treatises at the opening and included the nonscientific articles to which I have referred in the body of the bibliography. For a complete list of Nicolle's scientific articles, see the *AIPT* 26 (1937): 209–48. I have used my own translation of Nicolle's famous Nobel Prize lecture; however, it may also be found in full, and in English translation, at the Nobel Foundation's Nobel Prize Web site: http://nobelprize.org/medicine/laureates/1928/nicolle-lecture.html. Finally, all quotations from Nicolle's books, except those from his *Introduction à la Carrière de la Médecine Expérimentale*, are taken from the original editions. For the *Introduction,* I have instead used the 1981 reissue, published by the Maison Tunisienne de l'Edition (Tunis). The volume includes an introductory essay by the IPT's longtime director Prof. Amor Chadli, another central contributor to the preservation of Nicolle's legacy. The book was given to me by Prof. Dellagi. I am grateful to both men for their kind assistance and support.

Bibliography

Scientific and Philosophical Books by Nicolle:

Biologie de l'Invention. Paris: Félix Alcan, 1932.
Destin des Maladies Infectieuses. Paris: Félix Alcan, 1933.
La Destinée Humaine. Paris: Félix Alcan, 1936.
L'Expérimentation en Médecine. Paris: Félix Alcan, 1934.
Introduction à la Carrière de la Médecine Expérimentale. Paris: Félix Alcan, 1932.
Naissance, Vie et Mort des Maladies Infectieuses. Paris: Félix Alcan, 1930.
La Nature: Conception et Morale Biologique. Paris: Félix Alcan, 1934.
Responsabilités de la Médecine, 2 vols. Paris: Félix Alcan, 1935–36.

Novels by Nicolle:

Les Contes de Marmouse et de Ses Hôtes. Paris: Reider, 1930.
Les Deux Larrons. Paris: Calmann-Lévy, 1929.
Les Feuilles de la Sagittaire. Paris: Calmann-Lévy, 1920.
Marmouse et Ses Hôtes. Paris: Reider, 1927.
Les Menus Plaisirs de l'Ennui. Paris: Calmann-Lévy, 1924.
La Narqoise. Paris: Calmann-Lévy, 1922.
Le Pâtissier de Bellone. Paris: Calmann-Lévy, 1913.

Other Sources:

Abdel-Hameed, Ahmed Awad. "The Wellcome Tropical Research Laboratories in Khartoum (1903–34): An Experiment in Development." *Medical History* 41 (1997): 30–58.

Adas, Michael. *Machines as the Measure of Men: Science, Technology, and Ideologies of Western Dominance*. Ithaca, NY: Cornell University Press, 1989.
Allen, Garland E. *Life Sciences in the Twentieth Century*. Cambridge: Cambridge University Press, 1978.
———. "Naturalists and Experimentalists: The Genotype and the Phenotype." In *Studies in the History of Biology*, edited by William Coleman and Camille Limoges, 179–209. Baltimore: Johns Hopkins University Press, 1979.
Amsterdamska, Olga. "Medical and Biological Constraints: Early Research on Variation in Bacteriology." *Social Studies of Science* 17 (1987): 657–87.
———. "Stabilizing Instability: The Controversy over Cyclogenic Theories of Bacterial Variation During the Interwar Period." *Journal of the History of Biology* 24 (1991): 191–222.
———. "Standardizing Epidemics: Infection, Inheritance, and Environment in Prewar Experimental Epidemiology." In Gaudillière and Löwy, *Heredity and Infection*, 135–79.
Anderson, Benedict. *Imagined Communities: Reflections on the Origin and Spread of Nationalism*. Rev. ed. London: Verso Press, 1993.
Anderson, John F., and Joseph Goldberger. "The Relation of So-Called Brill's Disease to Typhus Fever." *Public Health Reports* 27 (1912): 149–60.
Anderson, Lisa. *The State and Social Transformation in Tunisia and Libya, 1830–1980*. Princeton: Princeton University Press, 1986.
Anderson, Warwick. "Disease, Race, and Empire." *BHM* 70 (1996): 62–67.
———. "How's the Empire? An Essay Review." *JHM* 58 (2003): 459–65.
———. "Immunities of Empire: Race, Disease, and the New Tropical Medicine, 1900–1920." *BHM* 70 (1996): 94–118.
———. "Natural Histories of Infectious Disease: Ecological Vision in Twentieth-Century Biomedical Science." *Osiris* 19 (2004): 39–61.
Anker, Peder. *Imperial Ecology: Environmental Order in the British Empire, 1895–1945*. Cambridge, MA: Harvard University Press, 2001.
Annabi-Ben Nefissa, Kmar. "L'Organisation Sanitaire en Tunisie à la Veille de la Création de l'Institut Pasteur de Tunis." *AIPT* 71 (1994): 345–49.
Antliff, Mark. *Inventing Bergson: Cultural Politics and the Parisian Avant-Garde*. Princeton: Princeton University Press, 1993.
Arnold, David. *Colonizing the Body: State Medicine and Epidemic Disease in Nineteenth Century India*. Berkeley: University of California Press, 1993.
———, ed. *Imperial Medicine and Indigenous Societies: Disease, Medicine, and Empire in the Nineteenth and Twentieth Centuries*. Manchester: Manchester University Press, 1988.
———. "Medicine and Colonialism." In *Companion Encyclopedia of the History of Medicine*, edited by W. F. Bynum and Roy Porter. 2 vols., 2: 1393–1416. London: Routledge, 1993.
Association pour l'Extension des Études Pastoriennes. Paris: R. Tancrède, 1921.
Bacon, Francis. *The New Organon*. Edited by Fulton H. Anderson. Indianapolis: Bobbs-Merrill, 1960.
Balfour, Andrew. "Introduction." *First Report of the Wellcome Research Laboratories at the Gordon Memorial College, Khartoum*. Khartoum: Department of Education, Sudan Government, 1904.

Balinska, Marta Aleksandra. "The Rockefeller Foundation and the National Institute of Hygiene, Poland, 1918–45." *Studies in History and Philosophy of Biological and Biomedical Sciences* 31 (2000): 419–32.
Baltazard, M. "Le Respect des Conditions de la Nature dans l'Expérimentation." *AIPT* 43 (1966): 35–46.
Barykine, W., S. Minervine, and A. Kompaneez. "Le Typhus Exanthématique Inapparente et Son Importance Epidemiologique." *AIPT* 19 (1930): 422–32.
Bell, Catherine. *Ritual: Perspectives and Dimensions.* New York: Oxford University Press, 1997.
Benenson, Abram S., ed. *Control of Communicable Diseases in Man.* 14th ed. Washington, DC: American Public Health Association, 1985.
Bernard, Noel. *La Vie et l'Oeuvre d'Albert Calmette.* Paris: La Colombe, 1961.
Bertholon, Lucien Joseph. "Étude Statistique sur la Colonie Française de Tunisie, 1881–1892." *Revue Tunisienne* 1 (1894): 362–78.
———. "Mentalité Française et Colonisation Tunisienne." *Revue Tunisienne* 8 (1901): 379–406.
Bertholon, Lucien Joseph, and Ernest Chantre. *Recherches Anthropologiques dans la Berberie Orientale, Tripolitaine, Tunisie, Algérie.* Lyon: A. Rey, 1912–13.
"Biographie du Professeur Amor Chadli à l'Occasion de Son Election à l'Académie de Médecine de France." *AIPT* 61 (1984): 247–49.
Birn, Anne-Emanuelle. "Wa(i)ves of Influence: Rockefeller Public Health in Mexico, 1920–50." *Studies in History and Philosophy of Biological and Biomedical Sciences* 31 (2000): 381–95.
Black, Max. "Metaphor." In *Models and Metaphors: Studies in Language and Philosophy.* Ithaca, NY: Cornell University Press, 1962.
Blaizot, Ludovic, and E. Gobert. "Deux Epidémies de Fièvre Récurrente en Tunisie: Leur Origine Tripolitaine." *AIPT* 6 (1911): 278–80.
Blanc, Georges, J. Caminopetros, and E. Manoussakis. "Mémoires: Quelques Recherches Expérimentales sur la Dengue." *BSPE* (1928): 525–37.
Bliss, Michael. *The Discovery of Insulin.* Chicago: University of Chicago Press, 1982.
Bowler, Peter J. *Evolution: The History of an Idea.* 3rd ed., rev. Berkeley: University of California Press, 2003.
———. *The Mendelian Revolution: The Emergence of Hereditarian Concepts in Modern Science and Society.* London: Athlone Press, 1989.
Brandt, Allan M. *No Magic Bullet: A Social History of Venereal Disease in the United States since 1880.* Expanded edition. New York: Oxford University Press, 1987.
Breinl, Frederic. "Sur les Relations du Virus Exanthématique et des Bacilles Proteus X." *AIPT* 13 (1924): 208–11.
Brill, Nathan. "An Acute Infectious Disease of Unknown Origin: A Clinical Study Based on 221 Cases." *American Journal of the Medical Sciences* 139 (1910): 484–502.
———. "The Form of Typhus Fever That Is Now Endemic in New York City." *Medical Record* 88 (1915): 914–17.
———. "On the Identity of Typhus Fever and Brill's Disease." *Medical Record* 81 (1912): 1037–38.
———. "Pathological and Experimental Data Derived from a Further Study of an Acute Infectious Disease of Unknown Origin." *American Journal of the Medical Sciences* 142 (1911): 196–218.

Brill, Nathan. "A Study of Seventeen Cases of a Disease Clinically Resembling Typhoid Fever, But Without the Widal Reaction." *New York Medical Journal* 67 (1898): 48–54, 77–82.

Brunschwig, Henri. *French Colonialism, 1871–1914: Myths and Realities.* New York: Frederick A. Praeger, 1966.

Bulloch, William. *The History of Bacteriology.* London: Oxford University Press, 1938.

Burgdorfer, Willy, and Robert L. Anacker, eds. *Rickettsiae and Rickettsial Diseases.* New York: Academic Press, 1981.

Burian, Richard M., Jean Gayon, and Doris Zallen. "The Singular Fate of Genetics in the History of French Biology, 1900–1940." *Journal of the History of Biology* 21 (1988): 357–402.

Burke, Timothy. "Colonialism, Cleanliness, and Civilization in Colonial Rhodesia." In Conklin and Fletcher, *European Imperialism,* 86–95.

Burnet, Etienne. "Charles Nicolle." *AIPT* 43 (1966): 91–97.

Burnet, F. Macfarlane. *Biological Aspects of Infectious Disease.* Cambridge: Cambridge University Press, 1940.

Butler, Thomas. "Relapsing Fever." In *Hunter's Tropical Medicine and Emerging Infectious Diseases.* 8th ed., edited by G. Thomas Strickland, 448–52. Philadelphia: W. B. Saunders, 2000.

Calmette, Albert. *Les Missions Scientifique de l'Institut Pasteur et l'Expansion Coloniale de la France.* Paris, 1923.

Calmette, Albert, H. Parenty, and A. Wits. "Protestation des Savants de Lille contre les Actes de Barbarie des Allemands." *Presse Médicale* 26 (1918): 557–58.

Cannon, Walter B. *The Wisdom of the Body.* London: Kegan Paul, 1932.

Carter, Edward C., Robert Forster, and Joseph N. Moody, eds. *Enterprise and Entrepreneurs in Nineteenth- and Twentieth-Century France.* Baltimore: Johns Hopkins University Press, 1976.

Carter, K. Codell. "The Development of Pasteur's Concept of Disease Causation and the Emergence of Specific Causes in Nineteenth-Century Medicine." *BHM* 65 (1991): 528–48.

———. *The Rise of Causal Concepts of Disease: Case Histories.* Aldershot, England: Ashgate, 2003.

"La Célébration du 25me Anniversaire du Docteur Charles Nicolle à la Direction de l'Institut Pasteur de Tunis, 28 Avril 1928." *Revue Tunisienne des Sciences Médicale* 22 (1928): 119–48.

"Le Centenaire de Pasteur: Une Exposition Pastorienne au Palais des Sociétés Françaises." *Dépêche Tunisienne,* December 26, 1922.

Chadli, Amor. "Charles Nicolle et les Acquis de sa Periode Scientifique." *AIPT* 63 (1936): 3–14.

Chambers, David Wade. "Does Distance Tyrannize Science?" In Home and Kohlstedt, *International Science and National Scientific Identity,* 19–38.

Charle, Christophe, and Eva Telkès. *Les Professeurs du Collège de France: Dictionnaire Biographique, 1901–39.* Paris: Institut National de Recherche Pédagogique, 1988.

Charvet, Patrick Edward. *A Literary History of France: The Nineteenth and Twentieth Centuries.* New York: Barnes and Noble, 1967.

Chatelain, Yves, *La Vie Littéraire et Intellectuelle en Tunisie de 1900 à 1937*. Paris: Guenther, 1937.
Chatton, E. "Le Laboratoire Militaire de Bactériologie du sud-Tunisien (à Gabès): Organisation Rendement du 1er Août 1916 au 1er Juillet 1918." *AIPT* 10 (1917–18): 199–242.
Coleman, William. "Koch's Comma Bacillus: The First Year." *BHM* 61 (1987): 315–42.
Collard, Patrick. *The Development of Microbiology*. Cambridge: Cambridge University Press, 1976.
Comité d'Histoire du Service de Santé. *Historie de la Médecine aux Armées*. 3 vols. Paris: Charles-Lavauzelle, 1982–87.
"Compte Rendu de la Réception faite le 22 Octobre 1927, à l'Hôtel de Ville, par M. le Maire et le Conseil Municipal, en l'Honneur du Dr. Charles Nicolle, Lauréat du Prix Osiris." Pamphlet.
Comte, Charles. "Contribution à l'Historie du Rôle du Pou dans la Transmission du Typhus Exanthématique." *Revue Moderne de Médecine et de Chirurgie* 30 (1932): 303–6, 331–34.
———. "Contribution à l'Historie du Typhus Exanthématique." *Revue Moderne de Médecine et de Chirurgie* 30 (1932): 83–85.
Conklin, Alice L. *A Mission to Civilize: The Republican Idea of Empire in France and West Africa, 1895–1930*. Stanford, CA: Stanford University Press, 1997.
Conklin, Alice L., and Ian Christopher Fletcher, eds. *European Imperialism, 1830–1930: Climax and Contradiction*. Boston: Houghton Mifflin, 1999.
———. "Introduction." In Conklin and Fletcher, *European Imperialism*, 1–9.
Conry, Yvette. *L'Introduction du Darwinisme en France au dix-neuvième siecle*. Paris: J. Vrin, 1974.
Conseil, Ernest. "Discours du Docteur Conseil." *Revue Tunisien des Sciences Médicales* 22 (1926): 123–31.
———. "Rapport du Chef du Bureau d'Hygiène, 1910." *Bulletin Officiel Municipal de la Ville de Tunis* 3 (1911): 91–166.
———. "Rapport du Chef du Bureau d'Hygiène de Tunis pour l'Année 1909." *Bulletin Officiel Municipal de la Ville de Tunis* 2 (1910): 125–96.
———. "Résultats de la Prophylaxie du Typhus Exanthématique à Tunis de 1909 à 1912." *Tunisie Médicale* 2 (1912): 401–2.
———. "Le Typhus Exanthématique en Tunisie." *AIPT* 2 (1907): 145–54.
———. "Le Typhus Exanthématique en Tunisie Pendant l'Année 1909." *AIPT* 5 (1910): 19–42.
———. "Le Typhus Exanthématique en Tunisie Pendant l'Année 1910." *AIPT* 6 (1911): 134–49.
Cooper, Frederick, and Ann Laura Stoler, eds. *Tensions of Empire: Colonial Cultures in a Bourgeois World*. Berkeley: University of California Press, 1997.
Crawford, Elisabeth. *The Beginnings of the Nobel Institution: The Science Prizes, 1901–1915*. Cambridge: Cambridge University Press, 1984.
———. "The Prize System of the Academy of Sciences, 1850–1914." In Fox and Weisz, *Organization of Science and Technology*, 283–307.
Creager, Angela N. H. *The Life of a Virus: Tobacco Mosaic Virus as an Experimental Model, 1930–1965*. Chicago: University of Chicago Press, 2002.

Crosby, Alfred W. *America's Forgotten Pandemic: The Influenza of 1918*. Cambridge: Cambridge University Press, 1989.
Cross, Stephen J., and William R. Albury. "Walter B. Cannon, L. J. Henderson, and the Organic Analogy." *Osiris* 3 (1987): 165–92.
Curtin, Philip D. *Death by Migration: Europe's Encounter with the Tropical World in the Nineteenth Century*. Cambridge: Cambridge University Press, 1989.
———. *Disease and Empire: The Health of European Troops in the Conquest of Africa*. Cambridge: Cambridge University Press, 1998.
Dana, Raoul. "La Société des Sciences Médicales de Tunisie de 1902 à 1952." In *Médecine et Médecins de Tunisie de 1902 à 1952*. Edited by the Société des Sciences Médicales de Tunisie. Tunis, 1952.
de Kruif, Paul. *Microbe Hunters*. San Diego: Harvest/HBJ, 1926, 1954.
Debré, Patrice. *Louis Pasteur*. Translated by Elborg Forster. Baltimore: Johns Hopkins University Press, 1998.
Delattre, A. L. "Documents pour Servir à l'Histoire de la Pathologie Infectieuse de l'Afrique Mineure: La Peste à Carthage en 253." *AIPT* 3 (1908): 133–38.
Delaunay, Ablert. *l'Institut Pasteur des Origines à Aujourd'hui*. Paris: France-Empire, 1962.
Deleuze, Gilles. *Bergsonism*. Translated by Hugh Tomlinson and Barbara Habberjam. New York: Zone Books, 1988.
Dible, J. Henry. *Recent Advances in Bacteriology and the Study of the Infections*. 2nd ed. London: J. & A. Church, 1932.
"Discussion, Nicolle, 'Unité ou Pluralité des Typhus.'" *BSPE* 26 (1933): 331–40.
Dostoevsky, Fyodor. "Dream of a Ridiculous Man." Translated by Constance Garnett, www.ellopos.net/politics/eu_dostoyiefsky.html
Douglas, Mary. *Purity and Danger: An Analysis of Concepts of Pollution and Taboo*. London: Routledge, 1966, 1984.
Doury, Paul. "Henry Foley et la Découverte du Rôle du Pou dans la Transmission de la Fièvre Récurrente et du Typhus Exanthématique." *Histoire des Sciences Médicales* 30 (1996): 363–69.
Drayton, Richard. *Nature's Government: Science, Imperial Britain, and the 'Improvement' of the World*. New Haven: Yale University Press, 2000.
Duclaux, Emile. *Pasteur: Histoire d'un Esprit*. Sceaux: Charaire, 1896.
———. *Pasteur: The History of a Mind*. Edited and translated by Erwin F. Smith and Florence Hedges. Philadelphia: W. B. Saunders, 1920; Metuchen, NJ: Scarecrow Reprint Corporation, 1973.
———. "Preface." *BIP* 1 (1903): 1–3.
———. *Traité de Microbiologie*. 4 vols. Paris: Masson et Cie, 1898.
Duhamel, Georges. *Civilization, 1914–1917*. Translated by E. S. Brooks. New York: The Century Co., 1919.
———. *L'Humaniste et L'Automate*. Paris: Hartmann, 1933.
———. *Light on My Days*. Translated by Basil Collier. London: J. M. Dent & Sons, 1948.
———. *Le Prince Jaffar*. Paris: Mercure de France, 1924, 1946.
———. *Scènes de la Vie Future*. Paris: Mercure de France, 1930.
———. "Voies de Communication." *Mercure de France* 280 (1937): 5–8.
Dutton, J. Everett, and John L. Todd. "The Nature of Tick Fever in the Eastern Part of the Congo Free State." *BMJ* 2 (1905): 1259–60.

Dyer, R. E. "A Virus of the Typhus Type Derived from Fleas Collected from Wild Rats." *Public Health Reports* 46 (1931): 334–38.
Edel, Leon. *Writing Lives: Principia Biographica.* New York: Norton, 1959, 1984.
Eliot, T. S. "The Hollow Men." In *Poems, 1909–25.* London: Faber and Gwyer, 1925.
Elwitt, Sanford. *The Third Republic Defended: Bourgeois Reform in France, 1880–1914.* Baton Rouge: Louisiana State University Press, 1986.
Espie, A. "Fonctionnement du Laboratoire Régional de Sfax (Année 1925)." *AIPT* 15 (1926): 194–96.
Ettling, John. *The Germ of Laziness: Rockefeller Philanthropy and Public Health in the New South.* Cambridge, MA: Harvard University Press, 1981.
"Experimental Transmission of Typhus to Man." *Lancet* 1 (1922): 445.
Eyquem, André, and Jacqueline de Saint Martin. "Hommage à Charles Nicolle: Naissance, Éclipse et Résurgence du Concept et des Maladies par Auto-immunisation." *AIPT* 64 (1987): 5–14.
Fabiani, G. "Genèse et Signification du Concept d'Infection Inapparente dans l'œuvre de Charles Nicolle." *La Semaine des Hôpitaux* 48 (1946): 2879–88.
———. "L'Intérêt Toujours Actuel des Infections Inapparentes." *Annales d'Hygiène de Langue Française* 3 (1967): 58–67.
———. "Un Problème de Pathologie Générale: La Définition de l'Infection Inapparente." *Revue de Pathologie Comparée et de Médecine Expérimentale* 68 (1968): 217–22.
Falk, Raphael. "What Is a Gene?" *Studies in History and Philosophy of Science* 17 (1986): 133–73.
Farley, John, and Gerald L. Geison. "Science, Politics and Spontaneous Generation in Nineteenth-Century France: The Pasteur–Pouchet Debate." *BHM* 48 (1974): 161–98.
Felsenfeld, Oscar. *Borrelia: Strains, Vectors, Human and Animal Borreliosis.* St. Louis: Warren H. Green, 1971.
Fleck, Ludwig. *Genesis and Development of a Scientific Fact.* Edited by Thaddeus J. Trenn and Robert K. Merton, translated by Fred Bradley and Thaddeus J. Trenn. Chicago: University of Chicago Press, 1979.
"Fonctionnement du Laboratoire Régional de Sousse (Année 1922)." *AIPT* 12 (1923): 254–59.
Foster, Gaines M. "Typhus Disaster in the Wake of War: The American–Polish Relief Expedition, 1919–1920." *BHM* 55 (1981): 221–32.
Foucault, Michel. *The Birth of the Clinic. An Archaeology of Medical Perception.* Translated by A. M. Sheridan Smith. [London]: Tavistock, 1973.
———. *Discipline and Punish: The Birth of the Prison.* Translated by Alan Sheridan. London: Allen Lane, 1977.
Fox, Robert. "The *Savant* Confronts His Peers: Scientific Societies in France, 1815–1914." In Fox and Weisz, *Organization of Science and Technology,* 241–82.
Fox, Robert, and George Weisz, "Introduction: The Institutional Basis of French Science in the Nineteenth Century." In Fox and Weisz, *Organization of Science and Technology,* 1–28.
———, eds., *The Organization of Science and Technology in France, 1808–1914.* Cambridge: Cambridge University Press, 1980.
Frank, Joseph. *Dostoevsky: The Mantle of the Prophet, 1871–81.* Princeton: Princeton University Press, 2002.

Friéderich, Jean. "Un Grand Savant Français: Une Heure avec le Docteur Charles Nicolle." *Journal de Rouen,* February 1, 1932.
Fussell, Paul. *The Great War and Modern Memory.* New York: Oxford University Press, 1989.
Galison, Peter. "History, Philosophy, and the Central Metaphor." *Science in Context* 2 (1988): 197–212.
Gallagher, Nancy. *Medicine and Power in Tunisia, 1780–1900.* New York: Cambridge University Press, 1983.
Galperin, Charles. "Le Bactériophage, la Lysogénie et Son Déterminisme Génétique." *History and Philosophy of the Life Sciences* 9 (1987): 175–224.
Garnham, P. C. C. "Charles Nicolle and Inapparent Infections." *American Journal of Tropical Medicine and Hygiene* 26 (1977): 1101–4.
Garrett, Laurie. *The Coming Plague: Newly Emerging Diseases in a World Out of Balance.* New York: Farrar, Straus and Giroux, 1994.
Geison, Gerald. "Pasteur." In *Dictionary of Scientific Biography,* edited by Charles Coulston Gillispie. 16 vols., 10: 350–416. New York: Scribner and Sons, 1972.
——— . "Pasteur, Roux, and Rabies: Scientific *versus* Clinical Mentalities." *JHM* 45 (1990): 341–65.
——— . *The Private Science of Louis Pasteur.* Princeton: Princeton University Press, 1995.
Geison, Gerald, and Manfred D. Laubichler. "The Varied Lives of Organisms: Variation in the Historiography of the Biological Sciences." *Studies in the History and Philosophy of Biology and the Biomedical Sciences* 32 (2001): 1–29.
Gellner, Ernest. *Nations and Nationalism.* Ithaca, NY: Cornell University Press, 1983.
Gheorghiu, Marina. "Le BCG, Vaccin Contre la Tuberculose: Leçons du Passe pour Aujourd'hui." In Moulin, *L'Aventure de la Vaccination,* 219–28.
Gildea, Robert. *The Past in French History.* New Haven: Yale University Press, 1994.
Giroud, Paul. "Eloge: Charles Nicolle (1866–1936)." *Bulletin de l'Académie Nationale de Medecine* 45 (1961): 714–22.
Giroud, Paul, and J. B. Jadin. "Les Maladies Inapparentes de Charles Nicolle, les Affections Superposées sont à la Base des Faillites de l'Immunité." *AIPT* 63 (1986): 97–99.
Giroud, Paul, and H. Plotz. "Etude Expérimentale des Infections, Déterminées par les Cultures des Virus Typhiques Historique ou Murin, et des Immunités Qu'elles Déterminent vis-à-vis de Ces Virus ou de Leurs Cultures." *AIPT* 24 (1935): 420–34.
Grandsire, G. "L'Hôpital Sadiki de 1902 à 1915 sous la Direction de Brunswic-le-Bihan." *Tunisie Médicale* 25 (1931): 240–48.
Grmek, Mirko D. "A Plea for Freeing the History of Scientific Discoveries from Myth." In *On Scientific Discovery,* edited by M. D. Grmek, R. S. Cohen, and Guido Cimino, 9–42. Dordrecht, Holland: R. Reidel, 1980.
Guégan, A. "L'Evolution de l'Assistance Médicale en Tunisie." *Tunisie Médicale* 3 (1913): 150–53.
Guégan, F.-J. "La Station Sanitaire de La Goulette: Son Fonctionnement Pendant la Dernière Campagne Anticholérique." *AIPT* 7 (1912): 53–60.
Guénel, Annick. "The Creation of the First Overseas Pasteur Institute, or the Beginning of Albert Calmette's Pastorian Career." *Medical History* 43 (1999): 1–25.
Hadley, Philip. "Microbial Dissociation." *Journal of Infectious Disease* 40 (1927): 1–312.
Hamburger, Viktor. "Wilhelm Roux: Visionary with a Blind Spot." *Journal of the History of Biology* 30 (1997): 229–38.

Hanna, Martha. *The Mobilization of Intellect: French Scholars and Writers During the Great War.* Cambridge, MA: Harvard University Press, 1996.
Hannaford, Ivan. *Race: The History of an Idea in the West.* Baltimore: Johns Hopkins University Press, 1996.
Harant, H. "Charles Nicolle, 'Inventeur' de l'Ecologie Médicale." *AIPT* 43 (1966): 323–30.
Harden, Victoria. "Koch's Postulates and the Etiology of Rickettsial Diseases." *JHM* 42 (1987): 277–95.
———. *Rocky Mountain Spotted Fever: History of a Twentieth-Century Disease.* Baltimore: Johns Hopkins University Press, 1990.
Harrison, Mark. *Climates and Constitutions: Health, Race, Environment, and British Imperialism in India, 1600–1850.* New Delhi: Oxford University Press, 1999.
———. *Public Health in British India: Anglo-American Preventive Medicine, 1859–1914.* Cambridge: Cambridge University Press, 1994.
Haynes, Douglas M. *Imperial Medicine: Patrick Manson and the Conquest of Tropical Disease.* Philadelphia: University of Pennsylvania Press, 2001.
Headrick, Daniel R. *The Tools of Empire: Technology and European Imperialism in the Nineteenth Century.* New York: Oxford University Press, 1981.
Hildreth, Martha Lee. *Doctors, Bureaucrats, and Public Health in France, 1888–1902.* New York: Garland, 1986.
Hirsch, August. *Handbook of Geographical and Historical Pathology.* 3 vols., 2nd ed., translated by Charles Creighton. London: New Sydenham Society, 1883–86.
Hobsbawm, Eric. *The Age of Empire, 1875–1914.* New York: Vintage Books, 1989.
Holmes, Frederic L. "Claude Bernard, the 'Milieu Intérieur,' and Regulatory Physiology." *History and Philosophy of the Life Sciences* 8 (1986): 3–25.
———. *Investigative Pathways: Patterns and Stages in the Careers of Experimental Scientists.* New Haven: Yale University Press, 2004.
Home, R. W., and Sally Gregory Kohlstedt, eds. *International Science and National Scientific Identity: Australia between Britain and America.* Dordrecht, Holland: Klewer, 1991.
Horder, T. J., J. A. Witkowski, and C. C. Wylie, eds. *A History of Embryology.* Cambridge: Cambridge University Press, 1985, 1986.
Hueber, J.-J., ed. *Entretiens d'Humanistes: Correspondance de Charles Nicolle et Georges Duhamel, 1922–1936.* Rouen: Académie des Sciences, Belles-Lettres et Arts de Rouen, 1996.
Huet, Maurice. "L'Expérimentation Humaine au Temps de Charles Nicolle." *Histoire des Sciences Médicales* 34 (2000): 409–14.
———. *Le Pommier et l'Olivier: Charles Nicolle, une Biographie (1866–1936).* Paris: Sauramps Médical, 1995.
Hughes, H. Stuart. *Consciousness and Society: The Reorientation of European Social Thought, 1890–1930.* New York: Vintage, 1961, 1977.
L'Institut Pasteur: Cinquantenaire de la Fondation. Paris: J. Demoulin, 1939.
Keating, L. Clark. *Critic of Civilization: Georges Duhamel and His Writings.* Lexington: University of Kentucky Press, 1965.
Keating, Peter. "Vaccine Therapy and the Problem of Opsonins." *JHM* 43 (1988): 275–96.
Kennou, M. F. "Propos sur *Toxoplasma gondii.*" *AIPT* 63 (1986): 123–32.
Kevles, Daniel J. *In the Name of Eugenics: Genetics and the Uses of Human Heredity.* New York: Knopf, 1985.

Kevles, Daniel J., and Gerald L. Geison. "The Experimental Life Sciences in the Twentieth Century." *Osiris* 10 (1995): 97–121.

Kingsland, Sharon. "The Battling Botanist: Daniel Trembly MacDougal, Mutation Theory, and the Rise of Experimental Evolutionary Biology in America, 1900–1912." *Isis* 82 (1991): 479–509.

Knapp, Bettina L. *Georges Duhamel*. New York: Twayne Publishers, 1972.

Kohler, Robert E. "Bacterial Physiology: The Medical Context." *BHM* 59 (1985): 54–74.

———. "Innovation in Normal Science: Bacterial Physiology." *Isis* 76 (1985): 162–81.

———. *Lords of the Fly: Drosophila Genetics and the Experimental Life*. Chicago: University of Chicago Press, 1994.

Kolata, Gina. *Flu: The Story of the Great Influenza Pandemic of 1918 and the Search for the Virus That Caused It*. New York: Farrar, Straus and Giroux, 1999.

Kolle, W. "Aktive Immunisierung und Schutzimpfung." *Zentralblatt für Bakteriologie, Parasitenkunde und Infektionskrankheiten* 104 (1927): 90–115.

Kraut, Alan M. *Goldberger's War: The Life and Work of a Public Health Crusader*. New York: Hill and Wang, 2003.

LaBerge, Marie-Paule. "Les Instituts Pasteur du Maghreb: La Recherche Scientifique Médicale dans le Cadre de la Politique Coloniale." *Revue Français d'Histoire d'Outre-Mer* 74 (1987): 27–42.

LaChenal, Guillaume. "Le Centre Pasteur de Cameroun: Trajectoire Historique, Stratégies et Pratiques de la Science Biomédicale Post-Coloniale (1959–2002)." Thesis, University of Paris VII, n.d.

———. "Franco-African Familiarities: A History of the Pasteur Institute of Cameroon, 1945–2000." Manuscript.

Lagrange, Emile. *Monsieur Roux*. Bruxelles: Goemaere [1954?].

Laigret, Jean. *Titres et Travaux Scientifiques du Dr. J. Laigret, Chef de Laboratoire à l'Institut Pasteur de Tunis*. Tunis: J. Aloccio, 1936.

Lakoff, George, and Mark Johnson. *Metaphors We Live By*. Chicago: University of Chicago Press, 1980.

Latour, Bruno. *Pasteur: Une Science, un Style, un Siècle*. Paris: Perrin, Pasteur Institute, 1994.

———. *The Pasteurization of France*. Translated by Alan Sheridan and John Law. Cambridge, MA: Harvard University Press, 1988.

———. *Science in Action: How to Follow Scientists and Engineers through Society*. Cambridge, MA: Harvard University Press, 1987.

———. *We Have Never Been Modern*. Translated by Catherine Porter. New York: Harvester Wheatsheaf, 1993.

Lawrence, Christopher, and George Weisz, eds. *Greater Than the Parts: Holism in Biomedicine, 1920–1950*. New York: Oxford University Press, 1998.

Leavitt, Judith Walzer. *Typhoid Mary: Captive to the Public's Health*. Boston: Beacon Press, 1996.

Lebovics, Herman. *True France: The Wars over Cultural Identity, 1900–1945*. Ithaca, NY: Cornell University Press, 1994.

Lederer, Susan E. *Subjected to Science: Human Experimentation in America before the Second World War*. Baltimore: Johns Hopkins University Press, 1995.

Ledingham, J. C. G., and J. A. Arkwright. *The Carrier Problem in Infectious Diseases*. London: Edward Arnold, 1912.

Lefèvre, Frédéric [Charles Nicolle]. "Une Heure avec le Docteur Charles Nicolle, Professeur au Collège de France—Prix Nobel 1928. La Grande Misère de l'Institut Pasteur: Un Cri d'Alarme." *Nouvelles Littéraires,* February 3, 1934.

Leishman, William B. "An Experimental Investigation of *Spirochaeta duttoni*, the Parasite of Tick Fever." *Lancet* 2 (1920): 1237–44.

Lenoir, Timothy. "A Magic Bullet: Research for Profit and the Growth of Knowledge in Germany around 1900." *Minerva* 26 (1988): 66–88.

Leonard, Jacques. "Comment Peut-on être Pasteurien?" In Salomon-Bayet, *Pasteur et la Révolution Pastorienne,* 143–79.

Levere, Trevor H. "Romanticism, Natural Philosophy and the Sciences: A Review and Bibliographic Essay." *Perspectives on Science* 4 (1996): 463–88.

Levy, Stuart B. *The Antibiotic Paradox: How the Misuse of Antibiotics Destroys Their Curative Powers.* 2nd ed. Cambridge, MA: Perseus, 2002.

Liebenau, Jonathan, ed. *Pill Peddlers: Essays on the History of the Pharmaceutical Industry.* Madison, WI: American Institute of the History of Pharmacy, 1990.

Liebenau, Jonathan, and Michael Robson. "L'Institut Pasteur et l'Industrie Pharmaceutique." In *L'Institut Pasteur: Contributions à son Histoire,* edited by Michel Morange, 52–61. Paris: Editions la Découverte, 1991.

Limoges, Camille. "Natural Selection, Phagocytosis, and Preadaptation: Lucien Cuénot, 1886–1901." *JHM* 31 (1976): 176–214.

Loir, Adrien. "Démographie: Statistique de la Population de Tunis." *Revue Tunisienne* 5 (1898): 348–453.

———. "La Vaccination Obligatoire en Tunisie." *Revue Tunisienne* 4 (1897): 405–15.

Lot, Germaine. *Charles Nicolle et la Biologie Conquérante.* Paris: Editions Seghers, 1961.

Löwy, Ilana. "From Guinea Pigs to Man: The Development of Haffkine's Anticholera Vaccine." *JHM* 47 (1992): 270–309.

Löwy, Ilana, and Patrick Zylberman. "Introduction: Medicine as a Social Instrument: Rockefeller Foundation, 1913–45." *Studies in History and Philosophy of Biological and Biomedical Sciences* 31 (2000): 365–79.

"Ludovic Blaizot." *AIPT* 32 (1955): 11–15.

Mackie, F. Percival. "The Part Played by Pediculus Corporis in the Transmission of Relapsing Fever." *BMJ* 2 (1907): 1706–9.

MacLeod, Roy, and Milton Lewis, eds. *Disease, Medicine, and Empire: Perspectives on Western Medicine and the Experience of European Expansion.* London: Routledge, 1988.

Malinas, M., and M. Tostivint. "Mutualité Coopérative et Projet Général d'Assistance Médical Indigène." *Revue Tunisienne* 12 (1905): 283–304, 386–422, 480–515.

Markel, Howard. *Quarantine! East European Jewish Immigrants and the New York City Epidemics of 1892.* Baltimore: Johns Hopkins University Press, 1999.

———. *When Germs Travel: Six Major Epidemics that Have Invaded America since 1900 and the Fears They Have Unleashed.* New York: Pantheon, 2004.

Marks, Shula. "What Is Colonial about Colonial Medicine? and What Has Happened to Imperialism and Health?" *Social History of Medicine* 10 (1997): 205–19.

Marks, Shula, and Neil Andersson. "Typhus and Social Control: South Africa, 1917–50." In MacLeod and Lewis, *Disease, Medicine, and Empire,* 257–83.

Martineau, Harriet. *The Positive Philosophy of Auguste Comte.* Kitchener: Batoche Books, 2000; London: George Bell and Sons, 1896, http://socserv2.mcmaster.ca/~econ/ugcm/3ll3/comte/index.html

Mataud, Melanie, and Pierre-Albert Martin. *La Médecine Rouennaise à l'Époque de Charles Nicolle, de la Fin du XIXeme Siècle aux Années 1930.* Luneray: Editions Bertout, 2003.

Mathis, Constantin. *L'Oeuvre des Pastoriens en Afrique Noire.* Paris: PUF, 1946.

Maxcy, Kenneth F. "Clinical Observations on the Endemic Typhus (Brill's Disease) in Southern United States." *Public Health Reports* 41 (1926): 1213–20.

———. "An Epidemiological Study of Endemic Typhus (Brill's Disease) in the Southeastern United States, with Special Reference to Its Mode of Transmission." *Public Health Reports* 41 (1926): 2967–95.

Mazumdar, Pauline. *Species and Specificity: An Interpretation of the History of Immunology.* Cambridge: Cambridge University Press, 1995.

McNeill, William H. *Plagues and Peoples.* Garden City, NY: Anchor Press, 1976.

Meir, Yoelli. "Charles Nicolle and the Frontiers of Medicine." *New England Journal of Medicine* 276 (1967): 670–75.

Mendelsohn, J. Andrew. "Cultures of Bacteriology." Ph.D. dissertation, Princeton University, 1996.

———. "From Eradication to Equilibrium: How Epidemics Became Complex after World War I." In Lawrence and Weisz, *Greater Than the Parts,* 303–31.

———. "'Like All that Lives': Biology, Medicine and Bacteria in the Age of Pasteur and Koch." *History and Philosophy of the Life Sciences* 24 (2002): 3–36.

———. "Medicine and the Making of Bodily Inequality in Twentieth-Century Europe." In *Heredity and Infection: The History of Disease Transmission,* edited by Jean-Paul Gaudillière and Ilana Löwy, 21–79. London: Routledge, 2001.

———. "'Typhoid Mary' Strikes Again: The Social and the Scientific in the Making of Modern Public Health." *Isis* 86 (1995): 268–77.

Mesnil, Félix. "Notice Nécrologique sur M. Charles Nicolle." *Bulletin de l'Académie de Médecine* 115 (1936): 541–49.

Metchnikoff, Elie. *The Nature of Man: Studies in Optimistic Philosophy.* Edited and translated by P. Chalmers Mitchell. New York: Putnam, 1903.

Metchnikoff, Olga. *Life of Elie Metchnikoff, 1845–1916.* Boston: Houghton Mifflin, 1921.

Meyer, K. F. "Latent Infections." *Journal of Bacteriology* 31 (1936): 109–35.

Mollaret, Henri H., and Jacqueline Brossollet. *Alexandre Yersin, le Vainqueur de la Peste.* Paris: Fayard, 1985.

Mooser, Herman. "An American Variety of Typhus." *Transactions of the Royal Society of Tropical Medicine and Hygiene* 22 (1928): 175–76.

———. "Ein Beitrag zur Ätiologie des Mexikanischen Fleckfiebers." *Archiv für Schiffs-und Tropenhygiene* 32 (1928): 261.

———. "Contribución al Estudio de la Etiología Tifo Mexicano." *Gaceta Medica de Mexico* 59 (1928): 219.

———. "Contribution to the Etiology of Mexican Typhus." *JAMA* 91 (1928): 19–20.

———. "Essai sur l'Histoire Naturelle du Typhus Exanthématique." *AIPT* 21 (1932): 1–17.

———. "Experiments Relating to the Pathology and the Etiology of Mexican Typhus (*Tabardillo*)." *Journal of Infectious Diseases* 43 (1928): 214–60; 261–72.

———. "Reaction of Guinea-Pigs to Mexican Typhus (*Tabardillo*): Preliminary Note on Bacteriologic Observations." *JAMA* 91 (1928): 19–20.

Mooser, Herman. "*Rickettsia typhi* (Wolbach and Todd 1920) Philip 1943, a Synonym of *Rickettsia prowazeki* Rocha Lima 1916." *AIPT* 36 (1959): 301–6.

———. "Tabardillo, An American Variety of Typhus." *Journal of Infectious Diseases* 44 (1929): 186–93.

Mooser, Herman, Gerardo Varela, and Hans Pilz. "Experiments on the Conversion of Typhus Strains." *Journal of Experimental Medicine* 59 (1934): 137–57.

Morgan, T. H. "The Relation of Genetics to Physiology and Medicine." "Nobel Lecture," http://nobelprize.org/medicine/laureates/1933/morgan-lecture.html

Moulin, Anne Marie. "L'Apprentissage Pastorien de la Mosaïque Tunisie." In *La Tunisie Mosaïque: Diasporas, Cosmopolitisme, Archéologies de l'Identité*, edited by Jacques Alexandropoulos and Patrick Cabanel, 369–88. Toulouse: Presses Universitaires du Mirail, 2000.

———. "Bacteriological Research and Medical Practice in and out of the Pastorian School." In *French Medical Culture in the Nineteenth Century*, edited by Mordechai Feingold and Anne La Berge, 327–49. Atlanta: Rodopi, 1994.

———. "Charles Nicolle, Savant Tunisien." *AIPT* 71 (1994): 355–70.

———. *La Dernière Langage de la Médecine: Histoire de l'Immunologie de Pasteur au Sida*. Paris: Presses Universitaires de France, 1991.

———. "Une Généalogie Scientifique: l''Isnad' de Tunis (1883–1993)." In *La Mise en Mémoire de la Science: Pour une Ethnographie Historique des Rites Commémoratifs*, edited by P. G. Abir-Am, 207–24. Paris: Editions des Archives Contemporaines, 1998.

———. "Historical Introduction: The Institut Pasteur's Contribution." *Research in Immunology* 144 (1993): 8–13.

———. "L'Hygiène dans la Ville: La Médecine Ottoman à l'Heure Pastorienne (1887–1908)." In *Villes Ottomanes à la fin de l'Empire*, edited by Paul Dumont and François Georgeon, 186–209. Paris: Editions L'Harmattan, 1992.

———. "Les Instituts Pasteur de la Méditerranée Arabe: Une Religion Scientifique en Pays d'Islam." In *Santé, Médecine et Société dans le Monde Arabe*, edited by Elisabeth Longuenesse, 129–64. Paris: Editions l'Harmattan, 1995.

———. "La Métaphore Vaccine: De l'Inoculation à la Vaccinologie." *History and Philosophy of the Life Sciences* 14 (1992): 271–97.

———. "The Pasteur Institute and the Logic of Non-Profit." Unpublished paper delivered at the Third International Conference of Research on Voluntary and Non Profit Organizations, Indiana University Center on Philanthropy, Indianapolis, 1992.

———. "The Pasteur Institute's International Network: Scientific Innovations and French Tropisms." In *Transnational Intellectual Networks: Forms of Academic Knowledge and the Search for Cultural Identities*, edited by Christophe Charle, Jurgen Schriewer, and Peter Wagner, 135–64. Frankfurt: Campus Verlag, 2004.

———. "The Pasteur Institutes Between the Two World Wars: The Transformation of the International Sanitary Order." In *International Health Organizations and Movements, 1918–1939*, edited by Paul Weindling, 244–65. Cambridge: Cambridge University Press, 1995.

———. "Patriarchal Science: The Network of the Overseas Pasteur Institutes." In *Science and Empires: Historical Studies about Scientific Development and European Expansion*, edited by Patrick Petitjean, Catherine Jami, and Anne Marie Moulin, 307–22. Dordrecht, Holland: Kluwer, 1992.

Moulin, Anne Marie. "Tropical without the Tropics: The Turning-Point of Pastorian Medicine in North Africa." In *Warm Climates and Western Medicine: The Emergence of Tropical Medicine, 1500–1900*, edited by David Arnold, 160–80, Amsterdam: Clio Medica, 1996.

Moulin, Anne Marie, and Annick Guénel. "L'Institut Pasteur et la Naissance de l'Industrie de la Santé." In *La Philosophie du Remède*, edited by Jean-Claude Beaune, 91–109. Seyssel: Champ Vallon, 1993.

Murard, Lion, and Patrick Zylberman. "Seeds for French Health Care: Did the Rockefeller Foundation Plant the Seeds between the Two World Wars?" *Studies in History and Philosophy of Biological and Biomedical Sciences* 31 (2000): 463–75.

Nataf, R. "Charles Nicolle et les Maladies Oculaires Transmissibles." *AIPT* 43 (1966): 449–53.

Neill, M. H. "Experimental Typhus Fever in Guinea Pigs: A Description of a Scrotal Lesion in Guinea Pigs Infected with Mexican Typhus." *Public Health Reports* 32 (1917): 1105–8.

Nicolle, Charles. "Conférence du Docteur Charles Nicolle sur les Travaux qui Lui Ont Valu l'Attribution du Prix Nobel de Médecine." *AIPT* 19 (1930): 113–21.

———. "Discours de M. Nicolle: Inauguration d'un Buste de Pasteur à l'Institut Pasteur de Tunis." *Revue Tunisien des Sciences Médicales* 17 (1923): 264–66.

———. "Discours du Dr. Charles Nicolle; Les Journées Médicales Tunisiennes, 2–5 Avril 1926." *Revue Tunisienne des Sciences Médicales* 20 (1926): 6–11.

———. "Discours du Dr. Nicolle, Président Sortant." *Bulletin de la Société des Sciences Médicales de Tunis* 8 (1909): 8–10.

———. "Discours Prononcé aux Obsèques du Docteur Ernest Conseil le 6 Juin 1930." *AIPT* 19 (1930): 387–89.

———. [Frédéric Lefèvre]. "Une Heure avec le Docteur Charles Nicolle, Professeur au Collège de France—Prix Nobel 1928. La Grande Misère de l'Institut Pasteur: Un Cri d'Alarme." *Nouvelles Littéraires*, February 3, 1934.

———. "L'Institut Pasteur de Tunis." *AIPT* 1 (1906).

———. "Lettre aux Sourds" (1929). Extract.

———. "Maurice Nicolle." Tunis: Imprimerie J. Aloccio, 1935.

———. "Mon Camarade Habib." Manuscript.

———. *Notice sur l'Institut Pasteur de Tunis*. Tunis: J. Parlier, 1924.

———. "Notice sur l'Institut Pasteur de Tunis." *AIPT* 15 (1926).

———. "Un Nouvel Exemple d'Infections Inapparentes, à Propos de la Découverte, Faite par G. Blanc, J. Caminoptros et E. Manoussakis de la Dengue Inapparente de l'Homme et de Celle du Cobaye." *AIPT* 17 (1928): 356–62.

———. "L'Oeuvre de l'Institut Pasteur de Tunis." *Tunisie Médicale* 1 (1911): 253–63.

———. "Paroles Biologiques sur la Crise Actuelle." *Mercure de France*, January 1934: 5–30.

———. "À Propos de la Posologie des Vaccins Microbiens." *AIPT* 17 (1927): 400–11.

———. "À Propos du Mémoire de S. Ramsine sur l'Existence du Typhus Inapparent chez l'Homme." *AIPT* 18 (1929): 255–57.

———. "Rapport Présenté par le Docteur Charles Nicolle à S. E. Monsieur Clinchant, Ambassadeur de France auprès de la République Argentine." *AIPT* 20 (1931): 94–97.

———. "Rapport sur une Mission Scientifique en Argentine." *AIPT* 15 (1926): 166–72.

———. "Le Sillon de Pasteur." *Dépêche Tunisienne*, December 27, 1922.

Nicolle, Charles, and Brunswic-le-Bihan. *Une Pendaison à Tunis.* Paris: C. Naud, 1904.
Nicolle, Marcelle. "Charles Nicolle: 1866–1936." *Femmes Médecins* 11 (1966): 289–310.
Nicolle, Maurice. *Les Antigènes et les Anticorps: Caractères Généraux—Applications Diagnostiques—Applications Thérapeutiques.* Paris: Masson et Cie, 1920.
Nicolle, Pierre. "Alphonse Laveran et Charles Nicolle." *AIPT* 88 (1981): 265–79.
———. "Charles Nicolle et Louis Pasteur Vallery-Radot, d'après Leur Correspondance." *Académie des Sciences, Belles-Lettres et Arts de Rouen* 47 (1971): 9–14.
———. "Charles Nicolle, Homme de Caractère." *Précis Analytique des Travaux de l'Académie des Sciences, Belles-Lettres et Arts de Rouen,* 23–32. Fécamp: L. Durand et Fils, 1967.
———. "Un Evénement Capital dans la Vie Passionnée de Charles Nicolle: Le Prix Nobel de Physiologie ou Médecine." *BSPE* 74 (1981): 101–18.
———. "Les Premières Années de Charles Nicolle à la Direction de l'Institut Pasteur de Tunis" [1976?].
———. "La Vie et la Personnalité de Charles Nicolle." *Annales d'Hygiène de Langue Française* 3 (1967): 87–91.
Novy, Frederick G. "Disease Carriers." *Science* 36 (1912): 1–10.
Novy, Frederick G., and R. E. Knapp. "Studies on *Spirillum Obermeieri* and Related Organisms." *Journal of Infectious Diseases* 3 (1906): 291–393.
Nuttall, George H. F. "Bibliography of Pediculus and Phthirus, including Zoological and Medical Publications Dealing with Human Lice, Their Anatomy, Biology, Relation to Disease, etc., and Prophylactic Measures Directed Against Them." *Parasitology* 10 (1917): 1–42.
———. "The Part Played by *Pediculus humanus* in the Causation of Disease." *Parasitology* 10 (1917): 43–79.
Nye, Mary Jo. *Science in the Provinces: Scientific Communities and Provincial Leadership in France, 1860–1930.* Berkeley: University of California Press, 1986.
O'Donnell, J. Dean Jr. *Lavigerie in Tunisia: The Interplay of Imperialist and Missionary.* Athens: University of Georgia Press, 1979.
Omran, Abdel R. "The Epidemiological Transition: A Theory of the Epidemiology of Population Change." *Milbank Memorial Fund Quarterly* 49 (1971): 509–38.
Opinel, A., and G. Gachelin. "The Rockefeller Foundation and the Prevention of Malaria in Corsica, 1923–1951: Support Given to the French Parasitologist Emile Brumpt." *Parassitologia* 46 (2004): 287–302.
Ortony, Andrew, ed. *Metaphor and Thought.* Cambridge: Cambridge University Press, 1979.
Osborne, Michael A. *Nature, the Exotic, and the Science of French Colonialism.* Bloomington: Indiana University Press, 1994.
———. "Science and the French Empire." *Isis* 96 (2005): 80–87.
Osborne, Michael A., and Richard F. Fogarty. "Views from the Periphery: Discourses of Race and Place in French Military Medicine." *History and Philosophy of the Life Sciences* 25 (2003): 363–89.
Otto, R., and H. Munter. "Beitrage zur Immunität Beim Experimentellen Fleckfieber des Meerschweinchens." *Zeitschrift für Hygiene und Infektions-Krankheiten* 194 (1925): 408–35.
Pachter, Marc, ed. *Telling Lives: The Biographer's Art.* Philadelphia: University of Pennsylvania Press, 1985.

Palladino, Paolo, and Michael Worboys. "Science and Imperialism." *Isis* 84 (1993): 91–102.
Parkenham, Thomas. *The Scramble for Africa: The White Man's Conquest of the Dark Continent from 1876 to 1912.* New York: Random House, 1991.
Pasteur, Louis. *Œuvres de Pasteur.* Edited by Louis Pasteur Vallery-Radot. 7 vols. Paris: Masson et Cie, 1922–39.
Paul, Harry. *From Knowledge to Power: The Rise of the Science Empire in France, 1860–1939.* Cambridge: Cambridge University Press, 1985.
Pelis, Kim. "A Louse, Divided." Paper delivered at the Annual Meeting of the American Association for the History of Medicine, Birmingham, Ala., April 2005.
―――. " 'Mosaics of Power': The Virus-Vaccine and Imperialism in French North Africa." Society for the Sociology of Medicine Conference, "Colonialism and Medicine," Oxford University, Oxford, England, 1996.
―――. "Pasteur's Imperial Missionary: Charles Nicolle (1866–1936) and the Pasteur Institute of Tunis." Ph.D. dissertation, Johns Hopkins University, 1995.
―――. "Prophet for Profit in French North Africa: Charles Nicolle and the Pasteur Institute of Tunis, 1903–1936." *BHM* 71 (1997): 583–622.
―――. "Reservoir Docs." Paper delivered at a Lunchtime Seminar, Department of Public Health, Sydney University, Sydney, Australia, 1997.
―――. "The Tunisian Medical 'Cosmos' of Charles Nicolle?" Paper delivered at the Symposium, "Medicine in the Arab World," Hammamet, Tunisia, 1994.
Perkins, Kenneth J. *A History of Modern Tunisia.* Cambridge: Cambridge University Press, 2004.
Pieper, Josef. *Leisure: The Basis of Culture,* trans. Alexander Dru. New York: Mentor Books, 1963.
Pinkerton, Henry. "Rickettsia-like Organisms in the Scrotal Sac of Guinea-Pigs with European Typhus." *Journal of Infectious Diseases* 44 (1929): 337–46.
Pinkerton, Henry, and Kenneth Maxcy. "Pathological Study of a Case of Endemic Typhus in Virginia with Demonstration of Rickettsia." *American Journal of Pathology* 7 (1931): 95–104.
Plancke, J. "Hygiène dans les Ecoles Primaires de Tunis." *Tunisie Médicale* 1 (1911): 23–25.
Plotz, Harry. "The Etiology of Typhus Fever (and of Brill's Disease): Preliminary Communication." *JAMA* 62 (1914): 1556.
Plotz, Harry, Peter K. Olitsky, and George Baehr. "The Etiology of Typhus Exanthematicus." *Journal of Infectious Diseases* 17 (1915): 1–68.
Poirson, A. "L'Epidémie de Typhus du Goubellat (1912)." *AIPT* 7 (1912): 140–43.
Polanyi, Michael. *Personal Knowledge: Towards a Post-Critical Philosophy.* London: Routledge, 1958.
Porter, Roy. *The Greatest Benefit to Mankind: A Medical History of Humanity from Antiquity to the Present.* New York: Norton, 1998.
Potel, René. "Observations Cliniques et Etiologiques sur les cas de Typhus Soignés à l'Hôpital Permanent de la Marine de Sidi-Abdallah: Action du Sérum Exanthématique." *AIPT* 9 (1914–16): 245–85.
Power, Helen. "The Calcutta School of Tropical Medicine: Institutionalizing Medical Research in the Periphery." *Medical History* 40 (1996): 197–214.
Prévost-Barancy, Andre. *Charles Nicolle.* Paris: R. Foulon, 1950.

Rabinow, Paul. *French Modern: Norms and Forms of the Social Environment.* Cambridge, MA: MIT Press, 1989.
Ramsine, S. "Sur l'Existence de la Forme Inapparente du Typhus Exanthématique chez l'Homme." *AIPT* 18 (1929): 247–57.
Rather, L. J. *Addison and the White Corpuscles: An Aspect of Nineteenth Century Biology.* London: Wellcome Institute, 1972.
Reynolds, Sian. *France between the Wars: Gender and Politics.* London: Routledge, 1996.
Rheinberger, Hans-Jorg. *Toward a History of Epistemic Things: Synthesizing Proteins in the Test Tube.* Stanford, CA: Stanford University Press, 1997.
Rivers, Thomas M. "The Nature of Viruses." *Physiological Reviews* 12 (1932): 423–52.
———, ed. *Viral and Rickettsial Infections of Man.* Philadelphia: J. B. Lippincott, 1948.
Robson, Michael. "The French Pharmaceutical Industry, 1919–1939." In *Pill Peddlers: Essays on the History of the Pharmaceutical Industry*, edited by Jonathan Liebenau, 107–22. Madison: American Institute of the History of Pharmacy, 1990.
Roger, Jules. *Les Médecins Normands du XIIe au XIXe Siècle: Biographie et Bibliographie.* Paris: G. Steinheil, 1890.
Roll-Hansen, Nils. "Experimental Method and Spontaneous Generation: The Controversy between Pasteur and Pouchet, 1859–64." *JHM* 34 (1979): 273–92.
Rosenberg, Charles. *The Cholera Years: The United States in 1832, 1849, and 1866.* Chicago: University of Chicago Press, 1962.
———. "Explaining Epidemics." In *Explaining Epidemics and other Studies in the History of Medicine*, edited by Charles Rosenberg, 293–304. Cambridge: Cambridge University Press, 1992.
———. "Pathologies of Progress: The Idea of Civilization as Risk." *BHM* 72 (1998): 714–30.
Ross, Philip H., and A. D. Milne. "Tick Fever." *BMJ* 2 (1904): 1453–54.
Roussel, A. E. "Brill's Disease, a Comparison of Four Cases with Four Cases of Typhus Fever Treated by the Author." *Maryland Medical Journal* 57 (1914): 729–35.
Roux, Emile. "Sur les Microbes Dite 'Invisibles.'" *BIP* 1 (1903): 7–12.
Rucker, W. C. "Mild Typhus Exanthematicus (Brill's Disease), with Report of a Case." *New Orleans Medical and Surgical Journal* 82 (1929): 177–79.
Said, Edward W. *Orientalism.* London: Routledge and Kegan Paul, 1978.
Salomon-Bayet, Claire, ed. *Pasteur et la Révolution Pastorienne.* Paris: Payot, 1986.
Savoor, Sadashivarao R., and Roberto Velasco. "The Survival of Varieties of Typhus Virus in Mouse Passage, with Particular Reference to the Virus of Brill's Disease." *Journal of Experimental Medicine* 60 (1934): 317–22.
Sergent, Edmond. "Le Pou, Inoculateur de Maladies Humaines (Aperçu historique)." *AIPT* 36 (1959): 307–10.
———. "Réflexions sur les Modalités de l'Infection." *AIP d'Algérie* 26 (1948): 91–104.
Sergent, Edmond, and H. Foley. "Recherches sur la Fièvre Récurrente et Son Mode de Transmission, dans une Epidémie Algérienne." *AIP* 24 (1910): 337–73.
Sergent, Edmond, H. Foley, and Ch. Vialatte. "Transmission à l'Homme et au Singe du Typhus Exanthématique par les Poux d'un Malade Atteint de Fièvre Récurrente et par les Lentes et Poux issus des Précédents." *CRAS* 158 (1914): 964–65.
———. "Transmission de Laboratoire du Typhus Exanthématique par le Pou." *AIPAN* 1 (1921): 218–30.

Sergent, Edmond, and Henri Foley. "Fièvre Récurrente du Sud-Oranais et *Pediculus vestimenti*: Note Préliminaire." *BSPE* 1 (1908): 174–76.
Shinn, Terry. "The Genesis of French Industrial Research, 1880–1940." *Social Science Information* 19 (1980): 607–40.
Shortland, Michael, and Richard Yeo, eds. *Telling Lives in Science: Essays on Scientific Biography.* Cambridge: Cambridge University Press, 1996.
Silverstein, Arthur. *A History of Immunology.* San Diego: Academic Press, 1989.
Simon, Pierre-Henri. *Georges Duhamel, où le Bourgeois Sauvé.* Paris: Editions du Temps Présent, 1946.
Smith, Dale C. "Gerhard's Distinction between Typhoid and Typhus and Its Reception in America, 1833–1860." *BHM* 54 (1980): 368–85.
———. "The Rise and Fall of Typhomalarial Fever: I. Origins." *JHM* 37 (1982): 182–220.
Smith, E. F. "Endemic Typhus Fever (Brill's Disease): A Case in Sussex County." *Delaware State Medical Journal* 2 (1930): 139–40.
Smith, Theobald. *Parasitism and Disease.* Princeton: Princeton University Press, 1934.
Snyder, John C. "Typhus Fevers." In Rivers, *Viral and Rickettsial Infections of Man,* 462–92.
Snyder, William H. *Quality and Quantity: The Quest for Biological Regeneration in Twentieth-Century France.* New ed. Cambridge: Cambridge University Press, 2002.
Soderqvist, Thomas. "Existential Projects and Existential Choice in Science: Science Biography as an Edifying Genre." In Shortland and Yeo, *Telling Lives in Science,* 45–84.
Sorin, Gerald. *A Time for Building: The Third Migration, 1880–1920 (The Jewish People in America).* Baltimore: Johns Hopkins University Press, 1992.
Starling, Ernest. "The Chemical Correlation of the Functions of the Body." *Lancet* 2 (1905): 339–41, 423–25, 501–3, 579–83.
Stephen, Martin, ed. *Poems of the First World War: 'Never Such Innocence.'* London: Everyman, 1988, 1993.
Stocking, George W. *Race, Culture, and Evolution: Essays in the History of Anthropology.* New York: Free Press, 1968.
Stoler, Ann Laura, and Frederick Cooper. "Between Metropole and Colony: Rethinking a Research Agenda." In *Tensions of Empire: Colonial Cultures in a Bourgeois World,* edited by Frederick Cooper and Ann Laura Stoler, 1–56. Berkeley: University of California Press, 1997.
Strong, Richard P., George C. Shattuck, A. W. Sellards, Hans Zinsser, and J. Gardner Hopkins. *Typhus Fever with Particular Reference to the Serbian Epidemic.* Cambridge, MA: The American Red Cross at the Harvard University Press, 1920.
Strouse, Solomon. "Brill's Disease, Mild Typhus Fever, in the Michael Reese Hospital." *Illinois Medical Journal* 23 (1913): 37–41.
Summers, William C. *Félix d'Herelle and the Origins of Molecular Biology.* New Haven: Yale University Press, 1999.
———. "From Culture as Organism to Organism as Cell: Historical Origins of Bacterial Genetics." *Journal of the History of Biology* 24 (1991): 171–90.
Sutphen, Mary P., and Bridie Andrews, eds. *Medicine and Colonial Identity.* London: Routledge, 2003.
Sutton, Michael. *Nationalism, Positivism and Catholicism: The Politics of Charles Maurras and French Catholics, 1890–1914.* Cambridge: Cambridge University Press, 2002.

Tansey, E. M., and Rosemary C. E. Milligan. "The Early History of the Wellcome Research Laboratories, 1894–1914." In Liebenau, *Pill Peddlers,* 91–106.
Tauber, Alfred I., and Leon Chernyak. *Metchnikoff and the Origins of Immunology: From Metaphor to Theory.* New York: Oxford University Press, 1991.
Theiler, Max. "Studies on the Action of Yellow Fever Virus in Mice." *Annals of Tropical Medicine and Parasitology* 24 (1930): 249–72.
Tilley, Helen. "Ecologies of Complexity: Tropical Environments, African Trypanosomiasis, and the Science of Disease Control in British Colonial Africa, 1900–1940." *Osiris* 19 (2004): 21–38.
Todes, Daniel P. *Darwin without Malthus: The Struggle for Existence in Russian Evolutionary Thought.* New York: Oxford University Press, 1989.
———. *Pavlov's Physiology Factory: Experiment, Interpretation, Laboratory Enterprise.* Baltimore: Johns Hopkins University Press, 2002.
Todorov, Tzvetan. *On Human Diversity: Nationalism, Racism, and Exoticism in French Thought.* Translated by Catherine Porter. Cambridge, MA: Harvard University Press, 1993.
Tomes, Nancy. *The Gospel of Germs: Men, Women, and the Microbe in American Life.* Cambridge, MA: Harvard University Press, 1998.
Topley, W. W. C., and G. S. Wilson. *The Principles of Bacteriology and Immunity.* 2 vols. London: Edward Arnold, 1929.
de la Tribonnière, X. "Edmond Sergent (1876–1969) et l'Institut Pasteur d'Algérie." *BSPE* 93 (2000): 365–71.
"La 'Tunisie Médicale.' " *Tunisie Médicale* 1 (1911): 1–2.
Vallery-Radot, René. "Pourquoi le Monde Entier Glorifie Pasteur." *Dépêche Tunisienne,* December 24, 1922.
———. *La Vie de Pasteur.* Paris: E. Flammarion, 1900.
van Helvoort, Ton. "Bacteriological and Physiological Research Styles in the Early Controversy on the Nature of the Bacteriophage Phenomenon." *Medical History* 36 (1992): 243–70.
———. "Félix d'Hérelle en de Controverse Rond het Twort-d'Hérelle Fenomeen in de Jaren 1920: Ultrafiltreerbarr Virus of Lytisch Ferment." *Tijdschrift voor de Geschiedenis der Geneeskunde, Natuurwetenschappen, Wiskunde en Techniek* 8 (1985): 58–72.
———. "History of Virus Research in the Twentieth Century: The Problem of Conceptual Continuity." *History of Science* 32 (1994): 185–235.
———. "What Is a Virus? The Case of Tobacco Mosaic Disease." *Studies in History and Philosophy of Science* 22 (1991): 557–88.
Vaughan, Megan. *Curing Their Ills: Colonial Power and African Illness.* Oxford: Polity Press, 1991.
Vieuchange, J. "Les Recherches de Charles Nicolle sur l'Etiologie de la Grippe." *AIPT* 43 (1966): 481–90.
Virtanen, Reino. "Claude Bernard's Prophesies and the Historical Relation of Science to Literature." *Journal of the History of Ideas* 47 (1986): 275–86.
Walsh, D. M. "Chasing Shadows: Natural Selection and Adaptation." *Studies in History and Philosophy of Science Part C: Studies in History and Philosophy of Biological and Biomedical Sciences* 31 (2000): 135–53.

Ward, Lorraine. "The Cult of Relics: Pasteur Material at the Science Museum." *Medical History* 38 (1994): 52–72.
Waterson, A. P., and Lise Wilkinson. *An Introduction to the History of Virology*. Cambridge: Cambridge University Press, 1978.
Weber, Eugen Joseph. *The Hollow Years: France in the 1930s*. New York: Norton, 1994.
Weber, Eugene. *Peasants into Frenchmen: The Modernization of Rural France, 1870–1914*. Stanford, CA: Stanford University Press, 1979.
Weil, E., and F. Breinl. "Über die Erzeugung von inapparenten, zu Aktiven Immunität Fuhrended Fleckfieberinfektionen bei Passiv Immunisierten Meerschweinchen." *Wiener Klinische Wochenschrift* 35 (1922): 458.
Weindling, Paul Julian. *Epidemics and Genocide in Eastern Europe, 1890–1945*. Oxford: Oxford University Press, 2000.
———. " 'Victory with Vaccines': The Problem of Typhus Vaccines During World War II." In *Vaccinia, Vaccination, Vaccinology: Jenner, Pasteur and Their Successors*, edited by S. Plotkin and B. Fantini, 341–47. Paris: Elsevier, 1996.
Weisz, George. "A Moment of Synthesis: Medical Holism between the Wars." In Lawrence and Weisz, *Greater Than the Parts*, 68–93.
———. "Reform and Conflict in French Medical Education, 1870–1914." In Fox and Weisz, *Organization of Science and Technology*, 61–94.
Wernick, Andrew. *Auguste Comte and the Religion of Humanity: The Post-Theistic Program of French Social Theory*. Cambridge: Cambridge University Press, 2001.
Widal, G. F. I., and A. Sicard. "Recherches de la Réaction Agglutinante dans le Sang et le Sérum Desséchés des Typhiques et dans la Sérosité des Vésicatoires." *Bulletin des Membres de la Société des Médecins des Hôpitaux de Paris* 13 (1896): 681–82.
Wilson, Leonard G. "Fevers and Science in Early Nineteenth Century Medicine." *JHM* 33 (1978): 386–407.
Winslow, Charles-Edward Amory. *The Conquest of Epidemic Disease: A Chapter in the History of Ideas*. Princeton: Princeton University Press, 1943.
Wolbach, S. B. "The Filterable Viruses, a Summary." *Journal of Medical Research* 22 (1912): 1–25.
Wolbach, S. B., John L. Todd, and Francis W. Palfrey, *The Etiology and Pathology of Typhus: Being the Main Report of the Typhus Research Commission of the League of Red Cross Societies to Poland*. Cambridge, MA: League of Red Cross Societies at the Harvard University Press, 1922.
Woolgar, Steve. "Discovery: Logic and Sequence in a Scientific Text." In *The Social Process of Scientific Investigation: Sociology of the Sciences*, Vol. IV, edited by Karin D. Knorr, Roger Krohn, and Richard Whitely, 239–68. Dordrecht, Holland: D. Reidel, 1980.
Worboys, Michael. *Spreading Germs: Disease Theories and Medical Practice in Britain, 1865–1900*. Cambridge: Cambridge University Press, 2000.
Wright, Gwendolyn. *The Politics of Design in French Colonial Urbanism*. Chicago: University of Chicago Press, 1991.
Young, Robert M. *Darwin's Metaphor: Nature's Place in Victorian Culture*. Cambridge: Cambridge University Press, 1985.
Zinsser, Hans. *As I Remember Him: The Biography of R. S.* Boston: Little, Brown, 1940.
———. *Rats, Lice, and History: The Biography of a Bacillus*. Boston: Little, Brown, 1934, 1935.

Zinsser, Hans. "Recent Advances in the Study of Typhus Fever." *Transactions of the College of Physicians of Philadelphia,* 3rd ser. 1 (1934): 1–15.

———. "Sur la Maladie de Brill et le Réservoir Interépidémique du Typhus Classique." *AIPT* 23 (1934): 149–54.

———. "Varieties of Typhus Virus and the Epidemiology of the American Form of European Typhus Fever (Brill's Disease)." *American Journal of Hygiene* 20 (1934): 513–32.

Zinsser, Hans, and M. Ruiz Castenada. "On the Isolation from a Case of Brill's Disease of a Typhus Strain Resembling the European Type." *New England Journal of Medicine* 209 (1933): 815–19.

———. "Studies on Typhus Fever, II: Studies on the Etiology of Mexican Typhus Fever." *Journal of Experimental Medicine* 52 (1930): 649–58.

Zinsser, Hans, M. Ruiz Castaneda, and H. Mooser. "Notes on the Epidemiology of Typhus Fever and the Possible Evolution of the Rickettsia Disease Group." *Transactions of the Association of American Physicians* 47 (1932): 129–42.

Zitouna, Mohamed Moncef. *La Médecine en Tunisie 1881–1994.* Tunis [?]: Simpact, 1994 [?].

Zitouna, Mohamed Moncef, and S. Haouet. "Du Lazaret à l'Hôpital de la Rabta." *Tunisie Medicale* 76 (1998): 311–13.

Index

Abbaye de Créteil, 131
Abbaye de l'Ane d'Or, l', 133
Abdesselem, Habib ben, 37, 82, 133, 247, 309n107, 309n108, 309n110, 318n97
Abt, Georges, 117, 118
Académie de Médecine, 5, 86–87, 163
Académie des Sciences, 21, 44, 62, 63, 72, 135, 163, 164–65, 220–21, 302n166, 318n101, 318n102
American Red Cross Sanitary Commission. *See* World War I: typhus
Amsterdamska, Olga, 268n78
Anderson, Charles, 127, 138, 158, 175, 196, 203, 312n1
Anderson, John F., 194–95, 196
Anderson, Lisa, 276n86, 276n88, 277n93
Anderson, Warwick, 265n46, 321n5, 340n7
anthrax vaccine, 5, 262n26
Archives de l'Institut Pasteur de Tunis. *See* journals (medical)
Arcos, René, 132

Association pour l'Extension des Etudes Pastoriennes, 122, 125–27, 141, 210
attenuation. *See* virulence

Bacon, Francis (and Baconian philosophy), 4, 47, 48–49, 128, 240, 266n59, 340n5
bacterial dissociation (variability), 12, 25, 155–57, 173, 177, 185, 188, 250, 270n22, 323n46, 343n47
bacteriology (microbiology), 9, 12, 18, 21, 181, 208, 210–11, 253, 265n52, 266n57, 268n78, 323n46, 343n47; and clinical medicine, 21, 26, 270n19, 274n61. *See also* Pastorians: model
bacteriophage, 154, 155, 316n52
Balozet, Lucien, 203, 221
Baltazard, Marcel, 78, 292n1, 293n12
Bartholome (Director of Agriculture, Tunisia), 42
Barykine, W., 153
BCG. *See* Calmette: BCG
Bédier, Joseph, 209–10, 211
Behring, Emil, 23

373

374 Index

Beijerinck, Martinus, 286n46
Berdnikoff, Prof., 300n125
Bergson, Henri, 119, 160, 166, 217, 319n123, 335n54
Bernard, Claude, 27, 126, 208, 211, 212, 215, 332n13
Bernard, Léon, 143
Bertholon, Louis, xvi, 48, 53, 55, 276n89, 283n2, 285n31
Billon, François, 86–87, 109, 147
Blaizot, Ludovic, 71, 78, 88, 91, 123, 160, 253, 291n135, 292n9, 305n52; and relapsing fever, 79, 80, 82–83, 84, 175; and vaccine production, 72, 86, 109; wartime service, 92, 94, 95
Blanc, Georges, 78, 79, 98, 108, 110, 117, 129, 134, 163, 168, 178, 210, 292n1, 292n3, 296n75, 314n31; and inapparent infections, 151, 186; Nicolle's aspirations for, 90–91, 118–19, 131, 157, 160–61, 245, 304n24, 317n72, 318n93; and relapsing fever, 83, 96, 175, 184; typhus vaccine, 193, 313n24; wartime service, 92, 93, 94, 95
Blanchard, Raphaël, 71, 78
Bloch, Jean Richard, 137
Bordet, Jules, 155, 166
Borrel, Amédée, 80, 158
Bouhageb, Hassen, 284n11
Breinl, Friedrich, 155, 156, 223
Brill, Nathan, 54, 193–95, 197, 207, 243, 299n109, 326n117, 327n124, 327n126
"Brill's disease." *See* typhus: Brill-Zinsser disease
Brumpt, Emile, 71, 79, 116, 293n12, 306n53, 312n1, 331n184
Brunchwig, Henri, 261n15
Brunon, Raoul, 26–28, 274n59, 274n61, 274n63

Brunswic-le-Bihan (director, Sadiki Hospital) 41, 50–51, 52, 284n13, 284n14, 284n19
Buen, Sadi de, 175, 176
Bugnot, Georges, 71, 279n130
Burnet, Etienne, 7, 117, 121, 131, 163, 217, 220–21, 245, 305n43, 318n87, 343n43, 343n44; appointment to IPT, 119–20; departure from Tunis, 160
Burnet, Macfarlane F., 321n5
Burnet, Lydia, 245, 343n44

Caillon, Louis, 298n102
Calmette, Albert, 109, 117, 118, 119, 122, 125, 127, 130, 150, 163, 228, 230, 282n167, 282n168; and BCG, 161, 228–29; as colonial (Pastorian) liaison, 35, 44, 80, 276n82, 282n168; Pasteur Institute of Saigon, 7, 30
Camus, Albert, 269n2
Cannon, Walter B., 215
Carthage, 17, 97, 142, 247, 248, 300n121
Castaneda, M. Ruiz, 199, 200
Catholic Church, 3, 19, 133–34; in Pastorism, 6, 7, 37–38, 49, 85, 226–28, 263n31, 263n45
Catouillard, Gaston, 36, 41
Chadli, Amor, 249
Chagas, Carlos, 138
Chaltiel, J., 37
Chamberland, Charles, 55
Chamberland filter, 55
Chambers, David Wade, 265n47
chancre mou, 22, 25
Chatton, Edouard, 95, 117, 298n102, 298n106
Collège de France, 208–14, 230, 244–45, 258n2, 280n147, 332n1, 332n13, 332n14
colonialism, xvi, 3, 30, 249, 251, 261n12, 261n13; French, 261n15,

278n116; and medicine, xviii, 41–42, 52, 56, 73, 142–43, 159–60, 163, 166–67, 191, 248–49, 251, 261n21, 264n38, 264n39, 275n76, 280n138; metropole/periphery, 7–8, 29, 52, 88, 92–93, 123, 143, 144, 231–32, 260n3 265n46, 265n47, 283n4; and Nicolle (isolation), xviii, 9, 13, 14, 29, 87, 88–89, 131, 137–38, 153, 165, 166, 170, 208, 213, 247–48, 253, 265n48; "Scramble for Africa," xvi, 3, 31, 260n11. *See also* France: civilizing mission
Comte, Auguste, 3
Comte, Charles, 36, 41, 43, 71, 218, 280n147, 281n152, 291n134, 320n136; and typhus, 63, 65, 169
Conklin, Alice, 4, 261n12, 261n13, 261n15
Conor, Alfred, 61, 70–71, 72, 73, 84, 90, 120, 288n81, 292n142, 296n72
Conor, Marthe Bugnot, 71, 77, 84–85, 86, 88, 90, 91, 92, 94, 103, 108, 130–31, 219, 252, 253, 295n47, 300n121, 301n156, 307n86, 308n87, 309n107
Conseil, Ernest, 41, 52, 63, 69, 72, 108, 120, 121, 123, 133, 158–59, 163, 281n148, 287n51, 287n65, 287n69, 288n76, 288n77, 290n111, 305n52; death of, 192; and hygiene, 42–43, 59, 65–66; typhus, epidemiology and prophylaxis, 57–61, 65–68, 73, 96, 107, 143, 169, 189, 290n120; typhus transmission, questioning, 77–78; typhus vaccine, 150, 178; wartime service, 92, 93, 94, 297n80
Creager, Angela, 286n47
Cuénot, Lucien, 164, 246, 325n89, 343n52
cyclogenic theory. *See* bacterial dissociation

D'Arsonval, Jacques-Arsène, 209
Daudet, Leon, 309n112
Delabarre, Edouard, 208, 214, 235, 247
Delattre, Alfred-Louis, 18, 97, 131, 142, 300n121
Dellagi, Koussay, 249
Descartes, René, 128
Diancono, Hector, 121
Dible, Henry J., 266n57, 314n37, 315n51, 336n80
Dinguizli, Bechir, 34, 50, 158, 228–29, 278n109, 317n74
diphtheria, 22–23, 87, 272n40
disease theory, xviii, 13, 84, 147, 153, 177–92, 216, 221–26, 245, 271n25, 273n50, 323n46; adaptation/mutation, 155–56, 174, 177, 187–88, 223, 245, 286n45; antigens, 179, 180, 182, 215, 222; "birth" (emergence) and "death," xviii, 13, 183, 186–92, 224, 313n23, 325n85; demonstration, standards of, 64, 81–82, 205–7, 294n31, 310n129, 320n128, 331n191; in epidemics, 185–86; evolution and, 13, 84, 106, 154–57, 174–77, 181–92, 200, 221, 223–26, 245, 251, 271n28, 302n165, 316n66, 322n21, 325n89, 342n28 (*see also* relapsing fever; typhus); in individuals, 184–85; "mosaic of powers," xviii, 2, 13, 222–26, 227, 254; specificity, 181–83, 222
Dmégon. *See* vaccines: *fluorurés*
"Door of the Sadiki" narrative. *See* typhus: discovery narrative
Dostoevsky, Fyodor, 22, 77, 104, 241, 341n17
Dougga, 97, 142
"Dream of a Ridiculous Man" (Dostoevsky), 104–5, 241–42, 301n158
Dubos, René, 321n5, 340n7

Duclaux, Emile, 8–10, 174, 266n54, 321n2
Ducloux, Edouard, 34, 37–38, 279n123
Duhamel, Blanche, 134, 160, 253, 310n121, 310n140
Duhamel, Georges, 18, 99, 131–33, 134–38, 145, 146, 160, 174, 209, 210, 211, 215, 217, 229, 230, 245, 246, 247–48, 300n127, 308n94, 309n112; biographical background, 131–32, 308n99; Nicolle's advocate, 136, 234, 310n138, 339n153; Nicolle's confessor, 136–38, 213, 235; philosophy of, 10, 131–32, 170, 191, 216, 308n93, 308n96, 335n67
Dyer, R. E., 198

Eckert, Jack, 344n72
École de Médecine (Rouen), 20, 22, 28; bacteriology laboratory, 22–23, 24, 25, 26–27, 28; *Cours* (Nicolle's), 24, 25, 272n44
École Préparatoire des Sciences et des Lettres (Rouen), 20, 21, 270n21
ecology, disease, 271n25, 321n5, 340n7
Einthoven, Willem, 165, 319n116
Eliot, T. S., 238
emerging diseases. *See* disease theory
Epictetus, 228, 242, 341n25
Erlich, Paul, 272n29
Essor, l', 132, 134, 142, 160, 308n101
evolutionary theory, 11, 12, 22, 218, 324n55

Faculté de Médecine (Paris), 71, 78, 131, 142, 143, 144, 165, 210
Faculty of Medicine (Stockholm), 144
Felix, Arthur, 152, 314n37
Felsenfeld, Oscar, 293n12, 315n50, 322n9, 343n45
Fichet, Alexandre, 132, 133, 308n101, 309n111

filterable viruses. *See* inframicrobes; viruses
Flaubert, Gustav, 18, 311n154
Fletcher, Ian Christopher, 261n12
Foley, Henri, 63–64, 80, 81, 82, 129, 289n94, 289n97, 293n15
fondation Roux, 127
Fourneau, Ernest, 296n56
France, Anatole, 86
France: "civilizing mission," xvi, xvii, 3, 4, 7, 11, 39, 41–42, 46, 49, 70, 142, 143, 170, 190, 222, 225, 226, 240, 252, 340n5; Franco-Prussian War, xvi, 2, 4, 5, 260n4; Third Republic, xvi, xvii, 2–4, 254, 260n4, 260n7. *See also* colonialism: French
Fussell, Paul, 92

Gallagher, Nancy, 32, 277n99
Geison, Gerald, 174, 262n28, 266n64, 321n1
genetics, 11, 12, 223–24
Geniaux, Charles, 208
germ theory, xvi, 9, 30, 49, 55, 264; "Koch's Postulates," 9, 55, 147–48; specificity, 8–9, 11–12, 49, 174, 180, 181–83, 321n2, 321n3. *See also* disease theory
Giroud, Paul, 127, 213–14, 229, 244, 343n39
Gobert, Ernest-Gustave, 79, 120, 121, 293n11, 297n80
Gobineau, Joseph-Arthur de, 335n67
Goethe, Johann Wolfgang von, 217
Goldberger, Joseph, 194–95, 196
Green, Robert, 316n66
Guégan, F.-J., 42
Guy, M. (architect), 36, 279n120

Habib. *See* Abdesselem, Habib ben
Hadley, Philip, 156
Halipré, A., 159, 274n61

Harvard University, 198–200, 203, 250–51, 298n94, 329n151, 330n176
healthy carriers. *See* hidden disease carriers
Henle, Joseph, 9, 49
Herelle, Félix d', 154, 155, 269n5
hidden disease carriers, 12, 146, 315n44. *See also* inapparent infection; latent infections
Hirsch, August, 47, 53–54, 285n32, 285n37, 285n39, 286n40
homeostasis, 215, 334n44
Hue, François, 22
Hueber, J.-J., 308n100
Huet, Maurice, 24, 86, 280n147, 300n126, 308n87, 320n136, 343n43
Hugnon, M., 36
Husson, Albert, 42, 281n152
hygiene ("rational"), xvii, 67, 73, 78, 92, 96, 120, 290n165. *See also* Tunisia: hygiene in

immunity, theories of, 11, 22, 49, 99, 106, 179
"inapparent infection," xviii, 2, 97, 99, 106–8, 110, 135, 139, 145–53, 167, 168, 183, 213, 226, 242–44, 245, 267n73, 302n165, 320n128; and "birth"/"death" of disease, 173, 186, 189–90, 202; dengue, 151; and epidemiology, 149–50, 151–53, 185–86, 196–97, 205, 315n48; and etiology, 147–48; and latent infections (or hidden carriers), 146, 313n9, 341n26; and symptoms, 147, 149–50, 320n128; in vaccines, 148, 150, 178–80, 203–4, 242, 330n178. *See also* typhus: reservoirs; typhus: vaccines; virulence
influenza, 97, 154, 267n69, 267n70, 315n51

"inframicrobes," 153–57, 223, 225, 245, 267n70, 316n55, 316n65; and disease birth, 188–89; and relapsing fever, 178
Institut de Carthage, 33, 134, 278n107
Ivanovski, Dmitri, 286n46

Jenner, Edward, 5, 188, 262n25
journals (medical); *Archives de l'Institut Pasteur de Tunis*, 38, 45, 129, 144, 157, 282n176; *Archives des Instituts Pasteur de l'Afrique du Nord*, 121, 129–30, 141, 305n32; *Bulletin de la Société de Pathologie Exotique*, 45, 64; *Bulletin de l'Institut Pasteur*, 45, 55, 282n170; *CRAS*, 45; *Journal of Experimental Medicine*, 329n152; *Normandie Médicale*, 24–25, 26, 45; *Paris Médical*, 166; *Presse Médicale*, 50, 145–46, 166; *Revue Médicale de Normandie*, 26, 45; *Tunisie Médicale, La*, 51–52, 284n22
Journées Médicales Tunisienne, 141, 142–43, 144, 145, 312n163
Joyeux, Charles, 312n1

Kahena, La, 134, 310n119
kala-azar, 43–44, 70, 84, 139, 141, 282n168
Kevles, Daniel J., 266n64
Kingsland, Sharon, 325n89
Koch, Robert, 9, 49, 54, 146, 174, 321n3
Kohler, Robert E., 268n78
Kraxner, Stephen, 282n169

Lacroix, Alfred, 229–30
La Fontaine, Jean de, 19
Lagrange, Emile, 227, 252
Laidlaw, Patrick, 316n66
Laigret, Jean, 203–4, 206, 242, 331n178
latent infections, 107, 313n9

378 Index

Latour, Bruno, 5, 39, 262n26, 270n19, 275n76
Laveran, Alphonse, 45, 282n168
Lavoisier, 27, 126, 217
Leavitt, Judith Walzer, 312n6
Lebailly, Charles, 83, 97, 106, 119–20, 152, 154, 160, 298n102, 305n30
Lefèvre, Frédéric, 230
LeGouis, Catherine, 301n158
Leishman, William Boog, 83, 317n67; and granular theory of bacterial reproduction, 156
leishmaniasis, 43, 141
Leredde, Emile, 116, 303n10
Leriche, René, 245
Leudet, Robert, 22
Levaditi, Constantin, 210, 211, 221, 336n80
lice, 92–93, 115, 129–30, 150–51, 289n96; in relapsing fever, 63, 81–83, 289n97; in typhus, 1, 63, 64–65, 66–67, 77–78, 202, 289n101, 292n4, 298n94, 307n79
Lister, Joseph, 262n23
Loir, Adrien, 48, 229, 276n84, 277n95, 277n104, 278n105, 278n108, 278n113; director in Tunis, 30, 32; Nicolle criticizes, 33, 37–39, 141, 158, 159, 280n136; and Tunisian medicine, 33–34
Lot, Germaine, 269n2
Lyautey, Hubert, 279n120

Mackie, Percival F., 63, 64, 80, 81, 293n15
Madame Bovary (Flaubert), 18
Magendie, François, 208
malaria, 41, 80, 281n152, 293n11, 317n80
Mallon, "Typhoid" Mary, 146, 312n6
Martin, Albert, 132
Martin, Louis, 23, 230, 234

Mathis, Constantin, 117, 203, 322n22, 330n175
Maxcy, Kenneth, 196–99, 200, 328n136, 329n151
Mazumdar, Pauline, 174
Mazza, Salvadore, 144, 312n2
médecins tolérés. See Tunisia: medicine in
Meister, Joseph, xv, 5, 20
Mektouf, 37
Mendel, Gregor, 11, 217
Mendelsohn, Andrew J., 271n28, 321n3, 334n45
Mercure de France, 132, 229, 232
Mesnil, Félix, 80, 117, 121–22, 127, 210, 234, 282n168, 298n106, 304n12, 331n184, 339n149; colonial (Pastorian) liaison, 44–45, 46, 116, 282n169, 282n176; Nicolle's advocate in Paris, 163, 164–65, 319n110
Metchnikoff, Elie, 21–22, 44, 97–98, 105, 109, 110, 179, 195, 271n28, 272n29
Mexico, 153, 192, 220. *See also* typhus: varieties
Meyer, André, 210
microscope, dark-field, 71, 79, 82–83, 154, 156, 175, 184
milieu intérieur, 215
"missions" (Nicolle), xv–xviii, 9, 14, 18, 22, 27, 28, 37–38, 68, 70, 74, 79, 140, 143, 158, 170, 209, 210, 211–12, 225–26, 245, 251, 253, 254; Pasteur Institute, campaign for directorship, 229–32, 233–35; Pastorian mission, campaign to save, 113, 115, 116, 122–25, 138–39, 145, 158, 165–66, 190, 207, 227–28; Pastorian mission, redefined, 88, 98, 108, 109–10, 114, 123–24, 143, 162, 251; to South America and Mexico, 138–41, 201–2, 330n164

Mooser, Herman, 197–99, 200, 201, 202, 204–5, 206, 207, 242, 328n131, 328n144, 331n186
Morgan, Thomas Hunt, 223–24
Moulin, Anne Marie, 7, 49, 249, 262n25, 263n31, 263n33, 264n38, 269n3, 271n28, 275n80, 276n84, 277n96, 277n104, 277n105, 278n109, 278n110, 280n143, 304n13
mutation, 11, 12, 155, 156, 177, 187, 245, 250, 286n45

Nageotte, Jean, 211
natural history, 19, 21, 84, 174, 181, 273n50
Neill, M. H., 193, 195–96, 197, 326n117, 328n131
Neisser, Rudolf, 286n45
Netter, Arnold, 210, 211, 229, 338n128
Nicolle, Alice, 24, 89, 103, 181, 252
Nicolle, Avice, 19, 89
Nicolle, Charles: birth, early life, and education, 2, 18–22; career in Rouen, 22–28; conversion to Catholicism, 246; deafness, 20, 27, 28–29, 74, 89, 107, 135, 221, 295n41; death and burial of, 7, 247–48, 343n43; marriage and family, 23–24, 89–90; Nobel Prize, 1, 145, 165–66, 167–70, 211, 213, 217; prizes, 1, 44, 134, 158, 163–64, 317n73, 318n101, 318n102
Nicolle, Charles, works by: *Biologie de l'Invention*, 202–3, 212, 215–20, 222, 335n54; "Comme un Souvenir Qui ne Vieillit Point," 99–106, 241; *Destin des Maladies Infectieuses*, 136, 221–26, 334n47; *Destinée Humaine, La*, 246; *Introduction à la Carrière de la Médecine Expérimentale*, 212–13, 333n21; *Naissance, Vie et Mort des Maladies Infectieuses*, 136, 174, 181–92, 202, 211, 212, 216, 224; *Nature, La*, 186, 239–42, 246; novels, 85–86, 88, 90, 99–106, 131, 137–38, 211, 295n45, 300n126
Nicolle, Eugène, 19–21, 28, 140, 174, 181, 248, 270n19
Nicolle, Marcel, 19, 89, 318n87
Nicolle, Marcelle, 24, 90, 103, 133, 161, 209, 219, 244, 245, 246–47, 296n69, 318n95, 330n164, 343n43
Nicolle, Maurice, 19, 20, 21, 30, 34, 89–90, 106, 140, 174, 271n22, 318n97; "mosaic of antigens," 179, 181–82, 215, 222, 323n35, 327n124
Nicolle, Pierre, 24, 103, 130, 133, 181, 245, 272n42, 295n41, 303n3
"NNN," 44, 146, 282n166
Nobel, Alfred, 170
Nobel Prize. *See* Nicolle, Charles: Nobel Prize
Noelle, Eva, 133
Nouvelles Littéraires, Les, 230–32, 233, 338n136
Novy, Frederick G., 44, 146, 313n8, 315n44
Nuttall, George, 115, 303n8
Nutton, Vivian, 339n139
Nye, Mary Jo, 259n3

Oswaldo Cruz Institute, 139
Ottenberg, Reuben, 194, 327n119

Pasteur, Louis, xvi, xvii, 5–7, 21, 39, 45, 54, 116, 125, 126, 146, 173–74, 215, 262n22, 270n22, 321n3, 332n13; centenary of birth, 7, 113–14, 127–29, 130; death, 8; and Nicolle, xviii, 46, 113, 127–29, 167, 180, 217, 271n24. *See also* Rabies

Pasteur Institute of Paris, xvi, 6, 108;
Conseil Scientifique, 234–35, 242;
Cours, 21, 30, 45, 150; Lacroix
Commission, 230; mission to "save,"
109, 115, 117, 122, 125–27, 166,
177, 207, 210, 227–28, 229–32;
origins, 5, 20; social structure, 5–7,
163. *See also* Pastorians (Pastorism)

Pasteur Institute of Tunis, 22, 30–32,
34–39, 66, 73, 141–43, 161–62, 232,
247, 279n130, 281n150, 295n44;
functions and expansions, 39–40,
41–43, 121, 141, 161–62, 203,
255–56, 277n95, 279n122; "origin
myth," 37–39, 142, 280n133; and
Pastorian mission, 39–40, 41–42, 43,
44–45; staff, 36–37, 40–41, 61,
70–71, 78, 119, 161–62, 203, 245,
257–58, 292n3; and Tunisian
government, 7, 31, 32, 34, 36, 40,
41–42, 62, 70–71, 94, 119–20, 162;
and "typhus" (as signature disease), 46,
48, 56, 57, 59, 70, 73; veterinary
services, 36, 141, 203, 279n123,
330n174

Pasteur Institutes and laboratories
("filials"), 4, 7, 30, 39, 49, 115, 121,
125, 203, 231, 234, 252; Algeria, 30,
80, 115, 234, 293n17, 304n14;
Athens, 116–18, 134, 234;
Brazzaville, 203; Casablanca, 116,
161, 178, 234; Constantinople, 7, 30;
Dakar, 203; Lille, 30;
"Mediterranean," 115, 116, 121, 122,
123, 234–35, 275n80, 304n13,
305n43; Nhatrang, 30; Saigon, 7, 30,
203; Tangiers, 115, 235; Teheran,
292n1

Pastorians (Pastorism), xviii, 8, 49, 78,
163, 167, 210–11, 263n31; "mission,"
xvi, xvii, 2, 4–8, 9, 14, 30, 37, 39,
49, 64, 68, 88, 110, 143, 145, 190,
221, 226, 231–32, 240, 252, 254,
280n143, 282n170 (*see also* Pasteur
Institute of Paris: mission to "save");
model ("microbiology"), xvi, xvii, 7,
18, 21, 25, 27, 32, 39, 43, 46, 49, 51,
70, 109, 125, 175; profit, 6, 74,
87–88, 124–25, 263n32, 263n33,
263n34, 295n53. *See also* philosophy
(Nicolle's): profit

patents, for medicine. *See* Pastorians:
profit

Pellegrin, Arthur, 134

philosophy (Nicolle's), 98, 99, 147, 174,
177, 203, 212–13; civilization,
190–92, 216–20, 222, 226, 232–33,
239–42, 249; colonialism, 191, 240,
248–49; equilibrium, 13, 208, 215,
216–19, 223, 227, 232, 233, 240,
253; genius/intuition/discovery, 2,
110, 123, 128, 140, 143, 167–68,
170, 177, 181, 183, 213, 215,
216–20, 222, 226, 240, 242, 253,
254, 307n74, 324n57, 333n29,
334n47; mutation, 217, 221; power,
221–22, 224–26, 240, 253, 254;
profit, 52, 74, 86–88, 108, 109–10,
305n52; progress, 240–42; race,
140–41, 218–19, 248–49, 267n67,
315n44, 335n67, 345n76;
reason/logic/"science," xviii, 10, 64,
97–98, 99, 104–5, 110, 170, 217,
239, 245–46; "scientific medicine,"
48–52, 59–60, 63, 64, 67, 70, 98,
177–78, 266n59; women, 218, 219,
252–53, 269n7, 311n149, 318n97,
335n59, 339n144

Pichon, Stephen, 35, 36, 37

Pinkerton, Henry, 199–200, 204,
329n152

plague, 42, 281n154, 291n123,
300n121

Plancke, J., 285n26

Plato, 13
Plotz, Harry, 195, 214, 299n109, 327n125
Poirson, A., 66–67, 290n111, 299n114
Polignac, Comte de, 126–27
positivism, 2, 3, 97–98, 110, 260n9
Potel, René, 107, 299n114
Pouchet, Félix-Archimède, 21, 224, 248, 270n21, 271n22
Poulenc *frères*, 86–88, 91, 109, 147, 296n56, 305n52
Prince Jaffar, La (Duhamel), 132–33
profit, in medicine. *See* Pastorians: profit
Prowazek, Stanislas von, 53

Quixote, Don, 88, 227

Rabies, 220–21, 223, 286n48, 291n129, 336n80; Pasteur's work on, xvi, 5, 20, 220–21, 262n28
Rabinow, Paul, 279n120
Ramon, Gaston, 234, 343n43
Ramsine, S., 151–53, 186
Reenstierna, John, 143, 144–45, 165–66
Relapsing Fever, xviii, 63–64, 78–85, 174–78, 184–87, 203, 293n15, 294n31, 343n45; evolution in, 84, 175, 176, 184, 187, 293n13; inframicrobes ("filterable" stage), 82–84, 178, 184, 315n50; louse-borne, 79–80, 81–84, 129, 153–54, 176, 184, 205, 289n97, 321n9; spirochetes (*borrelia*) in, 82–84, 176, 184–86, 293n12, 293n13; tick-borne, 80, 174–78, 293n13, 322n11
Remlinger, Paul, 221, 234, 291n129, 336n80
Renan, Ernest, 335n67
reservoirs of disease, 44, 185. *See also* Relapsing Fever; typhus
Richet, Charles, 246

Ricketts, Henry, 53, 95
Rockefeller Foundation, 93, 126–27, 297n90, 306n67
Rocky Mountain Spotted Fever, 195, 196
Rogers, Stephen J., xix
Rosenberg, Charles, 275n76
Rouen, 2, 18, 22, 28, 29, 89, 164, 219–20, 247, 275n73; hospitals in, 22, 27, 274n67
Roux, Emile, 6, 9, 20–22, 23, 37, 44, 55, 62, 65, 70, 72, 80, 98, 116, 117, 154, 162, 163–64, 167, 168, 174, 213–14, 252, 288n84, 302n175; criticisms of, 108, 116, 117, 121–24, 230–32, 233, 234, 252; death of, 229; successor of, 130, 228, 229, 234; tensions with Nicolle, 86–88, 109, 124–25, 127, 214, 226–28
Roux, Wilhelm, 11

Sadiki Hospital, 1, 33, 39, 40, 41, 50–51, 58, 59, 284n19; and typhus, 1, 60, 62, 169
Saint, Lucien, 311n162
Sauvageau, Camille, 164–65, 319n110
Schaeffer (Collège de France candidate), 210
Sellards, A. W., 203–4, 298n94
Serbia, typhus epidemic. *See* World War I: typhus
Sergent, Edmond, 80, 115–16, 121, 218, 289n97, 292n4, 293n15, 297n84, 303n7, 305n32, 313n9, 341n26; and relapsing fever, 63–64, 81, 82, 205; tensions with Nicolle, 129–30, 218, 289n96, 292n7, 292n8, 318n87, 320n134
Shaffer, Morris, 250, 329n151, 344n69
Sidi bou Saïd, 17–18, 89, 110, 131, 200, 169n1
smallpox vaccine, 5, 161, 188, 327n124

Smith, Theobald, 321n5
Sociedad Argentina de Patología Medical del Norte, 139
Société de Pathologie Exotique, 45, 139
Société des Ecrivains de l'Afrique du Nord (SEAN), 134, 309n116
Société Tunisienne des Sciences Médicale (also known as la Société des Sciences Médicales de Tunisie), 34, 40, 45, 49–51, 114, 142, 276n89, 278n108
Society of Medical Sciences. *See* Société Tunisienne des Sciences Médicales
Sparrow, Hélène, 150–51, 201–2, 203, 219, 252; vaccine work, 151, 178, 314n31
specificity, bacterial. *See* germ theory
spontaneous generation, 21, 224
Stanley, Wendell, 12, 154, 245
Starling, Ernest, 215
Sternberg, George Miller, 146
Strong, Richard Pearson, 93, 297n90

Temps, Le, 124–25, 234
Theiler, Max, 203–4, 330n176
Themistocles, 231
Third Republic France. *See* France: Third Republic
tobacco mosaic disease, 12, 154, 245
Topley, W. W. C., 323n30
Tournadé, Andre, 210, 211
toxoplasmosis, 43, 282n164
Tunisia, xvii, 29, 31, 140, 249, 276n86, 276n88; Agriculture, Commerce, and Colonization, Department of, 31, 32, 34, 36, 41–42, 70–71, 94; disease in, 31, 48, 276n89, 283n2; history, 31, 97, 140; hospitals in, 33, 277n102, 280n140, 287n65 (*see also* Sadiki Hospital); hygiene in, 32, 42–43, 59, 66, 73, 119–20, 277n96, 293n11; medicine in, 32–33, 49–52, 249, 277n99, 277n100, 278n116, 283n8, 283n9, 287n69; protectorate status, 3, 30, 31–32, 48, 142, 249, 276n90, 277n93, 278n110, 309n111; typhus epidemics, 31, 48, 57, 59, 61, 95–96, 291n122
Twort, Frederick, 316n52
typhoid, 24, 47, 48, 54, 55, 59, 146, 156, 182, 193, 195, 287n61
typhus, xvii, 46, 187, 285n28; Brill-Zinsser disease, 54, 193–98, 201, 207, 214, 243–44, 326n115, 327n128, 342n33 (*see also* typhus: varieties); and civilization, 47, 54, 56, 68–70, 91, 93, 168, 169–70, 190–92; cultivation (laboratory animals), 56, 61–62, 63, 72, 96–97, 106–8, 147, 197, 199–200; diagnosis, 56, 58–59, 68, 95–96, 288n76, 288n77; discovery narrative ("Door of the Sadiki"), 1–2, 62–63, 167, 168–70, 218, 254, 287n70, 291n134, 319n104, 320n134; epidemiology of, 47–48, 53–54, 56, 57–61, 64, 285n32, 285n37; evolution of, 156–57, 200, 202, 204; and germ theory, 54, 55–56; murine, 107, 174, 197–98, 201–2, 204–7, 244, 328n131, 330n163, 331n189 (*see also* typhus: varieties); prophylaxis ("rational hygiene"), 65–68, 69, 91–93, 98–99, 290n111, 290n112; Proteus, 152, 155, 223; reservoirs, 56, 60–61, 67–68, 69, 95–96, 106, 107, 149–50, 151–53, 189, 190–91, 196–97, 201–2, 204–7, 242–43, 313n16, 315n44, 315n48; rickettsia, 53, 95, 155, 199–200, 205, 223, 285n29, 299n109 (*see also* typhus: varieties); symptoms, 52–53, 189, 285n27, 288n76, 288n77, 290n120; transmission, 63, 64–65, 77–78,

110, 129, 168, 285n39, 289n101, 292n7, 298n94, 307n79; in Tunisia, 31, 48, 54, 56, 57–61, 67, 69–70, 299n108; vaccines, 65, 71–73, 95, 96, 150, 193, 244, 313n24, 314n25; varieties, 96, 192–202, 204–7, 222–23, 299n115, 328n144, 329n161, 330n163, 331n184, 331n185, 331n186; in World War I, 11, 53, 92–93, 108, 170 (*see also* World War I: typhus). *See also* "inapparent infection"

ultramicrobes. *See* inframicrobes; viruses
ultramicroscope. *See* microscope, dark field
United States, 127, 153, 220, 308n96
United States Public Health Service, 193, 194, 196, 198

vaccines, 6, 88, 109, 178–79, 189, 262n25, 295n52, 295n56; diphtheria antitoxin, 23; *fluorurés*, 72–73, 86–88, 94; rabies, 220–21, 223 (*see also* Rabies); "virus-vaccine," 5, 7, 11, 13, 204, 220, 226, 242; yellow fever, 203–4. *See also* "inapparent infection"; typhus: vaccines; virulence
Vaillard, Louis, 229, 230, 234, 338n128
Vallery-Radot, Louis Pasteur, 114, 130, 210, 211, 214, 230, 244, 245, 248, 253, 338n130, 339n151; Nicolle's advocate, 165, 337n112; Pastorian mission (saving), 113, 115–16, 122, 124, 125, 138–39, 145, 166, 228, 229–30, 234, 338n127
Vallery-Radot, René, 8, 113–14, 215
venereal diseases, Nicolle's approach to patients, 27–28
Verne, Jules, 19
Virchow, Rudolf, 285n39

virulence, 146–48, 178–80, 254, 321n1, 321n3, 324n52, 325n83, 337n99; as adaptive power, 156, 179, 183, 224–26, 323n30, 324n54; attenuation, 5, 72, 107, 146–44, 173, 178, 189, 221; spirochetes (relapsing fever), 83–84, 184. *See also* vaccines: "virus-vaccine"
viruses, 11, 12, 55, 82, 153–54, 286n46, 286n47. *See also* "inframicrobes"
Vries, Hugo de, 11, 325n89
Vuillier, Mme (laboratory, Hôpital Civil Français), 121

Walsh, D. M., 334n44
Weigl, Rudolf, 150, 193
Weil, Edmund, 152, 155, 156, 223, 314n37
Weil-Felix test, 152, 153, 155, 196, 199, 273n46, 273n47, 314n37
Weindling, Paul, 285n28
Widal, Fernand, 24, 54, 115, 165, 273n45
Widal test (agglutination, for typhoid), 24–25, 54, 193, 273n46, 273n47
Wilson, G. S., 323n30
Wolbach, S. B., 195–96, 199, 286n47, 317n75, 328n131, 329n151
Wolfe, Richard, 250
World War I, xviii, 10, 11, 87, 91–97, 98, 105–6, 131–32, 140, 240, 252; and the Pasteur Institute of Paris, 98, 108, 122, 140; and the Pasteur Institute of Tunis, 92, 94, 108, 110, 298n103; relapsing fever, 91, 92; typhus, 91–94, 95–96, 107–8, 150, 168, 297n83, 297n88, 297n89, 299n114 (*see also* typhus)

yellow fever vaccine. *See* vaccines: yellow fever
Yersin, Alexandre, 23, 30

Zaharoff, Basil, 304n14
Zinsser, Hans, 52, 53, 93, 145, 197, 198, 214, 250, 285n27, 313n24, 321n5, 329n159, 331n191, 342n29, 344n72; and Brill-Zinsser disease, 207, 243–44, 342n33; *Rats, Lice, and History*, 193, 200, 242–43, 244, 250; on typhus varieties, 192–93, 199–202, 206–7, 243–44, 342n28

Zitouna, Mohamed, 33, 277n100, 278n107, 281n148, 284n22

www.ingramcontent.com/pod-product-compliance
Lightning Source LLC
Chambersburg PA
CBHW071436300426
44114CB00013B/1459